Marketing Public Health

Strategies to Promote Social Change

Michael Siegel, MD, MPH

Assistant Professor
Boston University School of Public Health
Boston, Massachusetts

Lynne Doner, MA

Social Marketing Consultant
Arlington, Virginia

JONES AND BARTLETT PUBLISHERS

Sudbury, Massachusetts

BOSTON   TORONTO   LONDON   SINGAPORE

World Headquarters
Jones and Bartlett Publishers
40 Tall Pine Drive
Sudbury, MA 01776
978-443-5000
info@jbpub.com
www.jbpub.com

Jones and Bartlett Publishers Canada
2406 Nikanna Road
Mississauga, ON L5C 2W6
CANADA

Jones and Bartlett Publishers International
Barb House, Barb Mews
London W6 7PA
UK

Production Credits
Publisher: Michael Brown
Associate Editor: Chambers Moore
Marketing Manager: Joy Stark-Vancs
Production Assistant: Carolyn F. Rogers
Production Specialist: Anda Aquino-Eisenberg
Manufacturing and Inventory Coordinator: Amy Bacus
Printing and Binding: Integrated Book Technology, Inc.

ISBN: 0-7637-2651-6

Printed in the United States of America
08 07 06 05 04   10 9 8 7 6 5 4 3 2 1

To my wife, Rebecca, for her love and support, and for sharing her gift—writing—to make mine ever so more tolerable.

M.S.

To my husband, Barry Lotenberg, for his infinite patience and support, and to my daughter, Sienna Rachel, for making every day a new joy.

L.D.

Table of Contents

Acknowledgments .... **xi**

Introduction .... **xiii**

**PART I—MARKETING PRINCIPLES FOR PUBLIC HEALTH
        PRACTICE** **1**

Section I—Marketing Social Change **3**

Chapter 1   **Emerging Threats to the Public's Health—
             The Need for Social Change** **5**
             Unhealthy Lifestyles and Behaviors 8
             Deteriorating Social and Economic Conditions 9
             A Crisis in Access to Quality Health Care 17
             Implications of the Chronic Disease Epidemic for
               Public Health Practice 18
             Conclusion 21

Chapter 2   **Marketing Social Change—A Challenge for the
             Public Health Practitioner** **29**
             A Unique Marketing Challenge 31
             Conclusion 39

Chapter 3   **Marketing Social Change—An Opportunity for the
             Public Health Practitioner** **42**
             Finding Out What the Consumer Wants: The Role of
               Formative Research 49

Redefining the Public Health Product.................................. 51
Repackaging, Repositioning, and Reframing the
    Public Health Product.. 52
Marketing Public Health Programs and Policies 57
Conclusion 61
Appendix 3–A   The Importance of Formative Research
    in Public Health Campaigns: An Example from the
    Area of HIV Prevention among Gay Men 66

Section II—Marketing Public Health 71

Chapter 4   **Emerging Threats to the Survival of Public Health** 73
Misunderstanding of the Importance of Medical Treatment
    Compared with Population-Based Prevention 74
The Illusion of Health Care Reform as a Solution to the
    Public Health Crisis... 78
The Illusion of Managed Care as an Opportunity for
    Public Health 79
Political and Economic Factors That Directly Threaten
    Public Health Funding.. 83
The Lost Vision of Public Health 90
Conclusion 94
Appendix 4–A   Summary of Lobbying Regulations for
    Public Health Organizations.. 100

Chapter 5   **Marketing Public Health—A Challenge for the
    Public Health Practitioner** 102
An Unfavorable State of Demand for Public Health
    Programs.. 109
A Hostile Environment for Marketing Public Health
    Programs.. 111
Limited Capacity of Public Health Practitioners To
    Compete for Public Attention and Resources 113
Conclusion 114

Chapter 6   **Marketing Public Health—An Opportunity for the
    Public Health Practitioner** 117
Defining the Product: The Importance of Formative
    Research in Marketing Public Health Policies and
    Programs.. 118

Packaging and Positioning the Product: Framing Public
     Health Programs and Policies 122
Conclusion 136
Appendix 6–A   Exploring the Core Values of
     Policy Makers: Lessons from Public Health History 140
Appendix 6–B   An Example of Reframing a Public
     Health Policy Issue: Antismoking Ordinances 146

Section III—Marketing Public Health—Case Studies 149

Chapter 7   **Marketing Public Health Programs and Policies—**
     A Case Study **151**
          California 152
          Montana 155
          Massachusetts 157
          A Tale of Two States: Colorado and Arizona 163
          Summary 165
          Conclusion 168

Chapter 8   **Marketing Public Health as an Institution—**
     A Case Study **170**
          Conclusion 181
          Appendix 8–A   Excerpts from the Congressional Record,
               104th Congress 184

PART II—USING MARKETING PRINCIPLES TO DESIGN,
     IMPLEMENT, AND EVALUATE PUBLIC HEALTH
     INTERVENTIONS **193**

Section I—Planning **195**

Chapter 9   **Applying Marketing Principles to Public Health 197**
          The Roots of Marketing Social Change 197
          Key Concepts from Commercial Marketing 200
          Conclusion 218
          Appendix 9–A   Using Marketing Principles To
               Combat Telemarketing Fraud Victimization 220

Chapter 10   **The Planning Process 225**
          The Importance of Sound Strategy 227
          Planning Principles 229

The Role of Theory and Models of Behavior 230
The Outcome: A Strategic Plan 234
Analyzing the Situation 235
Setting Goals and Objectives 252
Selecting Primary and Secondary Audiences 255
Understanding Target Audiences 256
Putting It All Together: The Strategic Plan 257
Conclusion 258

Chapter 11   Formative Research **261**
The Role of Formative Research 261
Formative Research To Support Health Behavior
    Change 264
Formative Research To Support Public Health Policy
    Initiatives 273
Gaining Insights: The Qualitative Approaches 280
Conclusion 293
Appendix 11–A   Building Support for Coordinated
    School Health: Using Multiple Formative Research
    Techniques To Shape an Initiative 296
Appendix 11–B   Sample Recruitment Screener 303
Appendix 11–C   Sample Focus Group Moderator's
    Guide 306
Appendix 11–D   Information Resources 310

Chapter 12   **Framing the Message: Crafting Communication
    Strategies** **312**
The Communication Strategy 313
Conclusion 337
Appendix 12–A   Communication Strategy
    Development Worksheets 340

Section II—Development, Testing, and Implementation **343**

Chapter 13   **Translating Strategy into Tactics** **345**
What Is the Initiative Supposed To Accomplish? 346
Assessing Resource and Organizational Issues 347
Planning Changes in Products and Services 347
Planning Promotional Activities 350
The Development and Implementation Process 354

Conclusion 363
Appendix 13–A Selected National Health Observances
(by Month) 365

Chapter 14 **Working with Partners** 367
The Role of Partners 367
Types of Partners 368
Suggestions for Developing Successful Partnerships 369
Coalitions 374
Intermediaries 378
Conclusion 380

Chapter 15 **Mass Communication: Design and Implementation**
Issues 381
Use of Mass Communication 381
Planning Development Time 382
Assessing Proposed Materials and Activities 383
Establishing Identity 383
Print Materials 384
Electronic Media 387
Mass Media 392
Conclusion 413

Chapter 16 **Pretesting Messages and Materials** 415
The Role of Pretesting 415
Pretesting Messages: A Continuation of Communication
Strategy Development 416
Pretesting Materials 416
Common Pretesting Methodologies 418
Conclusion 435
Appendix 16–A Sample Central-Site Interview
Questionnaire 438

Section III—Assessing Progress and Making Refinements 447

Chapter 17 **Monitoring and Refining Implementation: Process**
Evaluation Tools 449
Planning and Conducting Process Evaluation Studies 450
Common Process Evaluation Activities 453
Tracking Target Audience Awareness and Reaction 472
Conclusion 475

Chapter 18   Issues in Outcome Evaluation **476**
The Role of Outcome Evaluation 476
Evaluating Social Change Initiatives: The Role of
    Experimental Designs 477
Considerations When Planning Evaluations 483
Conclusion 490

Epilogue—What Does the Future Hold? **494**

Appendix A—Hiring Agencies, Contractors, and Consultants **496**

Appendix B—Suggested Readings **504**

Appendix C—Glossary of Terms **506**

Index **510**

Acknowledgments

This book draws on the work of scholars and practitioners in a range of disciplines. Their inspiration, ideas, and experiences were invaluable to us.

Our editors at Aspen, Bob Howard, Kalen Conerly, and Denise Coursey, were supportive throughout the process of bringing this volume to fruition. Craig Schronz conducted much of the background research for the book and contributed greatly to Chapter 7. We would also like to thank those people who took the time to read portions of this manuscript and give us their comments: George Balch, Katharine Dusenbury, Jackie Haven, John Killpack, Kay Loughrey, Rebecca Sherman, Eve Siegel, Maureen Varnon, and the anonymous reviewers. While we take sole responsibility for the final product, their help was much appreciated in shaping our ideas and our presentation of them.

Finally, we are indebted to the many family members who put up with our distractions and mumblings during the year and a half we spent writing and revising this book.

Introduction

On January 9, 1995, U.S. House of Representatives Majority Whip Tom DeLay introduced HR450, a bill that would have placed a one-year moratorium on nearly all new federal regulations. Although the bill contained an exemption for regulations needed to address an "imminent threat" to public health or safety, it would have halted the promulgation of most federal public health regulations, especially those aimed at preventing disease, disability, and death. In essence, the implementation of population-based public health policies at the federal level would be dead.

In January 1996, Massachusetts Governor William Weld submitted to the state legislature plans to downsize state government by abolishing the Department of Health and Human Services in favor of a new Department of Family Services. As part of the plan, the Department of Public Health would be merged with the Department of Mental Health into an overall health services department. The state's focus on developing population-based preventive programs to reduce the burden of chronic disease would be lost; state public health functions would be blurred into a department that would focus on the provision of health and other services to individuals. The proposal would have put an end to the nation's oldest state public health department, established in 1869.

In January 1997, Massachusetts Representative Mary Jane Simmons introduced legislation that would have stripped local boards of health in Massachusetts of their ability to regulate exposure to secondhand smoke in restaurants. This would have been an unprecedented intrusion into the autonomy of boards of health, which have traditionally been given wide powers to protect public health in a state that prides itself on the principle of home rule.

As we approach the new millennium, the public health community faces unprecedented threats to its authority, role, and very existence at the national, state, and local levels. It is no longer enough for public health professionals to work to protect the health of the public. For the first time in history, public health practitioners must work to protect the survival of public health as an institution.

Changes in the health care delivery system and the social, political, and economic environments in which health care is delivered present a direct threat to the survival of public health. As managed care programs assume many of the functions formerly held by public health, the role of public health departments is no longer clear. Public health programs must now compete for public attention and resources. Funding for public health is declining due to budget cuts, block grants, and an increased level of scrutiny by policy makers, which requires public health to justify its funding by demonstrating long-term outcomes, even when such outcomes are difficult or impossible to measure. At the same time, the public's confidence in government interventions, including many public health programs, is falling, and a strong, anti-regulatory environment pervades all levels of government.

These same changes in health care delivery and the social, political, and economic environments also present a direct threat to the public's health. Unhealthy lifestyles and behaviors, deteriorating social and environmental conditions, and the growth of managed care programs, which are consumed by the effort to decrease costs at the expense of the provision of the most needed health interventions, threaten the public's health. As the chief causes of death in the United States have gradually shifted from communicable illnesses to chronic diseases, lifestyle and behavioral risk factors, as well as social and environmental conditions, have become the key determinants of the public's health. In contrast to its successes in controlling infectious diseases, the public health movement has been ineffective in controlling the emerging chronic disease epidemic. Programs to change individual behaviors and lifestyles have typically been ineffective, and public health professionals have not fully accepted the role of advocating for changes in social conditions and social policies. As a result, the public health community is equipped neither to confront existing public health crises, nor to prevent new ones.

Despite these threats, there are tools available to help the public health profession save itself and enable it to confront existing and emerging public health crises. There are public health initiatives that have successfully changed societal behaviors, improved social conditions, reformed social policies, and retained and even increased funding for public health programs and departments.

The common feature of these initiatives is public health practitioners' strategic use of marketing principles to promote social change. Understanding and applying marketing principles is essential for public health practitioners to successfully confront the imposing challenges they face, challenges to both the public's health and to the survival of the public health profession. However, public health practitioners are not typically trained in the principles of marketing.

Marketing Public Health: Strategies To Promote Social Change is designed to help public health practitioners understand basic marketing principles and strategically apply these principles in planning, implementing, and evaluating public health initiatives. We hope that this book will provide public health practitioners at all levels of government and in the private sector with a valuable tool to run more effective campaigns to change individual behavior, improve social and economic conditions, advance social policies, and compete successfully for public attention and resources.

We argue that the key to running effective public health programs is to abandon the traditional practice of deciding what policy makers or the public ought to want and then trying to sell it to them in the absence of significant demand. Instead, public health practitioners must first find out the needs and wants of their target audience (policy makers or the public) and then redefine their product (changes in individual behavior or the adoption of public health programs and policies) to satisfy an existing demand. Rather than appealing exclusively to the benefits of improved health, public health practitioners must learn to package, position, and frame their programs to appeal to more salient, powerful, and influential core values: freedom, independence, autonomy, control, fairness, democracy, and free enterprise.

The book is organized into two parts. Part I explains the reasons why both the public's health and the survival of public health itself are threatened and why an understanding of marketing principles is necessary for the public health practitioner to effectively confront these challenges. It outlines the major marketing principles that public health practitioners need to understand and illustrates the application of these principles to public health problems, through examples within the chapters and two case studies presented separately.

Part I is divided into three sections. The first section (Chapters 1–3) describes threats to the public's health and establishes that changing individual behavior, social and economic conditions, and social policy is important to successfully confront the chronic disease epidemic (Chapter 1). It illustrates the difficulties of promoting these social changes (Chapter 2), but also demonstrates how public health practitioners can use basic marketing principles to structure interventions that will facilitate social change (Chapter 3).

The second section (Chapters 4–6) describes threats to the survival of public health as an institution. It establishes that learning how to effectively market public health programs and policies and the idea of public health itself is essential to confront challenges to public health's survival. It shows why marketing public health programs and policies is profoundly difficult (Chapter 5), but demonstrates how public health practitioners can strategically apply basic marketing principles to promote public health programs and policies (Chapter 6).

The third section (Chapters 7 and 8) presents two case studies. In Chapter 7, we illustrate the use of marketing principles to promote adoption of a particular public health policy: increasing state cigarette excise taxes and earmarking the revenue to establish comprehensive anti-tobacco programs. In Chapter 8, we illustrate the use of marketing principles to promote increased funding for a major public health institution: the Centers for Disease Control and Prevention.

In essence, Part I answers three basic questions:

1. What is the problem?
2. What is the solution?
3. What do public health practitioners need to know to implement the solution?

Part II discusses how to apply the principles presented in Part I in planning, developing, implementing, evaluating, and refining public health efforts to change individual behavior or to promote the adoption of public health programs and policies.

Part II is divided into three sections that correspond to the stages of a marketing effort (planning; development, testing, and implementation; and assessment). Section I (Chapters 9–12) provides background on the basic marketing principles that a public health practitioner must understand and presents a process for planning public health efforts based on these principles. It begins by presenting key marketing concepts and discussing how they apply to individual and policy changes (Chapter 9). It then presents a strategic planning process (Chapter 10) and describes some commonly used formative research techniques and how they can be used to support the strategic planning process (Chapter 11). The final chapter in the section (Chapter 12) discusses how to frame messages about the social change so that they are believable, relevant, and compelling to target audiences.

Section II (Chapters 13–16) covers the process of developing, testing, and implementing the tactics, or components, involved in an initiative. Chapter 13 discusses translating the strategic plan into specific tactics and a carefully timed implementation. The next chapter describes the various roles that partners and intermediaries can play in an initiative and provides suggestions for developing productive partnerships (Chapter 14). Chapter 15 discusses some of the issues that may arise when developing and assessing mass communication activities and materials. The section closes with Chapter 16, which presents a variety of methods for pretesting tactics and materials before implementation.

Section III (Chapters 17 and 18) discusses tracking, evaluating, and refining social change efforts. Chapter 17 discusses the importance marketers place on monitoring and refining implementation, presents a range of process evaluation techniques for doing so, and discusses how to use the information to improve program implementation. Chapter 18 discusses issues in assessing the outcomes of marketing-based efforts using traditional approaches to summative evaluation and presents some techniques for assessing outcomes and using the results to make program refinements.

In essence, Part II answers three basic questions:

1. How do public health practitioners use marketing principles to plan a public health initiative?

2. What are some of the key issues to keep in mind as tactics are developed?
3. How can an initiative be monitored so that it can be refined as needed?

Although marketing principles have been applied to some efforts to change health-related behaviors for many years, their application usually is restricted to initiatives that focus on the behavior of individuals and ignore the larger issues of policy changes needed to aid and support individual efforts. The integration of marketing principles into day-to-day public health practice is a new concept, and one that has not yet been fully developed. These principles can provide powerful tools for influencing all the factors that contribute to social change: the individual, the environment, and social policy.

This book is a first attempt to describe how marketing principles might become part of public health practice and be used to develop and implement more effective public health initiatives. If our ideas stimulate further thought, research, and most important, experimentation among public health practitioners, we will have achieved our goal. It is our hope that the efforts that come from practitioners who read this book will provide far more answers to the difficult questions we pose here than the book itself does. For in the final analysis, the experience of public health practitioners will teach us all how to develop and implement more effective programs to promote social change and improve the quality of life today and tomorrow.

PART I

Marketing Principles for Public Health Practice

Marketing Social Change

To confront the chronic disease epidemic that threatens to dominate human health in the 21st century, public health practice must begin to focus on far more than providing basic medical care. To establish a favorable environment for human well-being, public health practitioners must concentrate on effecting social change by helping to modify individual behaviors and lifestyles, improve social and economic conditions, and reform social policies.

This section demonstrates that social change is essential to protecting the public's health and why creating social change presents a formidable task for public health practitioners. The ways that practitioners can use basic marketing principles to effectively confront this challenge are also explained.

This section focuses mainly on how to use marketing principles to accomplish the first task: modifying individual behavior. Using marketing principles to improve social and economic conditions and reform social policy is discussed in Part I, Section II.

CHAPTER 1

Emerging Threats to the Public's Health—The Need for Social Change

An epidemic of chronic disease threatens the public's health. Fueling this epidemic are unhealthy lifestyles and behaviors, deteriorating social conditions, and an increasingly hazardous environment, coupled with a crisis in access to quality health care. The emerging chronic disease epidemic poses both a threat to the public's health and a challenge to public health practice. As the turn of the millennium approaches, public health practice must focus on far more than the provision of medical care. It must, first and foremost, dedicate its efforts to modifying individual lifestyle and behavior, improving social and economic conditions, and reforming social policy to establish an environment that fosters optimal human health. In other words, the business of public health must focus on creating social change.

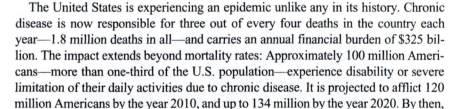

The United States is experiencing an epidemic unlike any in its history. Chronic disease is now responsible for three out of every four deaths in the country each year—1.8 million deaths in all—and carries an annual financial burden of $325 billion. The impact extends beyond mortality rates: Approximately 100 million Americans—more than one-third of the U.S. population—experience disability or severe limitation of their daily activities due to chronic disease. It is projected to afflict 120 million Americans by the year 2010, and up to 134 million by the year 2020. By then, the costs associated with the epidemic will approach $1 trillion per year.

Unlike previous epidemics, the historic proportions associated with chronic disease today are not reported as front-page news; efforts to confront the issues are not among the priority program activities of most local health departments; and policy makers allocate precious few resources to eliminate the epidemic or even to slow its spread. Improving sanitation and hygiene will do little to stem the tide. Even the medical profession is nearly powerless against it.

The primary and most urgent challenge to public health today is to find a way to halt the epidemic of chronic disease that threatens to dominate the population in the 21st century. Chronic disease—heart disease, cancer, stroke, injuries, chronic obstructive lung disease, diabetes, and liver disease—are the chief causes of death among Americans as we approach the end of the decade (Figure 1–1).

By far, the leading causes of death in the United States are heart disease, cancer, and stroke, which account for about 1.4 million (62%) of the nation's 2.3 million deaths each year (National Center for Health Statistics [NCHS], 1997). Injuries, including motor vehicle accidents, suicides, homicides, falls, and drownings, account for an additional 140,000 deaths annually (6.1% of all deaths). Violence, in particular, is an alarming part of the chronic disease epidemic. Homicide alone is the leading cause of death among Blacks ages 15 to 24, and is the second leading cause of death among all persons in this age group (NCHS, 1997; Rosenberg, Powell, & Hammond, 1997; Satcher, 1996). Chronic obstructive lung disease causes an additional 100,000 deaths annually (4.5% of all deaths).

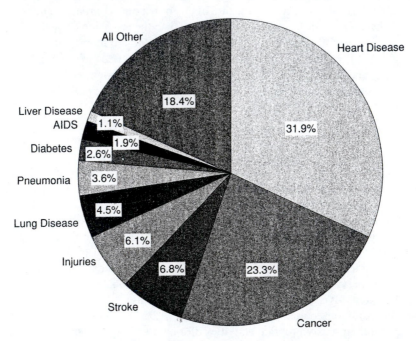

Figure 1–1 Causes of Death—United States, 1995. *Source:* Reprinted from NCHS, 1997.

Chronic diseases also cause a substantial amount of disability and suffering among Americans. Approximately 100 million people in the United States have one or more chronic medical conditions, such as heart disease, stroke, cancer, arthritis, diabetes, lung disease, osteoporosis, multiple sclerosis, and mental retardation; about 40% of this population has more than one chronic condition (Hoffman, Rice, & Sung, 1996). The direct medical costs—and indirect costs such as lost productivity—associated with these chronic conditions totaled $660 billion in 1990 (Hoffman et al., 1996). The direct medical costs associated with chronic diseases accounted for about 76% of all direct medical expenditures in the nation (Hoffman et al., 1996).

Despite advances in medical knowledge and treatment, little progress has been made in stemming the epidemic. Although stroke mortality rates declined by 59% and heart disease mortality rates declined by 46% from 1970 to 1995 (NCHS, 1997), only about one-third of the decline in mortality was due to a reduction in the incidence of cardiovascular disease (Sytkowski, Kannel, & D'Agostino, 1990), and the burden of disease morbidity is expected to increase, especially among the elderly (Bonneux, Barendregt, Meeter, Bonsel, & van der Maas, 1994). Although fewer people are dying of their disease, nearly the same proportion have cardiovascular disease and suffer from their chronic conditions (Bonneux et al., 1994; Centers for Disease Control and Prevention [CDC], 1993). Overall cancer death rates have remained essentially unchanged for the better part of the century (NCHS, 1997). There has been a modest decline in mortality from colorectal cancer, stomach cancer, uterine cancer, and liver cancer, but these changes have been more than offset by the striking increase in lung cancer mortality since 1930 (American Cancer Society, 1994). Although lung cancer death rates among men peaked in the early 1990s, rates are still increasing among women (NCHS, 1997). The rate of suicide among U.S. teenagers has more than tripled since 1950, and the homicide rate among teenagers has doubled in the past two decades alone, mostly due to the widespread availability of firearms (NCHS, 1997; Satcher, 1996). And the incidence of diabetes increased by 48% between 1980 and 1994 (CDC, 1997a). In 1994, the age-adjusted incidence of diabetes reached its highest level in one and a half decades (CDC, 1997a).

The chronic disease epidemic is taking a disproportionate toll on poor and underserved populations, and the nation has failed dismally in its efforts to reduce chronic disease mortality among these populations. While cancer death rates among White males and females have remained relatively stable during the past 25 years, rates among Black males have increased by 18% and among Black females by nearly 10% (NCHS, 1997). The disparity in overall mortality between higher and lower socioeconomic groups continues to increase in the United States (Pappas, Queen, Hadden, & Fisher, 1993). Between 1960 and 1986, overall mortality declined in all socioeconomic groups, but declines were significantly greater among persons with higher income and higher levels of education (Pappas et al., 1993). In communities that are particularly poor, death rates among Blacks have changed little since 1960 (Jenkins, Tuthill, Tannenbaum, & Kirby, 1977; McCord & Freeman, 1990; Pappas et al., 1993).

The disparity in health status between higher and lower socioeconomic class groups is itself a component of the chronic disease epidemic. Several studies have shown that the persistence of social class differences in health status is a stronger determinant of overall poor health than the level of poverty and disadvantage in a community (Henig, 1997; Kennedy, Kawachi, & Prothrow-Stith, 1995; Marmot, Bobak, & Smith, 1995; McCord & Freeman, 1990; Navarro, 1997; Townsend & Davidson, 1982; Wilkinson, 1990, 1992, 1997). As Johns Hopkins University professor Vincente Navarro (1997) pointed out,

> a poor person in Harlem, New York City, is likely to have worse health status than a middle-class person in Bangladesh (one of the poorest countries in the world), even though the former has, in absolute terms, more resources (monetary resources and goods and services) than the latter. Still, to be poor in Harlem is far more difficult (because of the social and psychological distance from the rest of society) than to be middle class in Bangladesh. It is not class structure but class relations that affect the levels of health of our populations. (p. 335)

The chronic disease epidemic must be viewed with no less urgency and concern than traditional infectious disease "epidemics" that have plagued society for centuries. As Dr. David Satcher, director of the CDC noted, chronic disease (violence, in particular) "can erode the well-being of neighborhoods and destroy communities with the same deadly impact as the outbreak of a fatal disease" (Satcher, 1996, p. 1707). And an *American Journal of Public Health* editorial argues that the problem of homelessness is equally applicable to all chronic disease: "We should be as much concerned about the thousands of people who are homeless in American cities and the thousands of children in residentially unstable families as we are when there is an epidemic of an infectious disease affecting a few hundred people, and we should respond with the same urgency" (Breakey, 1997, p. 153).

To understand why medical and traditional public health efforts have been virtually powerless in confronting chronic disease, we must understand the factors that are fueling the chronic disease epidemic: (1) unhealthy lifestyles and behaviors, (2) deteriorating social and economic conditions, and (3) a crisis in access to quality health care.

UNHEALTHY LIFESTYLES AND BEHAVIORS

A large body of medical and public health literature documents the role of individual behavior in disease, especially chronic disease. A series of large, population-based, cohort studies has identified behavioral risk factors for a variety of chronic diseases, most notably heart disease, stroke, and cancer (Slater & Carlton, 1985). The U.S. Department of Health and Human Services (USDHHS) estimates that of the 2.1 million annual deaths in the United States, more than 400,000 could be prevented by eliminating tobacco use; approximately 300,000 could be prevented through improved diet and physical activity; another 100,000 could be prevented by eliminating excess alcohol consumption; as many as 90,000 deaths could be prevented through improved vaccination; and an additional 30,000 could be prevented by eliminating unsafe sexual practices (CDC, 1995; USDHHS, 1995). Other behavior-related, preventable causes of death cited by the USDHHS report include workplace, home, recreational, and roadway injuries; firearms-related injuries; high blood pressure and high cholesterol levels (which are related to diet and physical activity); and breast and cervical cancer (where early screening could impact prognosis). In total, at least 1 million American lives, or about one-half of all deaths, could be saved each year by changes in individual health-related behaviors (Figure 1–2).

DETERIORATING SOCIAL AND ECONOMIC CONDITIONS

Poverty

The single best predictor of a person's health status is his or her socioeconomic status (Adler, Boyce, Chesney, Folkman, & Syme, 1997; Antonovsky, 1967; Gregorio, Walsh, & Paturzo, 1997; Hemingway, Nicholson, Stafford, Roberts, & Marmot, 1997; Kaplan & Lynch, 1997; Kawachi, Kennedy, Lochner, & Prothrow-Stith, 1997; Kitagawa & Hauser, 1973; Lynch, Kaplan, & Shema, 1997; Marmot et al., 1995; McDonough, Duncan, William, & House, 1997; Moss, 1997; Pappas et al., 1993; Patrick & Wickizer, 1995; Power, Hertzman, Matthews, & Manor, 1997; Satcher, 1996; Susser, Watson, & Hopper, 1985; Syme & Berkman, 1976; Yeracaris & Kim, 1978). Age-adjusted death rates for White males in 1986 ranged from 2.4 per thousand among men with an income greater than $25,000 to 16.0 per thousand among those with an income below $9,000 (Pappas et al., 1993). A similar pattern held for White females (1.6 versus 6.5 per thousand); Black males (3.6 versus 19.5 per thousand); and Black females (2.3 versus 7.6 per thousand). Even after controlling for differences in unhealthy behaviors and lifestyles (e.g., smoking, alcohol use, drug use) and for access to health care, poverty remains a strong, independent predictor of poor health (Haan, Kaplan, & Camacho, 1987). Controlling for baseline health status, race, income, employment status, access to medical care, health insurance coverage, smoking, alcohol consumption, physical activity, body mass index, and several other factors, persons living in poverty-stricken areas still have nearly twice as high a mortality rate as those who do not. As Henig (1997) concluded, "the very fact of being poor is itself an independent risk factor for getting sick" (p. 103).

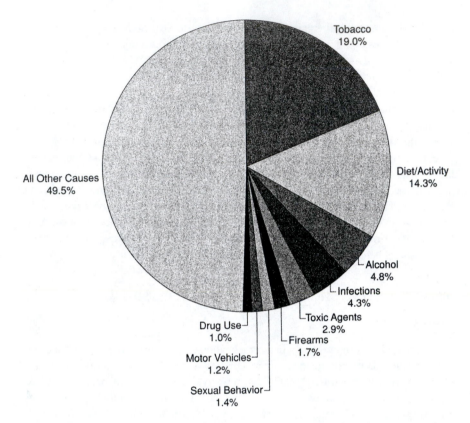

Figure 1–2 Behavior-Related Causes of Death—United States, 1990. *Source:* Data from McGinnis and Foege, 1993, NCHS, 1995, and Turnock, 1997.

Poverty is a particularly strong risk factor for disease and death among children. Children who grow up in poverty are eight times more likely to die from homicide; five times more likely to have a physical or mental disability; five times more likely to be subject to child abuse; three times more likely to die in childhood; and twice as likely to be killed in an accident (Children's Defense Fund, 1994).

Lisbeth Schorr (1989) summarized the problem succinctly: "Poverty is the greatest risk factor of all. Family poverty is relentlessly correlated with high rates of school-age childbearing, school failure, and violent crime—and with all their antecedents. Low income is an important risk factor in itself, and so is relative poverty—having significantly less income than the norm, especially in a society that places such a high value on economic success" (p. xxii).

Efforts to improve the public's health must therefore address the problem of poverty. Not only is poverty a social and economic problem, but it is also a fundamental threat to public health.

Despite the importance of poverty as a public health problem and in spite of the so-called War on Poverty during the Great Society reforms of the 1960s and President Lyndon Johnson's expressed national "commitment to eradicate poverty," poverty remains nearly as prevalent as it was during the late 1960s and has become more prevalent in recent years (Bok, 1996). The proportion of the population living below the official poverty line dropped from 22.4% in 1959 to 11.2% in 1974; however, it has increased since then, reaching 15.1% in 1993, the highest rate of poverty in the United States since the mid-1960s (Bok, 1996; NCHS, 1997). The proportion of people living in extreme poverty (income less than half the official poverty line) also has increased, rising from 30% in 1975 to 40% in the late 1980s (Bok, 1996).

Not only have rates of abject poverty increased, but the mean family income for the lowest 40% income segment in the country has declined since 1972 (Bok, 1996). Family income for the highest 40% income segment during the same period has increased, widening the gap in income disparity between the middle and upper class and the poor. Mean family income among the lowest 20% income segment decreased from $10,769 in 1972 (in constant 1992 dollars) to $9,708 in 1992, and among the second lowest 20% income segment from $23,725 to $23,337 (Bok, 1996). At the same time, mean family income among the highest 20% income segment increased from $82,534 to $99,252 and among the second highest 20% income segment from $47,588 to $53,365.

Hunger

The health consequences of hunger go beyond medical conditions associated with nutritional deficiencies and include inability to concentrate in school, feelings of worthlessness, and other psychological problems (Meyers, Sampson, Weitzman, Rogers, & Kayne, 1989; Pollitt, Gersovitz, & Garginlo, 1978; Rose & Oliveira, 1997; Sidel, 1997). Thus, hunger can significantly affect a person's physical and mental well-being. Recent estimates suggest that at least four million children under age 12 in the United States experience hunger daily and an additional 9.6 million may experience hunger at some point during the year (Sidel, 1997; Wehler, Scott, Anderson, Summer, & Parker, 1995).

Educational Attainment

Education is one of the most important determinants of health status. Age-adjusted death rates for White males in 1986 ranged from 2.8 per thousand among those with at least four years of college to 7.6 per thousand among those without a high school diploma (Pappas et al., 1993). Similarly, death rates for these educational groups ranged from 1.8 to 3.4 per thousand among White females; 6.0 to 13.4 per thousand among Black males; and 2.2 to 6.2 per thousand among Black females. Education is strongly related to unhealthy behaviors. For example, educational attainment is one of the best predictors of smoking status. In 1994, adult smoking prevalence ranged from 12.3% among adults with 16 or more years of education to 38.2% among those with only 9 to 11 years of education (CDC, 1996). Independent of its relation to behavior, education influences a person's ability to access and understand health information. For example, people who are illiterate will not be helped by written materials that public health practitioners produce to educate the public about health.

The United States has made little progress in improving the educational attainment of its population during the past two decades. The proportion of Americans ages 25 to 29 who have graduated from high school is approximately 83% and has remained stable at that level since the mid-1970s (Bok, 1996). Unless progress in this area is restored, the nation is unlikely to reach its goal of attaining a 90% high school graduation rate by the turn of the century. Perhaps of even more concern, the Department of Education estimates that about 35% of 18-year-olds in the nation are functionally illiterate (Harris, 1996; U.S. Department of Education, 1994).

Housing

The lack of adequate and stable housing is associated with a number of chronic and severe health problems. Homelessness is associated with tuberculosis, trauma, depression and other mental illnesses, alcoholism, drug abuse, sexually transmitted diseases, and poor nutrition (Breakey, 1997; Breakey & Fischer, 1995; Dellon, 1995; Greene, Ennett, & Ringwalt, 1997; Robertson, Zlotnick, & Westerfelt, 1997). The most recent national estimate suggests that the lifetime prevalence of homelessness (the percentage of persons who report having been homeless at some time in their lives) in the United States is about 7.4%, or 13.5 million people, and the five-year prevalence of homelessness was 3.1%, or about 5.7 million people (Breakey, 1997; Link et al., 1994). Although accurate estimates of trends in homelessness are not available, there is no evidence that the extent of homelessness is any less today than it was a decade ago (Breakey, 1997).

Even among those who do have housing, the quality of housing conditions is a significant concern. In 1991, 6.7% of all housing units had a leaking roof; 5.1% had open cracks in the ceiling or walls; and 5.0% had unusable toilets (Bok, 1996). The percentage of families eligible for federal assistance through public housing, subsidized housing, and rent supplements who receive such aid is only 30% (Bok,

1996). Although the federal government provides about $90 million in housing subsidies each year, $70 million of it is in the form of tax deductions for homeowners (Bok, 1996). For families not receiving subsidies or living in public housing, 77% pay more than half their income for rent (Bok, 1996).

The health consequences of poor-quality housing can be substantial. A recent study published in the *New England Journal of Medicine* found that exposure to cockroach debris may be the leading cause of asthma among inner-city children (Rosenstreich et al., 1997). Children who were exposed to higher levels of cockroach allergen not only had higher rates of hospitalization for asthma, but had more symptoms of wheezing, more physician visits, and more days of school absence than other asthmatic children. The high exposure to cockroaches in the inner city may explain both the high prevalence of asthma in the inner city and the increase in the incidence of asthma among inner-city children over the past 30 years (Platts-Mills & Carter, 1997).

Another example of important health consequences caused by poor housing is lead poisoning among children. Peeling lead-paint chips in older housing is still the chief cause of lead poisoning. Children living in houses built before 1946 are at greatest risk. From 1991 to 1994, about 16% of poor children living in such housing had elevated blood lead levels, putting them at risk for significant neurological and psychological impairment, including decreased school performance and IQ (CDC, 1997b).

Unemployment

Unemployment is recognized as a major predictor of morbidity and mortality in the population. Catalano (1991) has shown that for every 1% increase in unemployment during the 1980s, there was a 5% increase in mortality from heart disease and stroke and a 6% increase in homicide deaths. Economic strains associated with unemployment pose especially large health risks to disadvantaged people (Smith, 1987).

Overall unemployment rates in the United States have fallen slightly during the past two decades, from 8.5% in 1975 to 4.9% in 1997 (U.S. Department of Labor, 1997). However, unemployment rates among Black men and women during this period remained stable at about 14% to 15% (Office of the President of the United States, 1993; Sunstein, 1997). Moreover, fewer unemployed persons in the United States are receiving jobless benefits. Less than 30% of the unemployed received unemployment insurance during the 1990s, compared with more than 50% in the 1950s (General Accounting Office, 1992a) The General Accounting Office (1993) estimated that restrictions on unemployment insurance forced at least 250,000 people into poverty in 1990 alone.

Environmental Hazards

Exposure to environmental toxins is associated with a wide range of chronic health problems. Among the environmental hazards that cause the greatest disease burden are secondhand smoke (53,000 deaths per year) (Glantz & Parmley, 1991; Wells, 1988); indoor radon (7,000 to 30,000 deaths per year; Environmental Protection Agency, 1992; National Research Council, 1998); and arsenic in drinking water (about 4,700 deaths per year) (Smith et al., 1992). The CDC estimated that approximately 17% of all deaths in the United States could be prevented by reducing exposure to environmental hazards (CDC, 1995; USDHHS, 1995).

Despite improvements in environmental quality for the advantaged segment of the population, disadvantaged segments of the population still suffer from the adverse health effects of an unhealthy environment. A classic example of the disproportionate burden of environmental risk on the disadvantaged is the problem of childhood lead poisoning. Although the problem has been recognized for decades, the lead content in paint and gasoline has been regulated for many years, and the federal and state governments have spent millions of dollars on lead abatement programs, lead poisoning is still a significant health problem for poor, inner-city children (CDC, 1997b; General Accounting Office, 1992b). While only 1.0% of high-income children and 1.9% of middle-income children had elevated blood lead levels (>10 µg/dL) in the Third National Health and Nutrition Examination Survey (conducted between 1991 and 1994), 8.0% of low-income children had elevated blood lead levels (CDC, 1997b). Compounding the problem, more than 16% of low-income children who lived in houses built before 1946 had elevated blood lead levels, compared with 4.1% and 0.9% of middle- and high-income children, respectively. At least 3 to 4 million preschoolers in the United States have blood lead levels high enough to cause permanent nervous system or psychological impairment (Landrigan, 1992)

Crime and Violence

In 1984, former Surgeon General C. Everett Koop declared violence to be an epidemic and a public health problem: "Violence is as much a public health issue for me and my successors in this country as smallpox, tuberculosis, and syphilis were for my predecessors in the last two centuries" (Henig, 1997, p. 110). In 1988, CDC researchers Mercy and Houk called for a similar approach to the problem of violence: "The time has come for us to address this problem in the manner in which we have addressed and dealt successfully with other threats to the public health" (p. 1284). And most recently, CDC director David Satcher said, "If you look at the major cause of death today it's not smallpox or polio or even infectious diseases. Violence is the leading cause of lost life in this country today. If it's not a public health problem, why are all those people dying from it?" (Applebome, 1993, p. A7).

The disadvantaged communities in the United States have been ravaged by violence. Homicide is now the leading cause of death among young Black males, ages 15 to 24 and the second leading cause of death among all males in this age group (Satcher, 1996). The risk of homicide at some point in one's life is now 1 in 30 for Black males (U.S. Department of Justice, 1988). There are more than 200 million guns in private ownership throughout the United States and 5.5 million new ones introduced each year, of which 100,000 are carried by children to school each day (Bok, 1996). These firearms cause an estimated 35,000 deaths each year (USDHHS, 1995), and the link between the availability of firearms and the increasing homicide rate is "every bit as strong as the studies that linked cigarettes to lung cancer" (Taubes, 1992, p. 215). In addition, child abuse rates have increased from 10 per thousand children in 1976 to 45 per thousand in 1992; some of this increase may be attributable to increased reporting of abuse, but at least a portion is due to a real increase in incidence (Bok, 1996).

Between 1975 and 1991, rates of violent crime in the United States increased from 488 to 758 per 100,000 residents; rates of forcible rape increased from 26 to 42 per 100,000; and rates of aggravated assault increased from 231 to 433 per 100,000 residents (U.S. Department of Justice, 1992).

Social Support

The availability of a social support network—family, friends, and community programs to which an individual can turn to for help, advice, reassurance, and consolation—is a strong determinant of health status (Berkman, 1984; Berkman & Breslow, 1983; Berkman & Syme, 1979; Broadhead et al., 1983; Cassel, 1976; Corin, 1995; Patrick & Wickizer, 1995; Pilisuk & Minkler, 1985; Schorr, 1989). Even after controlling for most other known determinants of health—socioeconomic status, access to health care, and individual behaviors and lifestyle factors—the absence of social support remains a strong, independent predictor of disease (Berkman & Syme, 1979). As Schorr (1989) argued, "Formal social supports protect people from an amazing variety of pathological states, including destructive family functioning, low birthweight, depression, arthritis, tuberculosis, and even premature death" (p. 155).

The recent focus on what policy makers have termed "welfare reform" has taken a devastating toll on the availability and quality of social support networks in American communities. By reducing the level of government provision of basic needs—food, housing, transportation, child care, and health care—welfare "reform" has forced traditional social support networks, such as community support programs, to abandon their supportive tasks and instead scramble to find ways to meet the basic needs of their clients (Pilisuk & Minkler, 1985). As Pilisuk and Minkler (1985) argue, the primary value of welfare benefits is that it allows alternative support systems (families, friends, and community programs) to provide exactly the kind of support needed to keep people healthy.

> Family and community effectiveness in the provision of social support is heavily dependent upon the broader economic and social environment. . . . To build and maintain strong supportive ties, we must provide those programs, services, and policies on a societal level, which can help meet basic human needs. For it is only within this broader context of system-level support and commitment to people of all ages and places that social support on the individual and community levels can fulfill its potential. (p. 11)

The real threat that "welfare reform" poses to the public's health is that it renders ineffective the systems of social support in the family and community that are so closely tied to health status (Broadhead et al., 1983; Cassel, 1976; Cobb, 1976; Cohen & Syme, 1985; Pilisuk & Minkler, 1985). By forcing social support networks to concentrate on filling gaps in the basic needs of the poor rather than on providing a true social support system for those in distress, "welfare reform" as it is currently crafted makes it increasingly more difficult to achieve within communities the social conditions in which people can be healthy. Lisbeth Schorr (1989) summarized the problem:

> For those living in persistent and concentrated poverty, it is reformed services and institutions that will furnish the essential footholds for the climb out of poverty. Yet in the legislative, academic, and political forums where antipoverty strategies and welfare reform are debated, the spotlight is only on short-term measures to reduce the numbers now on welfare, now unable to work productively. The shocking deficiencies in the health, welfare, and education of poor children, the long-term investments that could help the vulnerable children of today to become the productive and contributing adults of tomorrow, are rarely on the agenda. . . . Children and families have needs that cannot be met by economic measures alone, and that cannot be met by individual families alone. (pp. xxiii, xxiv)

This is where community social support networks come into the picture.

The potential impact of the "welfare reform" provisions of the Personal Responsibility and Work Opportunity Act of 1996 (Pub. L. No. 104-193) has been evaluated by the Urban Institute (1996). According to the Urban Institute, the Act will lower 2.6 million people into poverty; 1.1 million of these will be children. Nearly 11 million families, or 10% of all families in America, will lose income; this includes more than 8 million families with children, which will lose an average of $1,300 per family.

In addition, most of the 800,000 legal immigrants who now receive supplemental security income (SSI) benefits and food stamps will be cut off, and new immigrants will not be eligible for any federal benefits, including welfare, SSI, food stamps, and Medicaid, for their first 5 years in the country (Edelman, 1997; Ladenheim, 1997). Several recent articles in the *American Journal of Public Health* suggest that these provisions will have profound public health implications, including health crises for persons with untreated diabetes, hypertension, and asthma and reduced control of communicable diseases (Ladenheim, 1997; Thamer, Richard, Casebeer, & Ray, 1997).

A CRISIS IN ACCESS TO QUALITY HEALTH CARE

Inadequate access to health care services is associated with increased burdens of economic hardship, poor health, and increased mortality (Blendon et al., 1994; Donelan et al., 1997; Franks, Clancy, & Gold, 1993; Henry J. Kaiser Family Foundation, 1994; Lurie, Ward, Shapiro, & Brook, 1984; Lurie et al., 1986; Weissman & Epstein, 1994). The CDC estimated that about 11% of all deaths could be prevented by improving the population's access to quality medical treatment (CDC, 1995; USDHHS, 1995). Approximately 15% of the population—more than 40 million people—lack health insurance (NCHS, 1997). In spite of the widespread recognition of this problem and the rhetoric about the importance of ensuring all citizens access to health care, the proportion of uninsured Americans increased from 13.6% in 1970 to 15.4% in 1995 (Bok, 1996; NCHS, 1997). As of 1995, 21% of all children less than 15 years old lacked private health insurance; 14% (10 million) neither had health insurance nor were enrolled in Medicaid (NCHS, 1997). Lack of insurance tends to be a problem of the poor. Of the uninsured, approximately one-third have incomes below the poverty line, and two-thirds have incomes at or below 200% of the poverty line (Bok, 1996). Nearly one-third of all persons living below the poverty line lack access to health insurance and to Medicaid (Bok, 1996).

The problem of access to quality health care among the poor is not limited to lack of insurance. Several studies have shown that disadvantaged populations tend to receive inferior health care, regardless of whether they have health insurance (Burstin, Lipsitz, & Brennan, 1992; Dalen & Santiago, 1991; Diehr, Richardson, Shortell, & LoGerfo, 1991; Goldberg, Hartz, Jacobsen, Krakauer, & Rimm, 1992; Kahn et al., 1994; Kasiske et al., 1991; Wenneker & Epstein, 1989; Yergan, Flood, LoGerfo, & Diehr, 1987). For example, even among those who are insured by Medicaid, access to high-quality health care is limited. Several studies have shown that Medicaid patients are less likely to receive preventive care and that their physical health fares worse under Medicaid managed care than under fee-for-service payment (Ware, Bayliss, Rogers, Kosinski, & Tarlov, 1996). Ware and associates (1997) found that during a four-year follow-up period, poor patients treated under Medicaid managed care suffered greater declines in physical health status than those treated under traditional, fee-for-service Medicaid. Even without managed care, Medicaid patients have less access to continuing care and preventive care than patients who are privately insured (Davidson, Klein, Settipane, & Alario, 1994; Kerr & Siu, 1993).

Similarly, poor elderly patients who are enrolled in Medicare managed care may be less likely to have access to the intensive rehabilitation and support services that are necessary to keep them self-sufficient and avoid institutionalization. Retchin, Brown, Yeh, Chu, and Moreno (1997) found that compared with fee-for-service Medicare patients, Medicare managed care patients who suffer a stroke are more likely to be discharged to nursing homes and less likely to be placed in rehabilitative settings or discharged to home. Access to home health care and outcomes under Medicare managed care have also been shown to be worse than under traditional, fee-for-service Medicare (Experton, Li, Branch, Ozminkowski, & Mellon-Lacey, 1997; Shaugnessy, Schlenker, & Hittle, 1994). And Ware and colleagues (1996) reported that elderly patients in health maintenance organizations (HMOs) had more significant declines in physical health compared with those who remained in fee-for-service settings over a four-year follow-up period.

The problem of inadequate access to health care has been exacerbated by recent initiatives, such as California's Proposition 187 (approved in 1994), which deny health care benefits (Medicaid) to children of illegal immigrants.

IMPLICATIONS OF THE CHRONIC DISEASE EPIDEMIC FOR PUBLIC HEALTH PRACTICE

During the nineteenth and early twentieth centuries, when the chief causes of preventable death were infectious diseases spread by contaminated water and food, the focus of public health practice was building a societal infrastructure for proper sanitation and hygiene and for the delivery of vaccines and treatments to the population. The chronic disease epidemic of the late twentieth century, however, is largely related to individual lifestyle and behavior and to deteriorating economic and social conditions and the failure of social policy to address problems such as affordable and accessible health care of high quality for all Americans. Thus, public health practice at the turn of the millennium must focus on modifying individual lifestyle and behavior, improving social and economic conditions, and reforming social policy.

To start, at least 1 million American lives, or about one half of all deaths, could be saved each year by changes in individual health-related behaviors (see Figure 1–2; CDC, 1995; USDHHS, 1995).

Although public health practice clearly has to focus on modifying individual lifestyle and behavior, it is important to note that personal behavior does not take place in a vacuum. Rather, it takes place within the context of a historical, cultural, and political environment and within communities with varying economic and social conditions. To effectively change individual behavior, one cannot ignore the conditions and environment in which that behavior takes place. In fact, some argue that focusing on the economic and social conditions that give rise to unhealthy behaviors is essential to change those behaviors. Because behavior is a product of the social conditions and social norms of the community in which a person lives (Tesh, 1994), "discussing changes in lifestyles without first discussing the changes in the social conditions which give rise to them, without recognizing that the lifestyle is derivative, is misleading" (Berliner, 1977, p. 119).

Not only do social and economic factors influence health behaviors and individual lifestyle, but also these factors are themselves independently related to health status. Several decades of research have demonstrated that lower social class, social deprivation, and lack of social support are among the most important determinants of health (Antonovsky, 1967; Berkman, 1984; Bright, 1967; Cassel, 1976; Conrad, 1994; Frey, 1982; Haan et al., 1987; Kitagawa & Hauser, 1973; Marmot, 1982; Morris, 1979, 1982; Rose & Marmot, 1981; Salonen, 1982; Stockwell, 1961; Syme & Berkman, 1976; Yeracaris & Kim, 1978). Moreover, the strong association between these socioeconomic factors and health is not entirely explained by differences in individual lifestyle and health behaviors between members of higher and lower social class groups (Haan et al., 1987; Rose & Marmot, 1981; Salonen, 1982; Slater & Carlton, 1985; Slater, Lorimor, & Lairson, 1985; Wiley & Camacho, 1980). Link and Phelan (1996) recently proposed a novel view of the relationship between socioeconomic status and disease, asserting that socioeconomic status must be viewed as a "fundamental cause" of disease.

The Institute of Medicine report (1988) on the future of public health, noting the importance of social and economic factors as determinants of health status, suggested that public health must take a much wider view of disease than in the past: "Public health programs, to be effective, should move beyond programs targeted on the immediate problem, such as teen pregnancy, to health promotion and prevention by dealing with underlying factors in the social environment. To deal with these factors, the scope of public health will need to encompass relationships with other social programs in education, social services, housing, and income maintenance" (p. 113).

The late Sol Levine noted that social factors "mean not only poverty but also social class, family, community, gender, ethnicity, racism, political economy, and culture. We have to learn how these interact with health, how, for example, culture, political economy, and racism may affect the community and family environment, which, in turn, may influence people's health. We have to look not only at individual characteristics but to the features of the society as well" (Henig, 1997, p. 102).

Because social and economic conditions are themselves a product of social policy, public health practice must also focus on changing social policy. Poverty is not a consequence of individual frailty, lack of responsibility, and lack of motivation, as some have argued. Rather, it is the product of social and economic conditions created and maintained by the historical, political, and cultural environment in which society has developed (Zaidi, 1988). Social policy contributes, at least in part, to the environment that determines social and economic conditions in the community. The availability of adequate food, housing, and jobs; the quality of the physical environment; access to medical services; the extent of social support in the community; and the amount of economic, employment, and educational opportunity are all influenced strongly by social policies. Former Harvard University president Derek Bok (1996) has argued that "current levels of poverty are not immutable but are the result of policy choices, choices that seem at odds with the stated desire of most Americans to do more for the deserving poor" (p. 351).

For example, government assistance for single mothers with no earned income is only 27% of the median family income in the United States, compared with 38% in France, 47% in Germany, 60% in Britain, and 64% in Sweden (Bok, 1996). The rate of poverty among single mothers in the United States is more than twice the rate in each of the other countries (Bok, 1996). Quite simply, social policy has a direct and understandable effect on social conditions.

To effectively confront threats to the public's health, the three major functions of public health must be (1) modifying individual behavior and lifestyle, (2) improving social and economic conditions, and (3) reforming social policies. All of these represent fundamental aspects of social change. Ultimately, then, public health is in the business of creating or facilitating social change (Figure 1–3).

It should be noted that although chronic diseases have replaced infectious diseases as the chief causes of death in the United States, the nation has recently experienced a reemergence of infectious diseases. After declining for decades, mortality rates from infectious causes are now increasing (Bartlett, 1997; Pinner et al., 1996). The rate of death from infectious diseases in the United States increased from 41 deaths per 100,000 persons in 1980 to 65 per 100,000 persons in 1992, a 58% increase (Pinner et al., 1996). The death rate among 25- to 44-year-olds increased by 630% during this period, from 6 to 38 deaths per 100,000 persons (Pinner et al., 1996). This increase was due primarily to the emergence of the acquired immunodeficiency syndrome (AIDS), which accounted for an estimated 43,000 deaths in 1995 (NCHS, 1997). The death rate among the elderly increased by 25%, from 271 to 338 deaths per 100,000 persons 65 years of age and older during the period 1980 to 1992; most of these deaths were attributable to respiratory tract infections. By 1992, infectious diseases combined represented the third leading cause of death in the nation (Pinner et al., 1996).

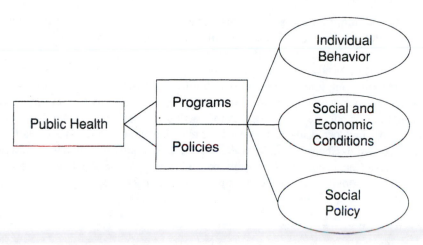

Figure 1–3 An Overview of the Functions of Public Health: Creating Social Change

The recent rise of infectious diseases as a major cause of mortality and the significant increases in the absolute rates of death from infectious diseases have led public health groups, including the CDC and the Institute of Medicine, to develop a new focus on what are termed *emerging infections* (Bartlett, 1997; CDC, 1994; Lederberg, Shope, & Oaks, 1992). These infections include the hantavirus pulmonary syndrome, Lyme disease, Ebola virus infection, and infection with group A ("flesh-eating") streptococcus (Bartlett, 1997). The emergence of new viral diseases is coupled with the recent rise of resistance to bacteria that were previously controlled easily.

The epidemic of emerging infectious diseases, like the chronic disease epidemic, is strongly related to individual lifestyles and behaviors, social and economic conditions, and social policy. Infection with the human immunodeficiency virus (HIV), for example, is precipitated by intravenous drug use. The spread of tuberculosis infection, especially multi–drug-resistant strains, is promoted by crowded and unsanitary living conditions. And the failure of society to develop rational policies to control the spread of HIV infection—such as needle exchange programs—that have been shown to be among the most highly effective interventions available has contributed to the AIDS epidemic (Lurie & Drucker, 1997).

CONCLUSION

The major implication of the chronic disease and emerging infectious disease epidemics for public health policy and practice is that public health must focus on far more than the provision of medical care. It must, first and foremost, focus on modifying individual lifestyle and behavior, improving social and economic conditions, and reforming social policy that contributes to an environment in which it is difficult for people to be healthy. Ultimately, then, public health is in the business of creating or facilitating social change.

The three-pronged attack that is necessary to control the epidemic of chronic disease and emerging infectious diseases in the United States—modifying individual lifestyle and behavior, improving social and economic conditions, and reforming social policy—is not one that public health practitioners have traditionally been well equipped to conduct. And it has not been one at which public health has been particularly successful. Chapter 2 explores the reasons that modifying individual lifestyle and behavior, improving social conditions, and reforming social policy represent a unique and formidable challenge to the public health practitioner.

REFERENCES

Adler, N.E., Boyce, W.T., Chesney, M.A., Folkman, S., & Syme, S.L. (1997). Socioeconomic inequalities in health: No easy solution. In P.R. Lee & C.L. Estes (Eds.), *The nation's health* (5th ed., pp. 18–31). Sudbury, MA: Jones and Bartlett.

American Cancer Society. (1994). *Cancer facts & figures—1994.* New York: Author.

Antonovsky, A. (1967). Social class, life expectancy, and overall mortality. *Milbank Memorial Fund Quarterly, 45,* 31–73.

Applebome, P. (1993, September 26). CDC's new chief worries as much about bullets as about bacteria. *The New York Times,* p. A7.

Bartlett, J.G. (1997). Update in infectious diseases. *Annals of Internal Medicine, 126,* 48–56.

Berkman, L.F. (1984). Assessing the physical health effects of social networks and social support. *Annual Reviews of Public Health, 5,* 413–432.

Berkman, L.F., & Breslow, L. (Eds.). (1983). *Health and ways of living: The Alameda County Study.* New York: Oxford University Press.

Berkman, L.F., & Syme, S.L. (1979). Social networks, host resistance, and mortality: A nine-year follow-up study of Alameda County residents. *American Journal of Epidemiology, 109,* 186–204.

Berliner, H. (1977). Emerging ideologies in medicine. *Review of Radical Political Economics, 9,* 116–124.

Blendon, R.J., Donelan, K., Hill, C.A., Carter, W., Beatrice, D., & Altman, D. (1994). Paying medical bills in the United States: Why health insurance isn't enough. *Journal of the American Medical Association, 271,* 949–951.

Bok, D. (1996). *The state of the nation.* Cambridge, MA: Harvard University Press.

Bonneux, L., Barendregt, J.J., Meeter, K., Bonsel, G.J., & van der Maas, P.J. (1994). Estimating clinical morbidity due to ischemic heart disease and congestive heart failure: The future rise of heart failure. *American Journal of Public Health, 84,* 20–28.

Breakey, W.R. (1997). Editorial: It's time for the public health community to declare war on homelessness. *American Journal of Public Health, 87,* 153–155.

Breakey, W.R., & Fischer, P.J. (1995). Mental illness and the continuum of residential stability. *Social Psychiatry and Psychiatric Epidemiology, 30,* 147–151.

Bright, M. (1967). A follow-up study of the Commission on Cultural Illness Morbidity Survey in Baltimore. II. Race and sex differences in mortality. *Journal of Chronic Diseases, 20,* 717–729.

Broadhead, W.E., Kaplan, B.H., James, S.A., Wagner, E.H., Shoenbach, V.J., Grimson, R., Heyden, S., Tibblin, G., & Gehlbach, S.H. (1983). The epidemiological evidence for a relationship between social support and health. *American Journal of Epidemiology, 117,* 521–537.

Burstin, H.R., Lipsitz, S.R., & Brennan, T.A. (1992). Socioeconomic status and risk for substandard medical care. *Journal of the American Medical Association, 268,* 2383–2387.

Cassel, J. (1976). The contribution of the social environment to host resistance. *American Journal of Epidemiology, 104,* 107–123.

Catalano, R. (1991). The health effects of economic insecurity. *American Journal of Public Health, 81,* 1148–1152.

Centers for Disease Control and Prevention. (1993). *Cardiovascular disease surveillance: Ischemic heart disease, 1980–1989.* Atlanta, GA: Centers for Disease Control and Prevention, National Center for Chronic Disease Prevention and Health Promotion, Division of Chronic Disease Control and Community Intervention.

Centers for Disease Control and Prevention. (1994). *Addressing emerging infectious disease threats: A prevention strategy for the United States.* Atlanta, GA: Centers for Disease Control and Prevention, National Center for Infectious Diseases.

Centers for Disease Control and Prevention. (1995). *1994: Ten leading causes of death in the United States.* Atlanta, GA: Centers for Disease Control, National Center for Injury Prevention and Control.

Centers for Disease Control and Prevention. (1996). Cigarette smoking among adults—United States, 1994. *Morbidity and Mortality Weekly Report, 45,* 588–590.

Centers for Disease Control and Prevention. (1997a). Trends in the prevalence and incidence of self-reported diabetes mellitus—United States, 1980–1994. *Morbidity and Mortality Weekly Report, 46,* 1014–1018.

Centers for Disease Control and Prevention. (1997b). Update: Blood lead levels—United States, 1991–1994. *Morbidity and Mortality Weekly Report, 46,* 141–146.

Children's Defense Fund. (1994). *Wasting America's future.* Washington, DC: Author.

Cobb, S. (1976). Social support as a moderator of life stress. *Journal of Psychosomatic Medicine, 38,* 300–314.

Cohen, S., & Syme, S.L. (Eds.). (1985). *Social support and health.* New York: Academic Press.

Conrad, P. (1994). Wellness in the workplace: Potentials and pitfalls of work-site health promotion. In H.D. Schwartz (Ed.), *Dominant issues in medical sociology* (3rd ed., pp. 556–567). New York: McGraw-Hill.

Corin, E. (1995). The cultural frame: Context and meaning in the construction of health. In B.C. Amick, III, S. Levine, A.R. Tarlov, & D.C. Walsh (Eds.), *Society and health* (pp. 272–304). New York: Oxford University Press.

Dalen, J.E., & Santiago, J. (1991). Insuring the uninsured is not enough. *Archives of Internal Medicine, 151,* 860–862.

Davidson, A.E., Klein, D.E., Settipane, G.A., & Alario, A.J. (1994). Access to care among children visiting the emergency room with acute exacerbations of asthma. *Annals of Allergy, 72,* 469–473.

Dellon, E.S. (1995). The health status of the Providence-area homeless population. *Rhode Island Medicine, 78,* 278–283.

Diehr, P.K., Richardson, W.C., Shortell, S.M., & LoGerfo, J.P. (1991). Increased access to medical care. *Medical Care, 10,* 989–999.

Donelan, K., Blendon, R.J., Hill, C.A., Hoffman, C., Rowland, D., Frankel, M., & Altman D. (1997). Whatever happened to the health insurance crisis in the United States? Voices from a national survey. In P.R. Lee, & C.L. Estes (Eds.), *The nation's health* (5th ed., pp. 283–291). Sudbury, MA: Jones and Bartlett.

Edelman, P. (1997, March). The worst thing Bill Clinton has done. *The Atlantic Monthly,* pp. 43–58.

Environmental Protection Agency. (1992). *A citizen's guide to radon* (2nd ed.). Washington, DC: Author.

Experton, B., Li, Z., Branch, L.G., Ozminkowski, R.J., & Mellon-Lacey, D.M. (1997). The impact of payor/provider type on health care use and expenditures among the frail elderly. *American Journal of Public Health, 87,* 210–216.

Franks, P., Clancy, C.M., & Gold, M.R. (1993). Health insurance and mortality: Evidence from a national cohort. *Journal of the American Medical Association, 270,* 737–741.

Frey, R.S. (1982). The socioeconomic distribution of mortality rates in Des Moines, Iowa. *Public Health Reports, 97,* 545–549.

General Accounting Office. (1992a). *Education issues.* Washington, DC: Author.

General Accounting Office. (1992b). *Environmental protection issues.* Washington, DC: Author.

General Accounting Office. (1993). *Decline in UI beneficiaries.* Washington, DC: Author.

Glantz, S.A., & Parmley, W.W. (1991). Passive smoking and heart disease: Epidemiology, physiology, and biochemistry. *Circulation, 83,* 1–12.

Goldberg, K.C., Hartz, A.J., Jacobsen, S.J., Krakauer, H., & Rimm, A.A. (1992). Racial and community factors influencing coronary artery bypass graft surgery rates for all 1986 Medicare patients. *Journal of the American Medical Association, 267,* 1473–1477.

Greene, J.M., Ennett, S.T., & Ringwalt, C.L. (1997). Substance use among runaway and homeless youth in three national samples. *American Journal of Public Health, 87,* 229–235.

Gregorio, D.I., Walsh, S.J., & Paturzo, D. (1997). The effects of occupation-based social position on mortality in a large American cohort. *American Journal of Public Health, 87,* 1472–1475.

Haan, M., Kaplan, G.A., & Camacho, T. (1987). Poverty and health: Prospective evidence from the Alameda County Study. *American Journal of Epidemiology, 125,* 989–998.

Harris, I.B. (1996). *Children in jeopardy: Can we break the cycle of poverty?* New Haven, CT: Yale University Press.

Hemingway, H., Nicholson, A., Stafford, M., Roberts, R., & Marmot, M. (1997). The impact of socioeconomic status on health functioning as assessed by the SF-36 questionnaire: The Whitehall II Study. *American Journal of Public Health, 87,* 1484–1490.

Henig, R.M. (1997). *The people's health: A memoir of public health and its evolution at Harvard.* Washington, DC: Joseph Henry Press.

Henry J. Kaiser Family Foundation (1994). Project LEAN idea kit for state and community programs to reduce dietary fat. Menlo Park, CA: Author.

Hoffman, C., Rice, D., & Sung, H.Y. (1996). Persons with chronic conditions: Their prevalence and costs. *Journal of the American Medical Association, 276,* 1473–1479.

Institute of Medicine, Committee for the Study of the Future of Public Health. (1988). *The future of public health.* Washington, DC: National Academy Press.

Jenkins, C.D., Tuthill, R.W., Tannenbaum, S.I., & Kirby, C.R. (1977). Zones of excess mortality in Massachusetts. *New England Journal of Medicine, 296,* 1354–1356.

Kahn, K.L., Pearson, M.L., Harrison, E.R., Desmond, K.A., Rogers, W.H., Rubenstein, L.V., Brook, R.H., & Keeler, E.B. (1994). Health care for Black and poor hospitalized Medicare patients. *Journal of the American Medical Association, 271,* 1169–1174.

Kaplan, G.A., & Lynch, J.W. (1997). Editorial: Whither studies on the socioeconomic foundations of population health? *American Journal of Public Health, 87,* 1409–1411.

Kasiske, B.L., Neylan, J.F., Riggio, R.R., Danovitch, G.M., Kahana, L., Alexander, S.R., & White, M.G. (1991). The effect of race on access and outcome in transplantation. *New England Journal of Medicine, 324,* 302–307.

Kawachi, I., Kennedy, B.P., Lochner, K., & Prothrow-Stith, D. (1997). Social capital, income inequality, and mortality. *American Journal of Public Health, 87,* 1491–1498.

Kennedy, B., Kawachi, I., & Prothrow-Stith, D. (1995). Income distribution and mortality: Cross-sectional ecological study of the Robin Hood Index in the United States. *British Medical Journal, 312,* 1004–1007.

Kerr, E.A., & Siu, A.L. (1993). Follow-up after hospital discharge: Does insurance make a difference? *Journal of Health Care for the Poor & Underserved, 4,* 133–142.

Kitagawa, E.M., & Hauser, P.M. (1973). *Differential mortality in the United States: A study in socio-economic epidemiology.* Cambridge, MA: Harvard University Press.

Ladenheim, K. (1997). Comment: Health insurance coverage of foreign-born US residents—The implications of the new welfare reform law. *American Journal of Public Health, 87,* 12–14.

Landrigan, P. (1992). Environmental disease—Preventable epidemic. *American Journal of Public Health, 82,* 941–943.

Lederberg, J., Shope, R.E., & Oaks, S.C., Jr. (Eds.). (1992). *Emerging infections: Microbial threats to health in the United States.* Washington, DC: National Academy Press.

Link, B.G., & Phelan, J.C. (1996). Review: Why are some people healthy and others not? The determinants of health of populations. *American Journal of Public Health, 86,* 598–599.

Link, B.G., Susser, E., Stueve, A., Phelan, J., Moore, R.E., & Struening, E. (1994). Lifetime and five-year prevalence of homelessness in the United States. *American Journal of Public Health, 84,* 1907–1912.

Lurie, N., Ward, N.B., Shapiro, M.F., & Brook, R.H. (1984). Termination from Medi-Cal: Does it affect health? *New England Journal of Medicine, 311,* 480–484.

Lurie, N., Ward, N.B., Shapiro, M.F., Gallego, C., Vaghaiwalla, R., & Brook, R.H. (1986). Termination of medical benefits: A follow-up study one year later. *New England Journal of Medicine, 314,* 1266–1268.

Lurie, P., & Drucker, E. (1997). An opportunity lost: HIV infections associated with lack of a national needle-exchange programme in the USA. *The Lancet, 349,* 604–608.

Lynch, J.W., Kaplan, G.A., & Shema, S.J. (1997). Cumulative impact of sustained economic hardship on physical, cognitive, psychological, and social functioning. *New England Journal of Medicine, 337,* 1889–1895.

Marmot, M., Bobak, M., & Smith, G.D. (1995). Explanations for social inequalities in health. In B.C. Amick, III, S. Levine, A.R. Tarlov, & D.C. Walsh (Eds.), *Society and health* (pp. 172–210). New York: Oxford University Press.

Marmot, M.G. (1982). Socioeconomic and cultural factors in ischemic heart disease. *Advances in Cardiology, 29,* 68–76.

McCord, C., & Freeman, H.P. (1990). Excess mortality in Harlem. *New England Journal of Medicine, 322,* 173–178.

McDonough, P., Duncan, G.J., William, D., & House, J. (1997). Income dynamics and adult mortality in the United States, 1972 through 1989. *American Journal of Public Health, 87,* 1476–1483.

McGinnis, J.M., & Foege, W. (1993). Actual causes of death in the United States. *Journal of the American Medical Association, 270,* 2207–2212.

Mercy, J.A., & Houk, V.N. (1988). Firearm injuries: A call for science. *New England Journal of Medicine, 319,* 1283–1285.

Meyers, A.F., Sampson, A.E., Weitzman, M., Rogers, B.L., & Kayne, H. (1989). School Breakfast Program and school performance. *American Journal of Diseases of Children, 143,* 1234–1239.

Morris, J.N. (1979). Social inequalities undiminished. *The Lancet, 1,* 87–90.

Morris, J.N. (1982). Epidemiology and prevention. *Milbank Memorial Fund Quarterly/Health and Society, 60,* 1–16.

Moss, N. (1997). Editorial: The body politic and the power of socioeconomic status. *American Journal of Public Health, 87,* 1411–1413.

National Center for Health Statistics. (1997). *Health, United States, 1996–97, and injury chartbook* (DHHS Publication No. PHS 97-1232). Hyattsville, MD: Author.

National Research Council. (1998). *Health effects of exposure to radon: BEIR VI.* Washington, DC: National Academy of Sciences, National Research Council, Committee on the Biological Effects of Ionizing Radiation (BEIR VI), Committee on Health Risks of Exposure to Radon.

Navarro, V. (1997). Topics for our times: The "Black Report" of Spain—The Commission of Social Inequalities in Health. *American Journal of Public Health, 87,* 334–335.

Office of the President of the United States. (1993). *Economic report of the President 1993.* Washington, DC: U.S. Government Printing Office.

Pappas, G., Queen, S., Hadden, W., & Fisher, G. (1993). The increasing disparity in mortality between socioeconomic groups in the United States, 1960 and 1986. *New England Journal of Medicine, 329,* 103–109.

Patrick, D.L., & Wickizer, T.M. (1995). Community and health. In B.C. Amick, III, S. Levine, A.R. Tarlov, & D.C. Walsh (Eds.), *Society and health* (pp. 46–92). New York: Oxford University Press.

Pilisuk, M., & Minkler, M. (1985, Winter). Social support: Economic and political considerations. *Social Policy,* 6–11.

Pinner, R.W., Teutsch, S.M., Simonsen, L., Klug, L.A., Graber, J.M., Clarke, M.J., & Berkelman, R.L. (1996). Trends in infectious diseases mortality in the United States. *Journal of the American Medical Association, 275,* 189–193.

Platts-Mills, T.A.E., & Carter, M.C. (1997). Asthma and indoor exposure to allergens. *New England Journal of Medicine, 336,* 1382–1384.

Pollitt, E., Gersovitz, M., & Garginlo, M. (1978). Educational benefits of the United States school feeding program: A critical review of the literature. *American Journal of Public Health, 68,* 477–481.

Power, C., Hertzman, C., Matthews, S., & Manor, O. (1997). Social differences in health: Life cycle effects between ages 23 and 33 in the 1958 British birth cohort. *American Journal of Public Health, 87,* 1499–1503.

Retchin, S.M., Brown, R.S., Yeh, S.J., Chu, D., & Moreno, L. (1997). Outcomes of stroke patients in Medicare fee for service and managed care. *Journal of the American Medical Association, 278,* 119–124.

Robertson, M.J., Zlotnick, C., & Westerfelt, A. (1997). Drug use disorders and treatment contact among homeless adults in Alameda County. *American Journal of Public Health, 87,* 221–228.

Rose, D., & Oliveira, V. (1997). Nutrient intakes of individuals from food-insufficient households in the United States. *American Journal of Public Health, 87,* 1956–1961.

Rose, G., & Marmot, M.G. (1981). Social class and coronary heart disease. *British Heart Journal, 45,* 13–19.

Rosenberg, M.L., Powell, K.E., & Hammond, R. (1997). Applying science to violence prevention. *Journal of the American Medical Association, 277,* 1641–1642.

Rosenstreich, D.L., Eggleston, P., Kattan, M., Baker, D., Slavin, R.G., Gergen, P., Mitchell, H., McNiff-Mortimer, K., Lynn, H., Ownby, D., & Malveaux, F. (1997). The role of cockroach allergy and exposure to cockroach allergen in causing morbidity among inner-city children with asthma. *New England Journal of Medicine, 336,* 1356–1363.

Salonen, J.T. (1982). Socioeconomic status and risk of cancer, cerebral stroke, and death due to coronary heart disease and any disease: A longitudinal study in eastern Finland. *Journal of Epidemiology and Community Health, 36,* 294–297.

Satcher, D. (1996). CDC's first 50 years: Lessons learned and relearned. *American Journal of Public Health, 86,* 1705–1708.

Schorr, L.B. (1989). *Within our reach: Breaking the cycle of disadvantage.* New York: Anchor Books.

Shaugnessy, P., Schlenker, R.E., & Hittle, D.F. (1994). Home health care outcomes under capitated and fee-for-service payment. *Health Care Financing Review, 16,* 187–222.

Sidel, V.W. (1997). Annotation: The public health impact of hunger. *American Journal of Public Health, 87,* 1921–1922.

Slater, C., & Carlton, B. (1985). Behavior, lifestyle, and socioeconomic variables as determinants of health status: Implications for health policy development. *American Journal of Preventive Medicine, 1,* 25–33.

Slater, C.H., Lorimor, R.J., & Lairson, D.R. (1985). The independent contributions of socioeconomic status and health practices to health status. *Preventive Medicine, 14,* 372–378.

Smith, A.H., Hopenhayn-Rich, C., Bates, M.N., Goeden, H.M., Hert-Picciotto, I., Duggan, H.M., Wood, R., Kosnett, M.J., & Smith, M.T. (1992). Cancer risks from arsenic in drinking water. *Environmental Health Perspectives, 97,* 259–267.

Smith, R. (1987). *Unemployment and health.* London: Oxford University Press.

Stockwell, E.G. (1961). Socioeconomic status and mortality in the United States. *Public Health Reports, 76,* 1081–1086.

Sunstein, C.R. (1997). *Free markets and social justice.* New York: Oxford University Press.

Susser, M., Watson, W., & Hopper, K. (1985). *Sociology in medicine* (3rd ed.). Oxford, England: Oxford University Press.

Syme, S.L., & Berkman, L.F. (1976). Social class, susceptibility and sickness. *American Journal of Epidemiology, 104,* 1–8.

Sytkowski, P.A., Kannel, W.B., & D'Agostino, R.B. (1990). Changes in risk factors and the decline in mortality from cardiovascular disease: The Framingham Heart Study. *New England Journal of Medicine, 322,* 1635–1641.

Taubes, G. (1992). Violence epidemiologists test the hazards of gun ownership. *Science, 258,* 215.

Tesh, S.N. (1994). Hidden arguments: Political ideology and disease prevention policy. In H.D. Schwartz (Ed.), *Dominant issues in medical sociology* (3rd ed., pp. 519–529). New York: McGraw-Hill.

Thamer, M., Richard, C., Casebeer, A.W., & Ray, N.F. (1997). Health insurance coverage among foreign-born US residents: The impact of race, ethnicity, and length of residence. *American Journal of Public Health, 87,* 96–102.

Townsend, P., & Davidson, N. (1982). *Inequalities in health: The Black Report.* Harmondsworth, England: Penguin.

U.S. Department of Education. (1994, April). *The reading report card, 1971–88.* Washington, DC: U.S. Department of Education, National Center for Education Statistics, National Assessment of Educational Progress.

U.S. Department of Health and Human Services. (1995). *Healthy people 2000: Midcourse review and 1995 revisions.* Washington, DC: U.S. Department of Health and Human Services, Public Health Service.

U.S. Department of Justice. (1988). *Report to the nation on crime and justice.* Washington, DC: Author.

U.S. Department of Justice. (1992). *Uniform crime reports for the United States 1992.* Washington, DC: U.S. Department of Justice, Federal Bureau of Investigation.

U.S. Department of Labor. (1997). *Employment and earnings.* Washington, DC: U.S. Department of Labor, Bureau of Labor Statistics.

Urban Institute. (1996). *Potential effects of Congressional welfare reform legislation on family incomes.* Washington, DC: Author.

Ware, J.E., Jr., Bayliss, M.S., Rogers, W.H., Kosinski, M., & Tarlov, A.R. (1996). Differences in 4-year health outcomes for elderly and poor, chronically ill patients treated in HMO and fee-for-service systems. Results from the Medical Outcomes Study. *Journal of the American Medical Association, 276,* 1039–1047.

Wehler, C.A., Scott, R.I., Anderson, J.J., Summer, L., & Parker, L. (1995). *Community childhood hunger identification project: A survey of childhood hunger in the United States.* Washington, DC: Food Research and Action Center.

Weissman, J.S., & Epstein, A.M. (1994). *Falling through the safety net: The impact of insurance on access to care.* Baltimore: Johns Hopkins University Press.

Wells, A.J. (1988). An estimate of adult mortality in the United States from passive smoking. *Environment International, 14,* 249–265.

Wenneker, M.B., & Epstein, A.M. (1989). Racial inequalities in the use of procedures for patients with ischemic heart disease in Massachusetts. *Journal of the American Medical Association, 261,* 253–257.

Wiley, J.A., & Camacho, T.C. (1980). Life-style and future health: Evidence from the Alameda County Study. *Preventive Medicine, 9,* 1–21.

Wilkinson, R.G. (1990). Income distribution and mortality: A "natural" experiment. *Sociology of Health and Illness, 12,* 391–412.

Wilkinson, R.G. (1992). Income distribution and life expectancy. *British Medical Journal, 304,* 165–168.

Wilkinson, R.G. (1997). Comment: Income, inequality, and social cohesion. *American Journal of Public Health, 87,* 1504–1506.

Yeracaris, C.A., & Kim, J.H. (1978). Socioeconomic differentials in selected causes of death. *American Journal of Public Health, 68,* 432–451.

Yergan, J., Flood, A.N., LoGerfo, J.P., & Diehr, P. (1987). Relationship between patient race and the intensity of hospital services. *Medical Care, 25,* 592–603.

Zaidi, S.A. (1988). Poverty and disease: Need for structural change. *Social Science and Medicine, 27,* 119–127.

CHAPTER 2

Marketing Social Change— A Challenge for the Public Health Practitioner

Public health aims to satisfy the human need for health by facilitating a series of individual and societal exchange processes. These exchanges include the adoption of individual behavior and lifestyle changes and the adoption of societal programs to improve social and economic conditions. Marketing is defined as "human activity directed at satisfying needs and wants through exchange processes." Thus, whether they realize it or not, public health practitioners are in the business of marketing. The basic public health product is social change, and the fundamental mission of the public health practitioner is to market social change.

Unlike most traditional products, however, those which public health must market tend to have negative demand, no demand, or unwholesome demand. People do not want the product, do not care about the product, or they desire an alternative product whose use is counterproductive to the goal of improving health. In addition, the environment is hostile to public efforts to stimulate demand for social change. Not only is the state of demand for social change unfavorable and the environment for marketing social change hostile, but the public health practitioner is not generally trained in the skills necessary to be an effective marketer. Thus, the need to market social change represents a formidable challenge to the public health practitioner.

——————— ❧ ———————

Marketing is defined as "human activity directed at satisfying needs and wants through exchange processes" (Kotler, 1976, p. 5). An exchange process is simply the transfer, between two parties, of something that has value to each party. The marketer's task is to facilitate exchanges so that customers can fulfill their needs and wants. Usually, the marketer benefits from the exchange by obtaining money, while the customers benefit by obtaining a good or service that satisfies a need or desire. Public sector and nonprofit marketers may, however, benefit in nonmonetary ways, through the fulfillment of their institutional mission, desires, and goals.

Health is certainly something that people need and want. However, it is not something that comes without paying a price. To achieve health, people must give up something of value: time, convenience, money, pleasure. For example, to achieve cardiovascular health, a person may have to give up the pleasure associated with smoking; pay for physician visits and blood pressure medication; accept the inconvenience of having to read food nutrition labels; and put in the time necessary to exercise and lose weight.

Similarly, on a societal level, a healthy population simply cannot be created without paying a price. We have to be willing to give up something of value—usually, public resources—to achieve a healthy society. For example, government may have to pay for health care for the uninsured, food and shelter for the poor, and public education programs to teach people the benefits of quitting smoking. Sometimes, the cost to society is not in dollars, but in something else of value, such as the desire to interfere as little as possible with the marketplace. To improve societal health, government may have to impose environmental health regulations on corporations, consumer product safety rules on manufacturers, or even professional practice guidelines on physicians.

In any case, achieving health, whether individual or societal, requires an exchange. And the role of the public health practitioner can be viewed as facilitating the individual and societal-level exchanges necessary to satisfy the human need and desire for health. Public health activity is directed at satisfying the human desire and need for health by promoting or facilitating the exchange of behaviors and lifestyles at the individual level and the exchange of social programs and policies at the societal level. Thus, public health, by its very nature, is in the business of marketing.

An exchange is necessary in order for the individual or society at large to obtain its need and desire for health because alternative methods of obtaining these wants are not readily available. Kotler (1976) described the three potential alternatives to an exchange as self-production, coercion, and supplication. For example, an individual is unable to create health for himself or herself (self-production), cannot forcibly obtain health from others (coercion), and cannot effectively plead for others to provide health to him or her (supplication). However, the individual can obtain health through an exchange. The individual can give up something valued in order to obtain health. He or she may give up cigarettes to improve cardiovascular health or may start exercising or reducing fat intake. He or she may trade the freedom of unprotected sex to obtain the promise of freedom from acquired immunodeficiency syndrome (AIDS).

Similarly, society cannot simply create healthy individuals, cannot somehow steal health for its people, and cannot effectively plead with individuals or businesses to provide for a healthy public. Instead, society can give up something of value—in this case, fiscal resources—to adopt a public health program that is designed to improve the health of its citizens.

In both examples, something of value is being exchanged for the promise of health. In the first case, the individual forfeits a valued behavior, like smoking, or a valued experience, like the pleasure of unprotected sex, in exchange for the prospect of improved health. In the second case, society exchanges fiscal resources for the prospect of improved population health.

Chapter 1 detailed the types of exchanges that public health practitioners must promote: the adoption of individual behaviors (or elimination of unhealthy behaviors) and the adoption of programs to improve social and economic conditions. The overall task is to create or facilitate social change. In other words, the primary challenge of the public health practitioner is to market social change.

Social change, then, can be viewed as the product public health is trying to sell. A product is simply "something that is viewed as capable of satisfying a want. . . . Anything capable of rendering a service, that is, satisfying a need, can be called a product" (Kotler, 1976, p. 5). And in the eyes of the public health practitioner, changes in behavior, social conditions, and social policy can help to satisfy the public's desire for health. That is, social change is a product because the public health practitioner views it as something that is capable of satisfying the individual and societal desire for healthy citizens and healthy communities.

Public health can be considered marketing because it involves a set of core activities directed at satisfying an important need and desire of the public—health—through a variety of individual and societal-level exchanges that take place continually. The product of public health—social change—may not be tangible, but it can be considered a product in a marketing sense because it is perceived by the public health practitioner as capable of satisfying the human desire for health.

A UNIQUE MARKETING CHALLENGE

The public health practitioner's fundamental task of marketing social change is a unique challenge for three reasons: (1) the unfavorable state of individual and societal demand for social change, (2) the hostile environment in which social change must be marketed, and (3) the limited training of public health practitioners in the skills necessary to market social change.

An Unfavorable State of Demand for Social Change

Protecting and promoting the public's health is a unique marketing challenge because of the special nature of the products that public health practitioners are asked to promote. These products fall into a particular niche in the marketing world that, although not exclusive to public health products, poses especially difficult barriers that must be overcome. Specifically, the products of public health—changes in behavior, social conditions, and social policy—tend to be unwanted, considered unimportant, or directly opposed to alternative products that people desire. The public and the policy makers generally do not want social change, do not care about social change, or are committed to social norms that directly oppose social change. This places public health in the initial stages of the product life cycle and creates a special challenge faced by marketers of traditional products only when they are first being introduced into the marketplace.

Kotler described eight states of the demand level for a product that require differing marketing tasks (Kotler, 1976). Most traditional products are in a state of full, overfull, faltering, irregular, or latent demand. Products in a state of full demand, where demand is at the desired level, simply require maintenance marketing. Products in a state of overfull demand, where demand is higher than the level at which the marketer is able to supply it, require demarketing: temporarily or permanently discouraging customers from using the product. Products in a state of faltering demand, where demand is less than its former level, require remarketing: altering the product, the target audience, or the marketing effort. Products in a state of irregular demand, where demand is seasonal or fluctuates widely, require synchromarketing: efforts to synchronize the fluctuations in demand and supply. Finally, products in a state of latent demand, where people share a strong need for a product that does not yet exist, require developmental marketing: creating and marketing a product to satisfy the existing demand. In all five cases, there is preexisting demand for the product; the marketer's task is simply to maintain, enhance, reform, or retime marketing efforts, or in the case of latent demand, to create a product to satisfy high levels of existing public demand.

Under these five demand states, it is reasonably possible to achieve significant changes in individual brand choices, product choices, and product use in the market. For example, within 3 years of introducing its Joe Camel marketing campaign in 1986, the youth market share for Camel cigarettes increased from less than 3% to 8%; after an additional 3 years, Camel's youth market share was up to 16% (Pollay et al., 1996; U.S. Department of Health and Human Services [USDHHS], 1994). Within 1 year of introducing a new 64-bit television video game system, Nintendo achieved a commanding 50% share of the market (Jensen, 1997). Within 4 years of an intensified marketing effort, Clorox increased its market share from 29% in 1992 to 40% in 1996 (Neff, 1997). And within 2 years of the initiation of their products in 1995, 17% of users of skin cream were buying Revitalist Plentitude antiaging cream (Zbar, 1997) and nearly 48% of Internet search engine users were using the Excite search engine (Heath, 1997).

In contrast, the public health product—social change—is generally in one of three demand states: negative demand, no demand, or unwholesome demand. Most commonly, public health products are in a state of negative demand, where the public dislikes the product, does not want the product, and is not willing to pay a price to obtain the product, regardless of its promised benefits. For example, people generally have a negative demand for low-fat foods. We enjoy the taste of high-fat foods and the convenience associated with their availability and easy access, and we would prefer not to give up the taste and convenience for the more distant promise of long-term health benefits. The high public demand for fast-food restaurants is a testament to the negative demand for healthy, low-fat diets. On a societal level, the adoption of programs to help people living in poverty by way of income redistribution is in negative demand. Policy makers stringently avoid the adoption of programs that would significantly redistribute income away from the wealthy and toward the poor. Policy makers often are more willing to pay the price of higher crime rates, more drug use, and higher rates of uncompensated medical care than to jeopardize their chances for reelection by increasing taxes on the wealthy and powerful.

Some public health products are in a state of no demand. People are simply uninterested in the product. For example, programs to provide job training for the homeless are not in great demand by policy makers. Officials are not necessarily making a conscious decision to avoid such programs—there simply is not a great deal of political pressure to address the needs of the homeless in the first place.

Other public health products must be marketed in an environment of unwholesome demand. These are products for which there are alternatives, under high demand by the public, that are considered unhealthy and undesirable by public health practitioners. On an individual level, tobacco, alcohol, and drugs are products for which there is unwholesome demand. On a societal level, there is an unwholesome demand among policy makers for "welfare reform" policies that cut social support for individuals without providing adequate job training, child care, and other support services. These programs are undesirable by public health standards because, as discussed in Chapter 1, they lead to adverse health outcomes. To reduce tobacco, alcohol, or drug use or to promote the adoption of programs that provide social support for poor individuals, public health practitioners must "demarket" popular alternative behaviors or social programs that run counter to the goals of improving health.

Unlike the traditional marketer, then, the public health marketer is almost always faced with a market in which there is no demand for his or her product, negative demand for his or her product, or an unwholesome demand for an alternative product whose use runs counter to the desires of the public health practitioner and the goals of improving health. All three of the public health practitioner's products—changes in lifestyle, changes in social and economic conditions, and changes in social policy—face this problem of an unfavorable state of preexisting demand.

Lifestyle Change

The most striking examples of the unfavorable state of demand for lifestyle change are the addictive behaviors. These unhealthy behaviors are, by definition, highly resistant to change. They represent an extreme example of unwholesome demand: They are behaviors that severely harm individual health but that are highly desired by those who are addicted to them. For example, demand for heroin among heroin addicts is extremely high. Despite the devastating effects of heroin on all aspects of the addict's life, the behavior is sustained at a high rate. Even among addicts who are successfully maintained on methadone for long periods of time, the overall relapse rate among patients who discontinue methadone is at least 50% (Weddington, 1990/1991). Similarly, despite the serious health consequences of smoking and the availability of a wide range of cessation programs ranging from hypnosis to acupuncture, the overall relapse rate for smokers who successfully graduate from cessation programs, even with nicotine replacement therapy, is about 80% (Fiore, Smith, Jorenby, & Baker, 1994; Orleans et al., 1994; Silagy, Mant, Fowler, & Lodge, 1994).

As a result of the unwholesome demand that exists for addictive behaviors, the public health movement has been relatively unsuccessful in reducing tobacco, alcohol, and illicit drug use. The decline in adult smoking prevalence from 42% in 1965 to 25% in 1990 was a result of 25 years of persistent antismoking messages (Giovino et al., 1995; Susser, 1995). Even so, smoking prevalence among adults has not declined further, remaining stable at 25% through 1995 (Centers for Disease Control [CDC], 1997a; National Center for Health Statistics [NCHS], 1997), and smoking prevalence among youth is increasing (CDC, 1996). The 40% reduction in alcohol-related traffic fatalities between 1980 and 1994 was the result of an intensive, 15-year public health campaign (Wald, 1996). Still, the annual number of alcohol-related traffic deaths is extremely high (17,000 per year), and in 1995, the number of alcohol-related fatal crashes increased for the first time in the 1990s (National Highway Traffic Safety Administration, 1997; Wald, 1996). And despite the adverse consequences of drug use and the highly publicized "Just Say No" campaigns, rates of cocaine and marijuana use among eighth-grade students more than doubled between 1991 and 1996 (NCHS, 1997), and the use of heroin by teenagers doubled during this period (Center on Addiction and Substance Abuse, 1997).

Public health interventions also have met with limited success in reducing high blood pressure, high cholesterol levels, and obesity. Several large-scale interventions conducted during the 1970s and 1980s to reduce heart disease risk factors failed to produce substantial differences in mortality rates in treated and comparison communities (Farquhar et al., 1990; Lefebvre, Lasater, Carleton, & Peterson, 1987; Luepker et al., 1994; Multiple Risk Factor Intervention Trial Research Group, 1982; Schwab & Syme, 1997).

Changes in Social and Economic Conditions

Changing the social and economic infrastructure of society to create conditions that will facilitate healthy individual behavior is a reform that tends to be under negative demand or no demand by the public and policy makers. Social and economic conditions are difficult to change, and investing the resources and effort to overcome barriers to change is not a priority for the general public or for most policy makers. Many politicians simply do not care about improving conditions for a segment of the population whose welfare will not affect their reelection chances (no demand). Among other policy makers, there has been a declining societal interest in providing support and resources to improve social and economic conditions for individuals living in poverty (negative demand).

The maximum level of AFDC (Aid for Families with Dependent Children) benefits for poor families fell by more than 17% between 1970 and 1996, after adjustment for inflation, in all 50 states (Kilborn, 1996). Nonwelfare human service benefits also have been reduced sharply. During the period 1994 to 1996 alone, federal subsidies for public housing declined by 11.1%; funding for programs to assist the homeless in finding and retaining housing was reduced by 31.3%; funding for food stamps dropped by 32.2%; emergency assistance to provide shelter for homeless families declined by 44.1%; and federal fuel assistance fell by 49.2% (John W. McCormack Institute of Public Affairs, 1997). Between 1990 and 1996, federal funding for the prevention of homelessness among families fell by 64.0%. There is clearly a negative demand among the public and policy makers for public investment in sincere efforts to improve social and economic conditions. If anything, demand for such an investment in society's social and economic infrastructure is declining.

Changes in Social Policy

The negative demand among the public and policy makers for the social policy reforms needed to create conditions in which people can be healthy is perhaps best illustrated by the 1995 Food and Drug Administration (FDA) regulations on the sale and promotion of tobacco products (FDA, 1996). The Clinton Administration's willingness, and the FDA's determination, to take on the tobacco industry by regulating tobacco for the first time in history represents the most positive political environment ever for social policy reform in the area of tobacco control. In asserting jurisdiction over tobacco products, the FDA found that nicotine is addictive, that cigarettes are a drug-delivery device, and that tobacco products kill more than 400,000 Americans each year (FDA, 1996). In spite of these findings, the FDA regulations did very little to change social policy regarding tobacco sale,

marketing, and use in the nation. Given the magnitude of this public health problem and the finding that cigarettes represented a drug-delivery device not unlike
others the FDA regulates, the most appropriate action, at least from a public health
perspective, would be to regulate the safety of the product. This might have taken
the form of regulating the production, sale, and marketing of tobacco: for example, making cigarettes and smokeless tobacco a prescription product, requiring
a reduction or elimination in the level of nicotine in tobacco products, or eliminating the marketing of these deadly products. Any of these actions would have represented a significant and profound change in social policy regarding tobacco.

However, due to perceived public and political opposition to meaningful social
policy reform, Clinton and the FDA decided to propose regulations that would
confront only the sale and marketing of tobacco to minors, which were already
either illegal or widely recognized as violating accepted social policy norms. The
FDA regulations leave the production, sale, and marketing of tobacco essentially
intact. They merely require enforcement of preexisting laws that restrict the sale of
tobacco to minors and place modest restrictions on forms of tobacco advertising
and promotion that appeal to youth. In this way, the FDA regulations do not represent a true change in social policy. They simply strengthen the enforcement of the
existing policy: that tobacco should not be sold or marketed to persons under the
age of 18.

The FDA's failure to provide a rational, public health justification for the decision to regulate tobacco only insofar as it represents an addictive threat to adolescents highlights the intensity of our policy makers' resolve not to alter deeply
ingrained norms of social policy.

As the FDA example demonstrated, changing social policy is under negative
demand in our society: Policy makers are willing to pay a price to avoid having to
tamper with longstanding social policy norms.

A Hostile Public Health Marketing Environment

Few marketers have to compete with high-intensity, well-financed campaigns
that aim to reduce demand for their products. There is no industry dedicated to
reducing the demand for Beanie Babies or to convincing people to avoid eating in
restaurants or to stop wearing shoes.

In contrast, public health practitioners often face high-intensity campaigns conducted specifically to counteract their marketing efforts. The marketer of public
health products must compete with industries whose prime objective is the promotion of unhealthy behaviors. At the same time that public health practitioners try to
convince people not to smoke and not to drink, the tobacco and alcohol industries
are spending $5 billion and $2 billion each year, respectively, for the sole purpose
of trying to get people to smoke cigarettes and drink alcohol (Federal Trade Commission, 1996; J. Mosher, personal communication, November 15, 1998). At the

same time that public health officials are trying to convince Congress and state legislators that firearms are a leading cause of death among young Americans, the National Rifle Association is spending $3 million to $6 million each year to influence legislators to vote against any proposals that would restrict the production, sale, or use of firearms (M. Gerkey, personal communication, 1997).

In addition to opposition to public health efforts by major industries and lobbying groups, the social environment itself, with its deeply ingrained social norms, often contributes to a hostile environment in which to market social change. For example, despite a vigorous campaign to increase physical activity among the population, and despite a high level of public demand for ways to increase physical activity, the social and occupational environments are hostile to this type of change. Workplace schedules generally are not designed to allow for a sufficient period of physical activity during the work day. Public transportation systems and urban planning are not developed well enough to allow large numbers of people to walk or bike to work. Intense marketing of and easy access to beer, fast food, and high-fat products undermine individual attempts to improve diet and reduce weight. As of 1994, about 30% of adults reported having no leisure-time physical activity, and close to 30% reported being overweight (CDC, 1997b).

The Limited Capacity of Public Health Practitioners To Market Social Change

The capacity of public health practitioners to market social change is limited by three factors: (1) inadequate emphasis on the advocacy role in public health, (2) limited expertise in advocacy skills among current public health practitioners, and (3) lack of training of public health students and practitioners in advocacy skills.

Inadequate Emphasis on Advocacy in Public Health Practice

The public health practitioner is, first and foremost, an advocate for social change. The historical roots of the public health movement lie in the efforts of visionaries whose lives were dedicated to advocating for social change. (See Chapter 4 for a more thorough discussion.) It was the social reforms advocated by these figures that gave public health its source, its mission, its foundation, and its original vision.

In recent years, the public health movement has lost its appreciation of advocacy as its primary tool and its sense of a common, unifying social mission that can serve as a rallying cry for the movement (Institute of Medicine, Committee for the Study of the Future of Public Health, 1988; Stevens, 1996). As discussed in Chapter 4, many public health officials have confused advocacy and lobbying, and in an effort not to violate federal laws that restrict lobbying by government and nonprofit agencies, they have completely renounced any semblance of a role in social advocacy. As the Institute of Medicine (1988) report on the future of public health showed, "although public health professionals have traditionally recognized influences of the physical environment on health status, they have been less adept at recognizing health-related influences in the business, economic, and social environment and in fashioning and advocating strategies to control these factors" (p. 113). The report later concludes that "too frequently, public health professionals view politics as a contaminant rather than as a central attribute of democratic governance" (p. 154).

Public health practitioners need a new job description: one that lists advocacy as the chief role and responsibility of the job and that calls on the public health practitioner to mobilize community support for societal efforts to produce social change. As Turnock (1997) concluded in his book, *Public Health: What It Is and How It Works,* "the public health system, from national to state and local levels, must recognize these circumstances and move beyond capably providing services to aggressively advocating and building constituencies for efforts that target the most important of the traditional health risk factors and that promote social policies that both minimize and equalize risks throughout the population. These represent a new job description for public health in the United States, but one that is both necessary and feasible" (pp. 355–356).

Limited Expertise in Advocacy among Current Public Health Practitioners

Even among public health agencies that still retain an advocacy role, few of the individual practitioners have been thoroughly trained in advocacy, and many of the skills necessary to advocate effectively are incompletely developed. As the Institute of Medicine (1988) noted, "effective public health action for many problems requires organizing the interest groups, not just assessing a problem and determining a line of action based on top-down authority" (p. 122). The Institute of Medicine found, however, that most public health workers have not received formal education in public health itself, much less in other critical areas needed for effective advocacy, including political science, community organizing, and management. Public health workers tend to lack skills that derive from education in these areas, including skills in media advocacy, political activity, community organizing, and coalition building.

Inadequate Training in Advocacy for Public Health Students and Practitioners

A convention of public health practitioners and academicians met in 1992 to develop a set of "universal competencies for public health professionals" (Sorenson & Bialek, 1992; Turnock, 1997). One of the competencies developed was "advocating for public health programs and resources" (Sorenson & Bialek, 1992). The Institute of Medicine (1988) recommended a set of political skills and capacities that should be essential components of training for all public health students and practitioners: "Public health agencies should be able to mobilize the support of important constituencies, including the general public, to compete successfully for scarce resources, to handle conflict over policy priorities and choices, to establish linkages with other organizations, and to develop a positive public image" (p. 154). These are essentially skills in advocacy.

Dr. Barry Levy, a former president of the American Public Health Association (APHA) wrote of the need for public health leaders who

> educate and inform, who facilitate grassroots advocacy to shape public policy. . . . Leaders with a holistic vision of public health, who appreciate the relevance of education, employment and housing to public health, who create horizontal integration of programs and services. . . . Leaders who do not fight to get a seat at the table, but who figuratively are the table—who set the stage, frame the issues, pose the questions and engage a wide range of people and organizations in the issues that affect them and their communities. Leaders who work for social justice. Leaders who empower the disadvantaged. (Levy, 1996, p. 2)

As a discipline, advocacy generally is not taught and certainly is not emphasized in schools of public health. For example, in 1997–98 less than one-third of accredited schools of public health in the United States offered a course in public health advocacy, and less than half offered a course in media advocacy or mass communication.

CONCLUSION

The combination of the unfavorable state of public demand for social change, the hostile environment in which public health practitioners must market social change, and the limited training of public health practitioners in marketing and advocacy makes confronting the emerging threats to the public's health a formidable marketing challenge for the public health practitioner. But the same marketing principles that help explain why social change is so difficult to create also can be used to redefine and reposition the public health product so that it is in demand by the public and by policy makers. Chapter 3 shows why marketing social change is both a challenge and an opportunity for the public health practitioner.

REFERENCES

Center on Addiction and Substance Abuse. (1997, August). *Substance abuse and the American adolescent.* New York: Author.

Centers for Disease Control and Prevention. (1996). Tobacco use and usual source of cigarettes among high school students—United States, 1995. *Morbidity and Mortality Weekly Report, 45,* 413–418.

Centers for Disease Control and Prevention. (1997a). Cigarette smoking among adults—United States, 1995. *Morbidity and Mortality Weekly Report, 46,* 1217–1220.

Centers for Disease Control and Prevention. (1997b). State- and sex-specific prevalence of selected characteristics—Behavioral Risk Factor Surveillance System, 1994 and 1995. *Morbidity and Mortality Weekly Report (CDC Surveillance Summaries), 46*(SS-3), 1–31.

Farquhar, J.W., Fortmann, S.P., Flora, J.A., Taylor, C.B., Haskell, W.L., Williams, P.T., Maccoby, N., & Wood, P.D. (1990). Effects of community-wide education on cardiovascular disease risk factors. *Journal of the American Medical Association, 264,* 359–365.

Federal Trade Commission. (1996). *Federal Trade Commission report to Congress for 1994: Pursuant to the Federal Cigarette Labeling and Advertising Act.* Washington, DC: Author.

Fiore, M.C., Smith, S.S., Jorenby, D.E., & Baker, T.B. (1994). The effectiveness of the nicotine patch for smoking cessation: A meta-analysis. *Journal of the American Medical Association, 271,* 1940–1947.

Food and Drug Administration. (1996, August 28). *Regulations restricting the sale and distribution of cigarettes and smokeless tobacco to protect children and adolescents: Final rule* (Fed. Reg., 21 C.F.R. Parts 801, 803, 804, 807, 820, and 897, pp. 44396–45318). Washington, DC: U.S. Department of Health and Human Services, Food and Drug Administration.

Giovino, G.A., Schooley, M.W., Zhu, B., Chrismon, J.H., Tomar, S.L., Peddicord, J.P., Merritt, R.K., Husten, C.G., & Eriksen, M.P. (1995). Surveillance for selected tobacco-use behaviors—United States, 1900–1994. *Morbidity and Mortality Weekly Report (CDC Surveillance Summaries), 43*(SS-3), 1–43.

Heath, R.P. (1997, June 30). The marketing 100: Excite. *Advertising Age, 68*(26), p. s10.

Institute of Medicine, Committee for the Study of the Future of Public Health. (1988). *The future of public health.* Washington, DC: National Academy Press.

Jensen, J. (1997, July 14). Nintendo plots fall ad campaign for its 64 system: Branding efforts for software, hardware will share message. *Advertising Age, 68*(28), pp. 3, 36.

John W. McCormack Institute of Public Affairs. (1997, January 10). *Over the edge: Cuts and changes in housing, income support, and homeless assistance programs in Massachusetts.* Boston: University of Massachusetts–Boston, John W. McCormack Institute of Public Affairs.

Kilborn, P.T. (1996, December 6). Welfare all over the map. *The New York Times,* p. 3E.

Kotler, P. (1976). *Marketing management: Analysis, planning, and control* (3rd ed.). Englewood Cliffs, NJ: Prentice-Hall.

Lefebvre, R.C., Lasater, T.M., Carleton, R.A., & Peterson, G. (1987). Theory and delivery of health programming in the community: The Pawtucket Heart Health Program. *Preventive Medicine, 16,* 80–95.

Levy, B.S. (1996, December). Putting the public back in public health. *The Nation's Health,* p. 2.

Luepker, R.V., Murray, D.M., Jacobs, D.R., Mittelmark, M.B., Bracht, N., Carlaw, R., Crow, R., Elmer, P., Finnegan, J., Folsom, A.R., Grimm, R., Hannan, P.J., Jeffrey, R., Lando, H., McGovern, P., Mullis, R., Perry, C.L., Pechacek, T., Pirie, P., Sprafka, J.M., Weisbrod, R., & Blackburn, H. (1994). Community education for cardiovascular disease prevention: Risk factor changes in the Minnesota Heart Health Program. *American Journal of Public Health, 84,* 1383–1393.

Multiple Risk Factor Intervention Trial Research Group. (1982). Multiple Risk Factor Intervention Trial: Risk factor changes and mortality results. *Journal of the American Medical Association, 248,* 1465–1477.

National Center for Health Statistics. (1997). *Health, United States, 1996–97, and injury chartbook* (DHHS Publication No. PHS 97-1232). Hyattsville, MD: Author.

National Highway Traffic Safety Administration. (1997, March). *Alcohol involvement in fatal traffic crashes 1995* (Tech. Rep. DOT HS 808-547). Washington, DC: Author.

Neff, J. (1997, June 30). The marketing 100: Clorox. *Advertising Age, 68*(26), p. s18.

Orleans, C.T., Resch, N., Noll, E., Keintz, M.K., Rimer, B.K., Brown, T.V., & Snedden, T.M. (1994). Use of transdermal nicotine in a state-level prescription plan for the elderly—A first look at "real-world" patch users. *Journal of the American Medical Association, 271,* 601–607.

Pollay, R.W., Siddarth, S., Siegel, M., Haddix, A., Merritt, R.K., Giovino, G.A., & Eriksen, M.P. (1996). The last straw? Cigarette advertising and realized market shares among youths and adults, 1979–1993. *Journal of Marketing, 60,* 1–16.

Schwab, M., & Syme, S.L. (1997). On paradigms, community participation, and the future of public health. *American Journal of Public Health, 87,* 2049–2051.

Silagy, C., Mant, D., Fowler, G., & Lodge, M. (1994). Meta-analysis on efficacy of nicotine replacement therapies in smoking cessation. *The Lancet, 343*(1), 139–142.

Sorenson, A.A., & Bialek, R.G. (Eds.). (1992). *The public health faculty/agency forum.* Gainesville, FL: University of Florida Press.

Stevens, R. (1996). Editorial: Public health history and advocacy in the money-driven 1990s. *American Journal of Public Health, 86,* 1522–1523.

Susser, M. (1995). Editorial: The tribulations of trials—Interventions in communities. *American Journal of Public Health, 85,* 156–158.

Turnock, B.J. (1997). *Public health: What it is and how it works.* Gaithersburg, MD: Aspen.

U.S. Department of Health and Human Services. (1994). *Preventing tobacco use among young people: A report of the Surgeon General.* Atlanta, GA: U.S. Department of Health and Human Services, Centers for Disease Control and Prevention, National Center for Chronic Disease Prevention and Health Promotion, Office on Smoking and Health.

Wald, M.L. (1996, December 15). A fading drumbeat against drunk driving. *The New York Times,* p. E5.

Weddington, W.W. (1990/1991). Towards a rehabilitation of methadone maintenance: Integration of relapse prevention and aftercare. *International Journal of the Addictions, 25,* 1201–1224.

Zbar, J.D. (1997, June 30). The marketing 100: Revitalift. *Advertising Age, 68*(26), p. s16.

CHAPTER 3

Marketing Social Change— An Opportunity for the Public Health Practitioner

The primary challenge facing public health practitioners is the need to market changes in behavior, societal conditions, and social policy in the absence of significant public demand for these changes. Through the strategic use of marketing principles, the public health practitioner can effectively confront these challenges. The key is for public health practitioners to abandon the traditional approach of deciding what they want the target audience to buy and then attempting to sell this product to an audience that has little demand for it. Instead, public health professionals must first find out what the consumer wants and then redefine, repackage, reposition, and reframe the product in such a way that it satisfies an existing demand among the target audience. The public health official must be able to offer a benefit that the audience appreciates and demands, to back up this offer with support, and to communicate an image of the product and its benefit that reinforces the most influential core values of the target audience.

———— ❧ ————

Chapter 2 demonstrated that the public health practitioner must market changes in behavior, social conditions, and policies under an unfavorable state of public demand for social change and in an environment that is hostile to social change. Fortunately, the same marketing principles that help explain why social change is so difficult to create can also provide the public health practitioner with powerful tools to facilitate social change.

This chapter explains how the strategic application of marketing principles can provide the public health practitioner with a unique opportunity to effect changes in individual behavior, social conditions, and social policies.

To see how the public health practitioner can use the principles of marketing to effect social change, we must return to the definition of *marketing*: "human activity directed at satisfying needs and wants through exchange processes" (Kotler, 1976, p. 5). At the very heart of marketing is the task of identifying and understanding the needs and wants of consumers. And at the very heart of public health is the task of identifying and understanding the individual's need for, and desire for, health.

What does it mean to people to be healthy? Why is it that people want to be healthy? How do people perceive health as a personal benefit? What about health makes it desirable? Is it the mere absence of disease that people desire, or does health have positive values that drive people's wants?

Perhaps the best way to find out what health means to people is to study what people miss most in the absence of health. To answer this question, we must turn to the field of medical sociology—the sociology of health and illness. And the first thing we must understand is the fundamental distinction between disease and illness.

As Conrad and Kern (1994) pointed out, disease and illness are not the same. Whereas disease is "the biophysiological phenomena that manifest themselves as changes in and malfunctions of the human body," illness is "the experience of being sick or diseased" (Conrad & Kern, 1994, p. 7). People might feel ill in the absence of disease, and they may be diseased without experiencing illness (Enthoven, 1980; Turnock, 1997). Because people experience illness, or the subjective experience of being sick, it is the illness experience rather than disease itself that best defines the nature of the value that individuals place on their health. Research on the illness experience can tell best what it means to people to be healthy.

In her classic ethnographic study of the experience of illness among gay and bisexual men with acquired immunodeficiency syndrome (AIDS), Rose Weitz (1994) found that the feeling of lack of control over one's life is the single most important and widely shared aspect of the illness experience. Weitz describes the critical importance to these men of learning to cope with uncertainty, to inject some degree of control over their lives. The great challenge to these men is dealing with the loss of control over their futures: Despite taking all the proper actions, they cannot control "what will happen to them, when it will happen, and why" (p. 138).

Perhaps the centrality of the concept of control to the illness experience was described best by one of the participants in the study by Weitz, who stressed the importance of "being active about this disease, whether it involves drinking a certain kind of tea or standing on your head twice a day or doing something, something that gives the patient a feeling of control over his own life that if you do these things, this might help you a little bit. . . . It's a sense of being in control, of being actively involved in your own health, which in itself produces health" (p. 145).

In fact, uncertainty is recognized as a central and common characteristic of all illness experiences (Conrad, 1987; Glaser & Strauss, 1968; Mishel, 1984; Mishel,

Hostetter, King, & Graham, 1984; Molleman et al., 1984; Weitz, 1994). In contrast to the uncertainty that accompanies other types of life crises, ill persons cannot necessarily alter the eventual outcomes of their situations (Weitz, 1994).

Weitz (1994) described the basic mechanism of coping with uncertainty in ill persons as constructing a framework to explain their situations that gives them some sense of control over their lives:

> These frameworks give people the sense that they understand what has happened and will happen to them. By making the world seem predictable, these frameworks help individuals to choose (albeit sometimes from among limited options) how they will live their lives. Thus . . . these frameworks reduce the stresses of uncertainty by enabling people to feel at least minimally in control of their lives. . . . [I]n the final analysis, it is this sense of control that enables people to tolerate uncertainty. (p. 139)

Thus, not the intrinsic presence of disease itself, but the loss of control associated with the illness experience brought on by that disease best characterizes the nature of the value people place on health. Weitz, for example, described one man with AIDS who lamented not being able to take a small trip for fear of having diarrhea while he was driving. Another man summarized his experience similarly: "AIDS has become my life. I live for AIDS. I don't live for me anymore, I live for AIDS. I'm at its beck and call and I'll do what it tells me when it tells me" (Weitz, 1994, p. 144). These examples illustrate the critical importance of values such as freedom, independence, autonomy, and control over one's life, above and beyond any value of health itself.

In *The Illness Narratives: Suffering, Healing, and the Human Condition*, psychiatrist Arthur Kleinman (1988) discussed the personal and social meaning of illness through the eyes of his patients. The themes of loss of control, loss of independence, and loss of freedom are repeatedly mentioned as the central source of personal suffering in the illness experience. For example, describing one severely disabled diabetic patient, Kleinman wrote, "It was not death that she feared, she would tell me, but the seemingly relentless march toward becoming an invalid. Loss of her leg forced the realization that she was now partially dependent and that one day she would be more completely so" (p. 35). And as the patient herself explains, "I began to see how terrible it would be to be incapacitated—to give up even the semblance of my independence, my control, my role in the family and in the community" (p. 37).

A large body of sociological research has revealed that health is of value to the individual not intrinsically, but because it assures a certain degree of personal freedom, independence, autonomy, and control over one's life. The disease experience is most difficult and dreaded not because it marks the absence of some ideal of the healthy state, but because it represents a loss of the individual's freedom, independence, autonomy, and control.

The diseased individual suffers mainly because of the loss of control over his or her life. Depending on the severity of the disease, a person may lose control over basic bodily functions (e.g., eating, breathing, urination), basic activities of daily life (walking, sitting, washing), or more advanced functions that contribute to emotional and occupational fulfillment (speaking, typing, running). Disability is most troubling because of the loss of personal freedom that comes with it. Individuals who are disabled may also lose a degree of independence; they may have to rely on others to help them with complex or even basic activities. Placing a loved one in a nursing home, for example, is difficult not because it represents the loss of some ideal healthy state, but because it represents a loss of the individual's ability to live independently and often, of the family's ability to adequately care for the individual.

As these examples show, it is not really health itself that people value most. Rather, it is the freedom, independence, autonomy, and control over their lives that come with being healthy for which people have the most fundamental need and desire. Therefore, the first lesson that the public health practitioner can learn by applying basic marketing principles to the fundamental task of marketing social change is that health itself is not the most effective product that the public health practitioner has to offer. The most compelling product of the public health practitioner is the freedom, independence, autonomy, and control over life that come with health.

If public health practitioners fail to make this subtle, yet critical, distinction in how they define and then market their product, they are unlikely to be successful. Why? Because it is not a disregard for health, but a desire for freedom, independence, autonomy, and control that leads to and sustains unhealthy behaviors and lifestyles in the first place. And if the public health practitioner ignores the role of the behavior in supporting these widely held core values, he or she can be sure that the industries promoting these unhealthy behaviors are fully aware of these core values and are using them to their advantage.

Although Americans certainly value health, they also hold other values that tend to be more important, more salient, and more influential on individual behavior. Often, these values are supported by maintaining, rather than changing, an unhealthy behavior. If an individual has firmly established a behavior in the first place, it must fulfill some core value for the individual. If the individual is aware that the behavior has undesirable health consequences, that awareness is less potent than the pull of the other values. The traditional public health approach to behavior change simply tries to reinforce the value of health, but in the process it conflicts with other deeply held values that are stronger and more influential.

The public health practitioner must realize that, as Andreasen (1995) described it, "target consumers in most behavior-change situations have very good reasons for maintaining the behavior patterns they have held—often for a lifetime" (p. 48). And as Salmon (1989) noted, public health campaigns "represent only one social force among many driving and restraining forces. For every campaign message intending to dissuade consumers from illegal drug use or cigarette smoking, there are literally dozens of forces . . . espousing competing philosophies, similarly at work" (pp. 44, 45).

For example, although public health practitioners try to convince adolescents not to smoke by appealing to their desire for health, other messages in the adolescent's world appeal to more salient and influential core values. Marlboro ads tell kids that smoking will make them free and independent, like a cowboy. Seeing adults smoking in bars and other places where kids are not allowed tells teenagers that smoking is a symbol of maturity and autonomy. The cigarette companies themselves, through campaigns that portray smoking as an adult decision and encourage youths to listen to their parents, tell kids that smoking is a way to exert independence from their parents and to give them, and not adult authority figures, control over their own lives.

The public health practitioner faces a similar challenge confronting alcohol consumption. As Winett and Wallack (1996) suggested, "given the social value placed upon recreational alcohol consumption, the availability and accessibility of alcoholic beverages, the environmental cues encouraging social drinking, and the pleasurable physical effects people often experience while drinking—the social marketing campaign designed to dissuade people from excessive drink by teaching them of the health risks faces a profoundly difficult task" (p. 179).

Although public health practitioners have not traditionally conducted marketing research to identify and understand the needs and desires of their target audiences, their opponents—for example, the cigarette industry—have long used marketing research to find out what consumers want, what is important to them, and what values are most salient, influential, and held most deeply by consumers. And although public health practitioners traditionally have relied solely on the individual's inherent value for health, their opposition has taken advantage of more compelling core values to sell their harmful products.

The tobacco industry, for example, conducted extensive research into the desires, needs, and values of adolescents and young adults. The consistent finding of this research was the importance of the themes of independence, freedom, autonomy, control, self-reliance, and rugged individualism. These themes have formed the basis for many of the tobacco industry's promotional campaigns during this century. As Surgeon General Joycelyn Elders concluded, "United States advertisers, too, have long thought that individualism and the stimulating notions of independence, self-reliance, and autonomy are important strategic concepts in ad development" (U.S. Department of Health and Human Services [USDHHS], 1994, p. 177).

As early as 1929, Edward Bernays, a public relations consultant for the American Tobacco Company, organized a group of women to smoke publicly in the New York Easter Parade and to carry placards identifying their cigarettes as "torches of liberty" (Bernays, 1965; Schudson, 1984; USDHHS, 1994). This strategy was based on the work of consulting psychoanalyst A.A. Brill, who advised the company to promote cigarettes as "symbols of freedom" (Bernays, 1965; USDHHS, 1994, p. 165).

Young and Rubicam conducted a series of motivational interviews of smokers in the 1950s (Smith, 1954; USDHHS, 1994). These studies revealed the importance of the themes of freedom and escape to smokers (USDHHS, 1994). They suggested that appeals based on health claims would offer only transient results, but to increase the cigarette market, companies would have to "tap the driving force of the real psychological satisfactions of smoking" (USDHHS, 1994, p. 171).

Imperial Tobacco Limited of Canada conducted research on adolescents that revealed that "the adolescent seeks to display his new urge for independence with a symbol, and cigarettes are such a symbol" (USDHHS, 1994, p. 175). The research also found that young males in particular are "going through a stage where they are seeking to express their independence and individuality under constant pressure of being accepted by their peers" (USDHHS, 1994). Another Imperial Tobacco Limited study provided guidelines "for the effective display of freedom and independence in advertising imagery" (USDHHS, 1994, p. 177) and recommended that cigarette brands designed for youth show someone "free to choose friends, music, clothes, own activities, to be alone if he wishes," who "can manage alone" with "nobody to interfere, no boss/parents" (USDHHS, 1994, p. 177). The research described the importance of developing imagery to tap into four core adolescent values: independence, self-reliance, autonomy, and freedom from authority (USDHHS, 1994).

Indeed, the Surgeon General noted that "the brands most successful with teenagers seem to be those that offer adult imagery rich with connotations of independence, freedom from authority, and/or self-reliance" (USDHHS, 1994, p. 176). Marlboro, the most popular brand among adolescents, epitomizes the stereotype of American independence. As the Surgeon General noted, the Marlboro man is "usually depicted alone, he interacts with no one; he is strikingly free of interference from authority figures such as parents, older brothers, bosses, and bullies. Indeed, the Marlboro man is burdened by no one whose authority he must respect or even consider" (USDHHS, 1994, p. 177). R.W. Murray, former president and chief executive officer of Philip Morris, observed that "the cowboy has appeal to people as a personality. There are elements of adventure, freedom, being in charge of your destiny" (as cited in Trachtenberg, 1987, p. 109) Jack Landry, a key advertising executive behind the Marlboro Man campaign, described the cowboy as "a perfect symbol of independence and individualistic rebellion" (as cited in Meyers, 1984, p. 70).

Unfortunately, the core values that tobacco and other corporate marketers are reinforcing with their advertising messages—freedom, independence, autonomy, and self-control—are precisely those most deeply ingrained in American society.

Once a person has recognized how an unhealthy behavior supports one or more of these core values, it will be most difficult to change the behavior, especially if one must rely solely on an appeal to the desire for health.

The importance of the core values of freedom, independence, autonomy, and control is apparent in the marketing campaigns of highly successful corporations. Nike, for example, has based its marketing of athletic footwear on the slogans "Just do it," and "I can." Nike is selling sneakers by telling people, essentially, that they can have control over their lives, they can be free, they can be independent. They can have control over their lives in much the same way as Michael Jordan has control over his body as he soars high over defenders to dunk the basketball while wearing Nike apparel. They can be independent, just as Michael Jordan is not dependent on others when making a spin move and body fake to break free and drive to the basket. And they can be autonomous, just as Bo Jackson has the ability to excel in any sport he chooses.

It is also instructive to note that when corporate marketers sell health products, they do not generally rely on the benefit of health to sell their products. Health clubs and exercise equipment are marketed to consumers not based on their ability to improve long-term health outcomes and prevent disease, but based on their ability to give people a feeling of control over how they look, how they feel, and how attractive they are to others. One doesn't usually see ads for health clubs that cite medical evidence about the benefits of physical activity in preventing chronic illness. More likely, one sees ads that show attractive people who seem to be in control of how they look, how they feel, and how others think about them.

Conrad and Kern (1994) conclude that "to understand the effects of disease in society, it is also necessary to understand the impact of illness" (p. 108). Perhaps it is the failure of the medical and public health professions to adequately understand the subjective meaning, experience, and impact of illness in addition to merely the objective phenomenon of disease that best explains the epidemic of unhealthy behaviors and lifestyles in the population. The advertisers of unhealthy products such as alcohol and tobacco have listened to the people, understood their feelings and experiences, and provided them with products to satisfy their subjective desires and needs. On the other hand, medical and public health professionals have tended to ignore the subjective meaning and experience of illness and to provide the public with what health professionals view as the needs of individuals. A public health practitioner's call for an individual to change his or her behavior may not be as compelling if it relies solely on the individual's intrinsic value of health as if it also feeds into the value that the individual places on personal freedom, independence, autonomy, and control over his or her life.

How can the public health practitioner begin to rely on these more influential core values to promote individual behavior change? The key is to redefine the public health product and its benefits in a way that appeals to the most compelling core values of the target audience. The public health practitioner must first abandon the traditional approach of deciding for himself or herself what product he or she wants the target audience to buy and then attempting to sell this product to an audience that has little demand for it. Instead, the public health practitioner must first find out what the consumer wants and then redefine, repackage, reposition, and reframe the product in such a way that it satisfies an existing demand among the target audience. All aspects of the marketing of the product must work together to reinforce, rather than conflict with, the most influential core values of the target audience.

In the remaining sections of this chapter, we review each of these steps in marketing individual behavior change to the public: (1) determining what the consumer wants; (2) redefining the public health product; and (3) repackaging, repositioning, and reframing the public health product.

FINDING OUT WHAT THE CONSUMER WANTS: THE ROLE OF FORMATIVE RESEARCH

What we are calling the "formative research" process in public health is not really a specific discipline, but a more general concept. The goal of "formative research" in public health is essentially to understand the consumer—in this case, the target audience for behavior change. Charlotte Vogel defined the purpose of formative research simply as "understanding consumers and what makes them tick" (Vogel, 1987, p. 31). Andreasen summarized the task as getting "inside the heads" of the target consumers (Andreasen, 1995, p. 47). Or as Marlboro Man creator Leo Burnett explains, "We have been able to get under (the consumers') skins a bit and find out what they really think about a product or the presentation of it and can't or won't express in words" (Burnett, 1961, p. 63).

There are many research fields that could potentially be used to help the public health practitioner accomplish this goal, including traditional marketing, political science, psychology, sociology, and anthropology. And there are many research methods that could help the public health practitioner understand what drives consumers' behavior. These methods include traditional marketing research methods, public opinion polling and surveys, clinical studies, behavioral research, cognitive and psychodynamic psychology research, focus groups, and ethnographic and other qualitative research methods.

It is not the method that is important, but the fact that some attempt is made to understand the consumer's needs, desires, and values before the public health program is designed and implemented. Andreasen emphasized the importance of this point by noting that John Sculley, former executive at Pepsi-Cola, had for years "been convincing consumers to buy his brand of colored sugar water over a competitor's colored sugar water with great success, mainly because he understood 'the Pepsi Generation' and how to speak to them" (Andreasen, 1995, p. 54).

While there is an abundance of quantitative articles in the medical and public health literature that consider why people do or do not engage in unhealthy behaviors, there is little qualitative research that allows the public health practitioner to learn "what makes them tick." For example, Weitz (1994) points out that "few published research studies have analyzed the experiences of persons with AIDS, and none has looked specifically at the issue of uncertainty. Instead, the social science literature on AIDS largely consists of quantitative studies regarding why people do or do not change their sexual behavior to protect themselves against infection" (p. 139).

Before public health practitioners can design programs that will be successful in changing individual behavior, they must attempt to get under the skin of their target audience and to explore core values such as freedom, autonomy, and control, and how they relate to the audience's perceptions of health, disease, behaviors, behavior change, and the experience of illness.

The existing biomedical paradigm for the practice of medicine and public health will not suffice for individual lifestyles to be changed in any significant way. Research that incorporates other models of behavioral and social change and provides a deeper understanding of the nature of illness and suffering—and not merely the presence or absence of disease—must become a central part of public health practice. "Whereas virtually all healing perspectives across cultures, like religious and moral perspectives, orient sick persons and their circle to the problem of bafflement, the narrow biomedical model eschews this aspect of suffering much as it turns its back on illness (as opposed to disease)" (Kleinman, 1988, p. 29).

One further essential element of the formative research process deserves emphasis. Even among a narrowly defined target group, such as gay men, there is a diversity of attitudes, beliefs, and values (see Appendix 3–A). Cultural differences between population groups make it imperative to conduct formative research among all the cultural subgroups that one is trying to reach. The values that are most important to gay White men, for example, may be quite different from those that are important to gay Black men, or to gay Latinos. When we speak about identifying the needs, desires, and values of the target audience, we are not assuming that these will be the same for all subgroups within the overall target audience. Depending on the extent of cultural differences within the audience, it may be necessary to intensively study various segments within the overall target population to identify their unique needs, desires, and culturally influenced values.

Flora, Schooler, and Pierson (1997) describe the importance of market segmentation, or breaking the target audience down into the smallest possible homogeneous groups, in formative research:

> A fundamental tenet of social marketing is that health promotion programs must be designed in response to audience needs, implemented to meet those needs, effective in satisfying those needs, and monitored both to ensure the program continues to meet these needs and to discover new or changing needs. Because a group's history, language, val-

ues, and beliefs influence group members' health-related knowledge, attitudes, and behavior, the values of a culture must be used as the foundation or building blocks of health promotion programs. Interventions or strategies that do not conform to cultural values (e.g., emphasizing long-term gains to a culture that prefers a present orientation) or worse, that actually challenge a group's values (e.g., assertive techniques in a society that values cooperative and fluid social relations) can be expected to fail. (p. 356)

REDEFINING THE PUBLIC HEALTH PRODUCT

In *Marketing Social Change: Changing Behavior To Promote Health, Social Development, and the Environment,* Alan Andreasen (1995) summarizes the importance of redefining the marketing product based on actual consumer needs and wants, rather than on the beliefs, wishes, or intuitions of the marketer. Andreasen (1995) explains that good marketers

do not seek to persuade target audiences to do what the marketer believes they ought to do. They do not try to make the audience accept the marketer's values and beliefs. Rather, they recognize that customers only take action when they believe that it is in their interests. Social marketing persuasion strategies therefore always start with an understanding of the target audience's needs and wants, their values, their perceptions. Social marketers do not start out with an assumption that their job is to change the customer to conform with the marketer. They recognize that they must often change their social marketing offerings and the way these are presented to meet target customer needs and wants. (pp. 14, 15)

Listening to the audience and changing the offering to meet its needs and wants means developing a new product based on the results of a formative research process. The marketer cannot decide in advance the product that he or she thinks the public will want and then try to sell it. Instead, the marketer must find out from the public what product it is seeking, and then design and present such a product to the public in a way that allows them to see how it will indeed provide the benefits being sought. As Andreasen (1995) explained it, "marketers know that they must understand where customers are coming from before they decide just what to try to sell" (p. 16).

The central task of redefining the public health product is to clearly identify the benefits that the public health practitioner has to offer the target audience. This task is so important to the ultimate success of a public health campaign that it must not depend only on the intuition of the practitioner. Formative research is essential to identify the needs and wants of the target audience. Only then can the practitioner decide what product benefits will be most likely to satisfy these needs and wants. David Ogilvy, the advertising wizard who founded the advertising agency known today as Ogilvy and Mather, told his agency staff, "your most important job is to decide what you are going to say about your product, what benefit you are going to promise. . . . The selection of the right promise is so vitally important that you should never rely on guesswork to decide it" (Ogilvy, 1964, p. 93).

For public health practitioners, this may mean a drastic change in the way the public health product is defined. For the most part, practitioners will no longer be able to sell health. Instead, they will have to sell the more compelling, salient, and deep core values that are widely held by their target audiences. This concept, although new to many public health professionals, is basic to marketers of many traditional products.

For example, at the most basic level, Philip Morris is not selling Marlboro cigarettes to youth. Instead, it is selling freedom and independence, control over one's life, risk and adventure. R.J. Reynolds is not selling Camel cigarettes to youth. It is selling style and character, coolness and slyness. Crompton and Lamb (1986) explain that marketers are not only selling a tangible product, but they are selling a meaning as well: "People buy things not only for what they do, but also for what they mean" (p. 403). The meaning, the image, the theme—everything that a product symbolizes and stands for—this is what defines the product more than anything.

In a similar way, Nike is not selling sneakers. It is selling control over one's life, a feeling of self-efficacy, a sense that you can do all the things you always wanted to do. The benefit—the promise that Nike is offering—is far more than a superior foot product or even superior athletic performance. The promise is control over your life and the fulfillment of your desires.

Public health practitioners must learn to redefine the public health product so as to offer a promise that appeals to people's core values. For example, the public health practitioner might try to prevent smoking initiation not by selling the idea of being a nonsmoker, but by selling freedom from nicotine addiction, independence from tobacco industry manipulation and victimization, and rebellion against an industry that is trying to trick you, seduce you, addict you, and ultimately, to kill you (Table 3–1). Instead of selling safe sex, the public health practitioner might redefine the product as freedom from AIDS, independence from the virus that is afflicting your friends and communities, and control over your destiny. And instead of selling exercise, the public health practitioner might sell control over your appearance, control over how you feel about yourself, control over how others think about you, and rebellion against feelings of unattractiveness.

REPACKAGING, REPOSITIONING, AND REFRAMING THE PUBLIC HEALTH PRODUCT

Once the product is defined, the public health practitioner must begin the process of packaging it, positioning it, and framing it in such a way that it offers the

Table 3–1 Product, Benefit, and Core Values for the Desired Action (Behavior Change) among the Target Audience—A Strategic Marketing Approach

Desired Action	Product/Benefits	Core Values
Prevent smoking initiation	Freedom from nicotine addiction Independence from tobacco industry manipulation Rebellion against an industry that is trying to trick you, seduce you, addict you, and kill you	Freedom Independence Control Rebellion
Practice safe sex	Freedom from AIDS Independence from the virus that is afflicting your friends and communities Control over your destiny	Freedom Independence Control Rebellion
Exercise more often	Identity as a physically strong and attractive person in control of your appearance Rebellion against feelings of unattractiveness and lack of control over your appearance	Freedom Independence Control Rebellion

benefits the target audience is seeking in a way that reinforces the audience's core values. At this stage, the process of developing an image for the product is central. This process involves the search for appropriate metaphors, symbols, words and phrases, visual images, and themes. All must work together to convince the consumer that the product will indeed fulfill his or her needs and desires, and in a way that is consistent with and reinforces his or her most salient core values.

Lauffer (1984) explains the significance of this task of framing, or image-building, as part of the strategic marketing process:

> In image building, symbols can be very important. In the United States, "welfare" tends to take on a negative connotation. To many, it means "cheating," "dependency," or a "drain on the taxpayers resources."
>
> But no one is against the "deserving poor." In a recessionary economy, who can be against "laid-off" workers, in contrast with the "unemployed," some of whom, at least, are blamed for their situation. Some people may be turned off by the term "runaway kids" but not by "troubled teens." People may be against the high cost of Medicare or Medicaid, but they won't be against serving crippled children or good

health care for impoverished senior citizens. They may be against welfare, but they are not against feeding hungry children. (p. 305)

For example, repackaging, repositioning, and reframing the product in a youth
antismoking campaign might focus on the adolescent core values of freedom, independence, control, identity, and rebellion (Table 3–2). Focus group research
conducted by the Centers for Disease Control and Prevention's (CDC's) Office on
Smoking and Health has revealed that "the desire of teenagers to gain control over
their lives would make them responsive to a counteradvertising strategy aimed at
exposing the predatory marketing techniques of the tobacco industry" (McKenna
& Williams, 1993, p. 85). The CDC research found that teens place a high value
on "self-determination and being in control" (p. 87) and concluded that "teenagers' rebellion can be viewed as a manifestation of asserting their independence
from adults' influence and control" (p. 87). The CDC researchers suggested that
the important adolescent values of independence and control could be used to
frame an antismoking message: "If you smoke, you are not in control; you are
being manipulated by the tobacco industry" (p. 87).

The potential effectiveness of such a reframing of the antismoking message can
be seen in the success of tobacco prevention initiatives among Black youth. In
1992, the percentage of Black high school seniors who smoked was 8.2%, four
times lower than the percentage who smoked two decades earlier (33.7% in 1974),

---

Table 3–2 Repositioning, Repackaging, and Reframing the Public Health Product:
Strategic Use of Marketing in a Smoking Prevention Campaign

Core Value	Message
Freedom	By not smoking, you can remain free of captivation by the addictive power of nicotine.
Independence	By not smoking, you can remain independent of the tobacco industry, which is trying to control you by fooling you into becoming a nicotine addict.
Control	By not smoking, you can maintain control over your social image, preventing being made a fool of by the tobacco industry.
Identity	Only the most mature youth are able to resist the tobacco industry's attempt to capture them; smoking is something that kids do because they are not mature enough to under-stand.
Rebellion	Rebel against an industry that is trying to deceive you, lie to you, manipulate you, seduce you, addict you, and kill you.

while smoking prevalence among White youth during this period remained essentially unchanged at 30% to 34% (USDHHS, 1994). One explanation for this difference is the development, in the Black community, of social norms that view smoking as an infringement of individual freedom and view promotion of tobacco as an effort to control and enslave Blacks. Several campaigns in the Black community, including successful efforts to end the tobacco industry's marketing of X cigarettes and Uptown cigarettes, both directed specifically at young Black people, infused the community with a spirit of rebellion against an industry that was portrayed as trying to enslave it. As Cass Sunstein (1997) describes it, the antismoking campaign was "symbolized most dramatically by posters in Harlem subways showing a skeleton resembling the Marlboro man lighting a cigarette for a black child. The caption reads, 'They used to make us pick it. Now they want us to smoke it.'" (p. 33)

Similar techniques could be used to reposition other public health "products" in ways that make their benefits to the audience more compelling (see Table 3–1). Fred Kroger, director of CDC's Office of Health Communication, summarizes: "Just as athletic footwear is sold as aids to 'soar through the air, slam dunk, in your face' feats of athleticism, rather than as canvas covers for the feet, such prevention products as condoms, monogamy, or abstinence still lack similar, consumer-oriented positioning" (Kroger, 1995, p. 46).

In reframing the public health product, public health practitioners must recognize that the most deeply ingrained core value—freedom—represents not only the absence of something, but the presence of something as well. Frances Moore Lappe (1989) asks, "Aren't there really two basic aspects of freedom—freedom *from* interference and freedom *to* do what we want?" (p. 21) Freedom includes both negative liberty, or the absence of interference and infringement of one's privacy, and positive liberty, or the presence of an individual's ability to control his or her own life (Gaylin & Jennings, 1996).

This distinction has profound implications for framing behavior change as a public health product. Sometimes, the pursuit of positive liberty—helping people to be able to gain control over their lives—requires placing some limitations on negative liberty. For example, men may perceive wearing a condom as an infringement on their personal lives and their privacy. But the behavior itself may help to ensure positive liberty for the individual by keeping him in control of his future and allowing him, not AIDS, to make his decisions.

Public health efforts to change individual behavior tend to run up against opposition because they are perceived as conflicting with the core value of freedom. Usually, though, this is because they conflict with the concept of negative liberty. Public health practitioners may be able to show individuals that the desired behavior change actually reinforces the core value of freedom by emphasizing the aspects of positive liberty that will be conferred to the individual by adopting the behavior.

Public health practitioners must demonstrate that people's behavior choices are not really free, that these decisions are strongly influenced by economic, social, and environmental constraints that do not allow the full expression of individual autonomy. By providing people with healthy alternatives, the public health marketer is actually providing people with a degree of autonomy and freedom that they may not have previously experienced. "Individuals may not be able to make the healthy choices they might wish to make when immediate constraints push them toward other choices, such as lower cost but less nutritious foods at the local supermarket, unavailable exercise sites, or nonsupportive attitudes among their peers. Individuals have little or no control over their surroundings and so are dependent on their communities to maintain healthful conditions and choices" (Milio, 1995, p. 96).

Not only must public health practitioners demonstrate to the audience how the behavior change will fulfill basic needs and desires, but they must also show that the alternative (maintaining the behavior) will conflict with basic needs and desires. Thus, it is not enough merely to promote the behavior change in isolation. The public health practitioner must research the reasons for the maintenance of the behavior in the population, the alternative messages being communicated, the sources of these messages, and the core values to which these messages appeal. Part of the process of packaging, positioning, and framing the public health product is finding a way to demonstrate to the target audience that the desired behavior change will fulfill important core values, while maintaining the behavior is actually conflicting with these values. "Any program seeking to moderate or eliminate this destructive behavior must recognize that it meets important needs and wants of the target audience. To effectively change the behavior, the social marketer must understand those needs and wants and show how the proposed behavior can either also meet those needs and wants or can meet other needs and wants that are subordinate" (Andreasen, 1995, p. 80).

For example, to promote increased physical activity, public health professionals must not only show why being physically active will fulfill some important needs and desires, but how remaining inactive will conflict with important needs. Not only must public health professionals offer benefits for adopting the desired behavior change, but they must identify and understand contradicting messages and confront them directly. Andreasen (1995) explains that marketers "recognize that every choice of action on the consumer's part involves giving up some other action. Thus, campaigns must keep in mind not only what the marketer is trying to get across but also what the customer sees as the major alternatives. Many times social marketers can bring about change as much by showing the deficiencies of an alternative as they can by emphasizing the benefits of the approach the marketer favors" (pp. 17, 18).

Part of demonstrating that a behavior will reinforce core target audience values is providing support to back up the promise. Traditionally, public health practitioners have relied on scientific evidence of the health benefits of a behavior change to support the promise of improved health from the behavior change. In contrast, successful corporate marketers tend to rely on much more compelling support for their promises. Nike, for example, backs up its offer of control over one's life with solid documentation: video footage of Michael Jordan—perhaps the most talented and successful athlete ever—in action. Ads for a health club might support their offer by showing a highly attractive, muscular, and self-confident individual using its facility.

Public health practitioners, too, must learn to provide equally compelling documentation or support for their promises. The increased use of peer as well as celebrity spokespersons is one approach that may be helpful. The source of the support is perhaps more important than the support message itself. People may be less likely to be convinced by documentation that comes from perceived public health authority, especially when there is now public skepticism about all the many public health messages that people are bombarded with, many of which present conflicting messages (e.g., fat is bad, some fat is good, polyunsaturated fat is good, alcohol is bad, some alcohol is good).

The components of the process of defining, positioning, packaging, and framing the public health product, then, are (1) defining the product; (2) determining the promise or the benefit that the product should offer; (3) developing an image for the product that is consistent with the promise; and (4) providing support for the promise (Figure 3–1).

MARKETING PUBLIC HEALTH PROGRAMS AND POLICIES

Marketing programs and policies for social change is similar to marketing behavior change, except that the target audience is not the individual but the public in general and policy makers in particular. The public health practitioner must market the policy to the policy makers who have the power to implement it, or in the case of initiatives or referenda, to the voters who will decide the fate of the ballot proposal. In either case, the public health practitioner must market the policy to the public at large, because public attitudes toward the policy will affect legislators' voting behavior, regardless of their personal opinions on the proposal.

The steps in marketing policies are identical to those in marketing behavior change: (1) find out what the target audience wants; (2) define the product to fulfill these needs and wants; and (3) package, position, and frame the product so as to reinforce the most important core values of the target audience. These steps are described in some detail in Chapter 6, which focuses on the strategic application of marketing principles to market public health programs and policies.

Product

Defined to offer a benefit desired by the target audience

Promise

Shows how the product will satisfy important needs and desires of the target audience

---

Image

Is a visual symbol of the product that reinforces core values of the target audience

---

Support

Documents how the product will deliver the promised benefit

Figure 3–1 Components of the Strategic Marketing Process for a Public Health Product

---

For now, it is important to point out that the needs and wants of policy makers regarding health and a healthy society are different from those of the individual. But as we will see in Chapter 6, the core values underlying policy makers' needs and wants regarding a healthy society are the same as those underlying the need for health among individuals. Policy makers desire a healthy population not because of a primary concern for the health of individuals, but because of a desire for their most powerful constituents to remain free of threats to their independence, autonomy, economic livelihood, and control over their destinies.

The case of Mothers Against Drunk Driving (MADD) and its campaign to advance policies to lower the legal blood alcohol limit for driving demonstrate the effective use of basic marketing principles to advance public health policy goals. Formed in 1980 by Candy Lightner, whose 13-year-old daughter was killed by a drunk driver, MADD has learned how to generate media coverage and how to use that coverage to not only inspire public sentiment, but to define and frame the issue of drunk driving in a way that advances policies to address the problem. MADD has helped to define drunk driving as an important social problem, to place the problem on the national agenda, and to successfully promote policies that regulate drinking and driving.

Defining the Product

MADD has consistently defined its public health policy product as far more than simply the reduction of alcohol-related motor vehicle fatalities. While saving lives is certainly an important benefit that MADD offers to policy makers through its proposed policies, a benefit that offers something even more compelling to policy makers is the creation of a society in which children and young adults are free to live their lives without being needlessly brought to their deaths by irresponsible behavior of others—behavior that is entirely preventable. By killing innocent victims, drunk driving interferes with the ability of individuals to have control over their lives, even if they themselves make wise and prudent choices. By defining the problem of drunk driving in this way, it can be seen to interfere with the powerful ethic of individualism and self-determination that lies at the very core of American culture. By focusing not only on reducing the number of fatalities, but on the nature of the fatalities that can and must be prevented, MADD has been able to define a product that truly offers to the policy maker a benefit that resonates deeply with his or her core values as a public official.

As the U.S. Department of Transportation explained in its analysis of the role of the media in drunk-driving interventions (Luckey et al., 1985), "when a person is killed or seriously injured as a result of someone else's drunken driving, the tragedy constitutes an obvious injustice as well. Such a clear affront to Americans' sense of fair play will sustain public attention longer than problems that appear more complex and ambiguous" (p. II-28). MADD has defined the problem of drunk driving in a way that appeals not merely to the policy maker's concern for the health of society's members, but to the widely shared principles of freedom, autonomy, fairness, and justice in society as a whole.

It is instructive to note that while public health efforts to reduce drunk-driving deaths have been quite successful (Ayres, 1994), efforts to address the problem of alcohol abuse itself have met with less success (DeJong & Wallack, 1992). To a large extent, this is due to the public health community's ability to define the problem of drunk driving in a way that offers a benefit that is highly important to policy makers—ensuring a society in which people, and especially children, have control over their lives. While reducing drunk-driving deaths is viewed as helping to ensure that parents can raise their children without the risk of having them taken away needlessly, reducing alcohol-related morbidity and mortality in its own right has not been defined in an equally compelling way. The public health product is still defined primarily as disease prevention. In light of the major public health successes observed in the area of policy regarding drunk driving, the lack of adequate prevention and treatment of alcohol abuse in society is a failure.

Positioning, Packaging, and Framing the Product

Not only has MADD been successful in defining its product in a way that offers a compelling benefit to policy makers, but the organization has been very effective in developing an overall campaign that packages the product such that it consistently reinforces the core values of policy makers. All components of MADD's marketing strategy—the product, the promise, the image, and the support—work together to reinforce these core values. The product is a society in which parents can raise their children free of the risk of having them taken away needlessly by other people's irresponsible behavior. The promise is that advancing MADD's policy goals—lowering the legal blood alcohol limit for driving, for example—will help policy makers to fulfill their need to ensure a society that provides freedom, independence, and autonomy to their constituents. The image that MADD has been able to consistently create is one of bereaved mothers mourning for a child who was killed by a drunk driver. This image has been created and reinforced by MADD's incredible ability to put a human face, an identified victim, to the policy issue. In this way, the support for MADD's promise is not merely scientific data about the reduction of alcohol-related traffic fatalities that result from lowering the legal blood alcohol limit, but documentation of the human suffering that results when a child is killed by a drunk driver.

An event staged by the Florida MADD chapter demonstrates these points vividly. To promote the creation of a state law that would reduce the legal blood alcohol limit for driving from 0.10 to 0.08 mg/dL, a candlelight vigil was held in the rotunda of the Florida Capitol building in Tallahassee. Hundreds of pairs of empty sneakers were placed in a circle around the rotunda, and the vigil participants joined hands around the sneakers. The sneakers represented children and adolescents whose lives were taken away by drunk drivers in Florida, and the number of pairs of sneakers corresponded with the statistics on drunk-driving fatalities in the state. In addition to being a moving experience for all the participants and creating an effective visual image for television cameras, the event successfully framed MADD's public health product in a way that reinforced the core values of freedom, independence, and autonomy. The product, promise, image, and support were all working together to market the public health policy.

Another effective image used in the campaign to promote stricter drunk-driving policies is the "red ribbon of memory," a collection of ribbons created by family members and friends of individuals killed by drunk drivers (National Highway Traffic Safety Administration [NHTSA], 1996). The ribbons are tied together to commemorate all victims of drunk driving in a community. A media event is organized around the ribbon ceremony that helps frame the issue of drunk driving as a threat to the safety, independence, and autonomy of the entire community (NHTSA, 1996).

The importance of using the identified victim, telling personal stories, and creating vivid images of the human suffering caused by drunk driving is emphasized in MADD's *How To Compendium*, a policy manual for public health advocates (Mothers Against Drunk Driving, 1991). The manual instructs advocates to "never underestimate your power or the power of a tragic true story to illustrate why the legislation is needed" (p. 138). The manual also instructs advocates to "utilize existing networks of victim service and victim rights organizations in your state. Be sure former victims who want to be involved and can make good presentations are given leading roles" (p. 138).

MADD's approach is effective not only because it appeals to the core values of policy makers, but because opponents of drunk-driving legislation are also trying to frame the issue as one of freedom and autonomy. The alcohol industry attempts to show policy makers that by tampering with the blood alcohol limit they will be imposing on the freedom of citizens to enjoy responsible, social drinking. Industry representatives have testified that lowering the blood alcohol limit to 0.08 will mean that an average-size woman can no longer drink two modest size glasses of wine if she is planning to drive. John Doyle of the American Beverage Institute, for example, argued that "they're trying to make .08 sound like some demonic level of consumption," when in fact "a 120-pound woman could reach .08 by drinking a couple of glasses of wine. . . . If you drop the legal limit to .08, that makes it illegal for a 120-pound woman to have two glasses of wine. You'll throw that 120-pound woman into jail, when she's not the problem" (McPhillips, 1997, p. A-22). The industry argues that the drunk-driving problem is one of a few individuals who drink extremely heavily and irresponsibly, and that by lowering the blood alcohol limit, society is imposing on the freedoms of the rest of our citizens, who are responsible people. If MADD were to frame the issue only as one of health and saving lives, then the alcohol industry would carry the theme of individual freedom to victory. By showing policy makers how failing to adopt 0.08 laws is what really represents an infringement of individual freedom, MADD has been able to effectively counter this argument and to win the marketing battle for the most important core needs, desires, and values of the policy maker. After all, the ultimate unfairness is not arresting people for drunk driving, but having innocent people killed by irresponsible drunk drivers.

CONCLUSION

If one looks at the major events that have led to the adoption of basic behavior change in the population, one finds that individual concern over one's health has rarely been the driving force. Instead, it has generally been the perception of lack of control over important aspects of one's life, loss of freedom, dependence, or striving for a certain identity that has prompted the most substantial health behavior changes. The significant declines in smoking prevalence observed during the 1970s and 1980s have been attributed largely to changes in societal norms that made the image of the smoker less socially desirable. The increased use of the designated driver was probably attributable more to the establishment of a social norm of behavior and the individual need to fit into this social pattern than any increased concern over the health impact of drunk driving. Changes in dietary habits and physical activity are most likely due more to the establishment of a desirable social image and identity associated with dieting, exercise, and slim and trim physical appearance than to people's increased concern about their long-term health and their desire to avoid chronic disease.

Public health practitioners must begin to sell something other than health itself, or health behavior change itself, if they are ever to be effective in addressing the chronic disease epidemic. First, they must begin to sell freedom, independence, control, identity, and rebellion. In other words, they have to redefine their product so that it offers benefits that will fulfill a clearly identified need or desire among their target audience. Second, they must package the product, position it, and frame it in a way that appeals to their audience's core values. This means they must place and promote the product in a way that will demonstrate to their audience how the product will fulfill their desires or needs. The perception that the unhealthy behavior in question is fulfilling or will fulfill basic needs and desires of the audience must be transformed into a realization that changing or not performing the behavior will actually satisfy these needs and desires to a far greater degree. The practitioner must define the product so that it offers a benefit desired by the target audience, offer a promise for how the product will satisfy important needs and desires of the target audience, present a visual image of the product that reinforces the audience's core values, and provide support or documentation that the product will indeed deliver the promised benefit. Each of these components of the marketing strategy must work together to reinforce the most important and compelling core values of the target audience.

In this new view of public health, epidemiologic surveillance and formative research (broadly defined as research to understand the consumer) will combine to form a basic foundation (Figure 3–2).

Surveillance identifies the most critical public health problems, the source of these problems, and the interventions that will be effective in solving the problems. These interventions can be translated into a set of specific behavior changes, changes in social and environmental conditions, and policy changes that are desired. Then, based on the findings of formative research, the most important

A. Public health surveillance

1. Identify and prioritize problems based on public health burden.
2. Identify effective interventions.
3. Identify specific behaviors, conditions, or policies to be changed (the object).
4. Identify the target population for each desired social change (the target).

B. Formative research

1. Identify and prioritize basic needs, desires, and values of target audience.
2. Identify attributes of the unhealthy behavior that satisfy or fulfill these needs, desires, and values.
3. Test ways of framing the desired behavior that will reinforce core values of target audience.

C. Strategic marketing for public health

1. Redefine the product so that it offers as a benefit fulfillment of important needs and desires (the product).
2. Package and position the product as a way to fulfill important needs and desires (the promise).
3. Show how the unhealthy behavior conflicts with fulfillment of underlying needs and desires.
4. Frame the communications in a way that reinforces, and does not conflict with, audience's core values.
5. Develop support for the promise: Demonstrate and convince audience that the product does and will fulfill their specific needs and desires (the support).

D. Assurance

1. Process monitoring.
2. Outcome evaluation.
3. Refinement of strategic marketing plan based on evaluation results.

Figure 3–2 A New Marketing Strategy for Public Health: Confronting Threats to the Public's Health

needs, desires, and values of the target audience can be identified. Next, the public health practitioner must define the product so that it will offer as a benefit the fulfillment of these desires and needs. Finally, the practitioner can package, position, and frame the product in an effort to demonstrate to the audience how it will indeed fulfill these desires and needs. The strategic marketing plan should be continuously assessed and refined based on the results of process and outcome evaluation.

REFERENCES

Andreasen, A.R. (1995). *Marketing social change: Changing behavior to promote health, social development, and the environment.* San Francisco: Jossey-Bass.

Ayres, B.D., Jr. (1994, May 22). Big gains are seen in battle to stem drunken driving. *The New York Times,* p. A1.

Bernays, E.L. (1965). *Biography of an idea: Memoirs of public relations counsel Edward L. Bernays.* New York: Simon & Schuster.

Burnett, L. (1961). *Communications of an advertising man.* Chicago: Burnett.

Conrad, P. (1987). The experience of illness: Recent and new directions. *Research in the Sociology of Health Care, 6,* 1–31.

Conrad, P., & Kern, R. (Eds.). (1994). *The sociology of health & illness: Critical perspectives* (4th ed.). New York: St. Martin's Press.

Crompton, J.L, & Lamb, C.W., Jr. (1986). *Marketing government and social services.* New York: John Wiley & Sons.

DeJong, W., & Wallack, L. (1992). The role of designated driver programs in the prevention of alcohol-impaired driving: A critical reassessment. *Health Education Quarterly, 19,* 429–442.

Enthoven, A. (1980). *Health plan.* New York: Addison-Wesley.

Flora, J.A., Schooler, C., & Pierson, R.M. (1997). Effective health promotion among communities of color: The potential of social marketing. In M.E. Goldberg, M. Fishbein, & S.E. Middlestadt (Eds.), *Social marketing: Theoretical and practical perspectives* (pp. 353–377). Mahwah, NJ: Lawrence Erlbaum Associates.

Gaylin, W., & Jennings, B. (1996). *The perversion of autonomy: The proper uses of coercion and constraints in a liberal society.* New York: The Free Press.

Glaser, B.G., & Strauss, A.L. (1968). *Time for dying.* Chicago: Aldine.

Kleinman, A. (1988). *The illness narratives: Suffering, healing, and the human condition.* New York: Basic Books.

Kotler, P. (1976). *Marketing management: Analysis, planning, and control* (3rd ed.). Englewood Cliffs, NJ: Prentice-Hall.

Kroger, F. (1995). Exhibit 1.1: Fred Kroger on HIV prevention: Communications success, marketing failure. In A.R. Andreasen (Ed.), *Marketing social change: Changing behavior to promote health, social development, and the environment* (pp. 45–46). San Francisco: Jossey-Bass.

Lappe, F.M. (1989). *Rediscovering America's values.* New York: Ballantine Books.

Lauffer, A. (1984). *Strategic marketing for not-for-profit organizations: Program and resource development.* New York: The Free Press.

Luckey, J.W., Jolly, D., Mills, K.C., McGaughey, K., Horn, D., & Richichi, E. (1985, December). *Role of media and public attention in drinking driver countermeasures* (Rep. No. DOT/OST/P-34/86/038). Washington, DC: U.S. Department of Transportation, Office of the Secretary of Transportation.

McKenna, J.W., & Williams, K.N. (1993). Crafting effective tobacco counteradvertisements: Lessons from a failed campaign directed at teenagers. *Public Health Reports, 108,* 85–89.

McPhillips, J. (1997, December 21). Fight looms over effort to toughen drunken-driving law. *The Providence Sunday Journal,* pp. A-1, A-22.

Meyers, W. (1984). *The image-makers: Power and persuasion on Madison Avenue.* New York: New York Times Books.

Milio, N. (1995). Health, health care reform, and the care of health. In M. Blunden & M. Dando (Eds.), *Rethinking public policy-making: Questioning assumptions, challenging beliefs* (pp. 92–107). Thousand Oaks, CA: Sage Publications.

Mishel, M.H. (1984). Perceived uncertainty and stress in illness. *Research in Nursing and Health, 7,* 163–171.

Mishel, M.H., Hostetter, T., King, B., & Graham, V. (1984). Predictors of psychosocial adjustment in patients newly diagnosed with gynecological cancer. *Cancer Nursing, 7,* 291–299.

Molleman, E., Krabbendam, P.J., Annyas, A.A., Koops, H.S., Sleijfer, D.T., & Vermey, A. (1984). The significance of the doctor-patient relationship in coping with cancer. *Social Science and Medicine, 18,* 475–480.

Mothers Against Drunk Driving. (1991, April 1). *How to compendium.* Irving, TX: Author.

National Highway Traffic Safety Administration. (1996, September). *National drunk and drugged driving prevention month program planner* (Rep. No. DOT HS 808-455). Washington, DC: U.S. Department of Transportation, National Highway Traffic Safety Administration.

Ogilvy, D. (1964). *Confessions of an advertising man.* New York: Atheneum.

Salmon, C.T. (1989). Campaigns for social improvement: An overview of values, rationales, and impacts. In C. Salmon (Ed.), *Information campaigns* (pp. 19–53). Newbury Park, CA: Sage Publications.

Schudson, M. (1984). *Advertising, the uneasy persuasion: Its dubious impact on American society.* New York: Basic Books.

Smith, G.H. (1954). *Motivation research in advertising and marketing.* New York: McGraw-Hill.

Sunstein, C.R. (1997). *Free markets and social justice.* New York: Oxford University Press.

Trachtenberg, J.A. (1987). Here's one tough cowboy. *Forbes, 139*(3), 108–110.

Turnock, B.J. (1997). *Public health: What it is and how it works.* Gaithersburg, MD: Aspen.

U.S. Department of Health and Human Services. (1994). *Preventing tobacco use among young people: A report of the Surgeon General.* Atlanta, GA: U.S. Department of Health and Human Services, Centers for Disease Control and Prevention, National Center for Chronic Disease Prevention and Health Promotion, Office on Smoking and Health.

Vogel, C.M. (1987). Putting research to work. In C. Degen (Ed.), *Communicators' guide to marketing* (pp. 31–42). New York: Longman.

Weitz, R. (1994). Uncertainty and the lives of persons with AIDS. In P. Conrad & R. Kern (Eds.), *The sociology of health & illness: Critical perspectives* (4th ed., pp. 138–149). New York: St. Martin's Press.

Winett, L.B., & Wallack, L. (1996). Advancing public health goals through the mass media. *Journal of Health Communication, 1,* 173–196.

The Importance of Formative Research in Public Health Campaigns: An Example from the Area of HIV Prevention among Gay Men

The public health effort to promote safe sex among gay men to prevent human immunodeficiency virus (HIV) infection illustrates the type of research and the type of understanding of the target audience that could provide meaningful insight to guide the development of more effective strategies to change individual behavior to improve health. It also shows how our current efforts to understand the target audience are woefully inadequate and often lead to prevention programs that conflict with the audience's core values.

Few published research studies have delved into the lives, the minds, and the hearts of gay and bisexual men to try to understand what love, relationships, and sex mean to them and how this is affected by the threat of AIDS and by public health admonitions to practice safe sex. As Weitz (1994) pointed out, most of the existing social science literature on AIDS consists of quantitative studies that examine factors related to sexual behavior practices. Complicating this problem is the fact that many AIDS prevention initiatives are based on the medical model, and, being viewed as medical interventions, fail to take the time and effort necessary to do formative research and find out the inner workings of the minds of the target audience. As Green explained in a 1996 article in *The New York Times Magazine,* "understandably eager to ingratiate themselves with the mainstream medical establishment on which they depend for funds, they have gravitated toward purely 'medical' interventions" (p. 54).

As a result of the shallow understanding of the feelings, attitudes, experiences, and values of gay men and the dynamics of the gay men's community, public health programs to prevent AIDS have often been at odds with some of the deepest core values of their target audience.

One example of a shortcoming of most HIV prevention programs that stems from a lack of insight into the lives, feelings, and experiences of gay men is the virtual disregard for risk reduction, as opposed to risk elimination strategies, and the reluctance to candidly discuss, rather than merely dismiss as deviant, unsafe sex. Public health programs have been characterized by what Green (1996) called "the unwavering focus of safe-sex campaigns on eternal condom use," (pp. 43–44) and what Rotello (1997) called "the condom code." As Odets (1995) pointed out, public health practitioners would never deliver this message—that people must use a condom every time they have sex for the rest of their lives—to the hetero-sexual community. Practitioners have respected the value heterosexuals place on long-term relationships, commitment, love, and marriage by acknowledging that heterosexuals do not need to use condoms to prevent AIDS after entering into a faithful marriage or monogamous relationship with a person who is free of infec-tion. The same understanding and respect for individual values has not been af-forded to homosexuals. Many gay men interpret this as a dismissal of the value of sex between men (Green, 1996).

As a consequence of this public health program failure, a sense of hopelessness and complete lack of control has arisen among gay men. Because they do not really believe that they will use a condom every time, many men assume that they are destined to become infected and therefore see no point in using condoms at all (Green, 1996). As Odets explained, "there's a difference between going out with a guy you've never met whose status you don't ask about, and a friend you've known 10 years who tells you he's negative. Education has refused to allow gay men even to think about that difference. It's like telling people that if they want to be safe drivers, they must always drive 35 miles per hour without regard to when, where or road conditions. Which any sane person will instantly reject" (Green, 1996, p. 45). Some men also feel that if the risk is so great that they cannot trust anyone, then there is no hope of obtaining a stable, long-term relationship. "If you can't trust, you can't love, so why even bother having a relationship?" (Green, 1996, p. 44).

A second failure of public health programs has been the inability to understand and acknowledge that for some gay men, it is the destructive nature of unprotected sex that motivates and supports the behavior in the first place. "For some—guilty, depressed, anxious, and living a life that often seems not worth living—the self-destructive aspects of unprotected sex are important incentives to practice it. This has nothing to do with complacency, nor will traditional AIDS education address it" (Odets, 1995, p. 47). As Odets added, "while our education and public policy continue to assume that unsafe sex is practiced despite its dangers, some men engage in it for precisely that reason" (p. 188).

Public health programs have failed, explains Odets, because they "have been guilty of ignoring the deepest root of gay men's unsafety: the psychological root, what they feel" (Green, 1996, p. 42). As Green's interviews with gay men re-vealed, at the deepest level of a gay man's psyche is a hole, a void, a loneliness, a feeling of guilt, and for those who have recently come out, a feeling of newfound freedom. Often, these men have experienced hatred, abuse, and lack of acceptance by their families, friends, communities, and society in general. And as Green (1996) concluded, "ignoring the role that homophobia plays in the psychology of AIDS means ignoring an element of disease at least as powerful as biology. If we care about public health, there is little choice but to care about people's feelings too" (p. 84).

Ultimately, the consequence of public health programs' failure to seek a deeper understanding of the reality of life for gay men in the "shadow of the epidemic," Odets (1995) argued, is that gay men feel a lack of control over their lives, a sense of being told what to do by people who do not understand what it is like to be gay in today's society, and of being told not only what to do, but who they are supposed to be. As Odets explained, gay men have "allowed [their] lives to once again slip from [their] grasp into the hands of those who too often believe, if quietly, that [they] should not even be what [they] are" (p. 264). And the public health practice of "simply instructing men in behaviors—'a condom every time'—actively obstructs the development of a capacity for informed judgment and perpetuates society's homophobic desire to simply dictate behaviors to gay men" (p. 194).

Instead of rendering gay men helpless, feeling a loss of independence, autonomy, and control, public health programs must find a way to offer gay men control over their lives. And rather than proscribing a course of action and even a lifestyle for these men and telling them how they should feel and what they should want, programs must help them to understand the epidemic and provide them with a realistic interpretation of the risks of HIV transmission, and must empower them to take control over their lives—lives that are respected, supported, and accepted and can therefore be meaningful and worthy of protecting and cherishing. The gay man can then discover and express the truth of his own feelings and develop new and independent desires.

Understanding the lack of control that many gay men feel may lead to prevention programs that place more control in the hands of the individual rather than the public health establishment. People must feel that their decisions are being left to them, that they are being given all the options and all the information, but that the final decision, and therefore the control of their future, is in their own hands. This means acknowledging, accepting, and even celebrating the meaning of love, relationships, and sex among gay men. It means discussing openly the differences in risk associated with sexual activities in different kinds of relationships. It means acknowledging the legitimacy of long-term relationships between men.

It also means providing true support, including counseling and other psychological services and benefits, to gay men and especially to gay youth. Instead of constantly telling these men what they should or should not be doing in the privacy of their homes, public health practitioners must begin to tell them that they care, that they understand, that they accept gay men for who they are, and that they are available to help. As Green (1996) asked, "in a world where financing for AIDS research keeps increasing but agencies that serve gay youths go begging for pennies, should we be surprised if gay men wonder whether the disease is more important than they are?" (p. 85).

Finally, public health efforts to change gay men's sexual behavior must include efforts to change the way society treats homosexuals and views homosexual relationships. Unless gay and lesbian relationships are acknowledged, celebrated, and respected in the same way that heterosexual relationships are, we cannot expect gay men to take messages about safe sex, stable relationships, and decreased promiscuity seriously.

Ultimately, public health practitioners must realize that "there is an epidemic beneath the epidemic we know about. Beneath and beyond. It predates AIDS and will probably outlast it and comes not from a virus but a vacancy. Like most minorities in America, gay men grow up feeling different, but uniquely they grow up both different and alone" (Green, 1996, p. 84). Only if public health practitioners take the time to go a little deeper beneath the surface of the gay man, to do the formative research necessary to understand his world, will they be able to design effective programs to confront the spread of AIDS among the gay population.

REFERENCES

Green, J. (1996, September 15). Flirting with suicide. *The New York Times Magazine,* pp. 39–45, 54–55, 84–85.

Odets, W. (1995). *In the shadow of the epidemic: Being HIV-negative in the age of AIDS.* Durham, NC: Duke University Press.

Rotello, G. (1997). *Sexual ecology: AIDS and the destiny of gay men.* New York: Penguin Books USA.

Weitz, R. (1994). Uncertainty and the lives of persons with AIDS. In P. Conrad & R. Kern (Eds.), *The sociology of health & illness: Critical perspectives* (4th ed., pp. 138–149). New York: St. Martin's Press.

Marketing Public Health

To confront the threats to the survival of public health as it approaches the 21st century, public health practitioners must extend their focus beyond the effort to protect the health of the public. They must now learn how to promote themselves and their institution. In other words, public health practitioners must enter the business of marketing public health.

This section shows why the survival of public health is threatened, why the task of marketing public health programs and policies is a formidable challenge for public health practitioners, and, finally, how practitioners can use basic marketing principles to confront this challenge effectively.

Section II also shows the public health practitioner how to strategically apply marketing principles to promote public health programs, public health policies, and the institution of public health itself.

CHAPTER 4

Emerging Threats to the Survival of Public Health

The survival of public health as a societal institution is threatened by emerging changes in the health care delivery system, the economy, the political climate, the public sentiment regarding public health and government in general, and the public health community itself. First, a misunderstanding of the relative importance of individual medical treatment compared with population-based prevention programs has led to a health system in which individual treatment rather than societal prevention is the dominant focus. This misunderstanding has fostered the illusion that health care reform is the solution to the nation's public health crisis and that managed care represents an important area of focus for public health. As a consequence, public health practitioners have been sidetracked from their mission as agents for social change. Also, political and economic forces directly threaten funding for public health departments and their policies and programs. These factors include budget cuts, block grants, the increasing influence of special interest groups, and the increasing antiregulatory sentiment in the nation. The greatest threat to the survival of the public's health, however, comes from within the public health movement itself. The public health community has lost a unified vision of its fundamental role and mission. To overcome these threats the public health movement must rediscover a strong, unifying model with a common vision, mission, and values to which the public and policy makers can relate. It will not be enough to promote the health of its constituents; the public health movement must now promote its own survival.

———— ❧ ————

Part I, Section I examined the factors that are responsible for the epidemic of chronic disease and emerging infectious diseases that threaten the health of the public. The key to confronting this epidemic is social change: changes in individual behavior, social conditions, and social policy. Public health practitioners are in the business of marketing social change, and the section demonstrated the ways they can use basic marketing principles to promote behavior and lifestyle change to the public.

Unfortunately, the attention of the public health practitioner cannot be focused entirely on improving the health of the public because the public's health is only one thing that the public health practitioner must save. Emerging changes in the health care delivery system, the economy, the political climate, public sentiment regarding government, and changes in the public health community itself now threaten the very survival of public health as a societal institution. In addition to promoting the health of its constituents, public health must now find a way to promote its own survival.

Part I, Section II broadens our perspective and considers not merely the need to protect the public's health, but also the need to ensure the survival of public health. The reasons that the survival of public health is threatened (Chapter 4), the challenge this threat poses to the public health practitioner (Chapter 5), and the potential role that the strategic application of basic marketing principles could play in helping the public health practitioner to confront this challenge (Chapter 6) are examined.

The survival of public health as a societal institution is threatened because of the adverse consequences of three major factors: (1) the persistent emphasis on individual rather than societal health and on treatment rather than prevention; (2) economic and political factors that directly threaten public health funding; and (3) the loss, among public health practitioners, of a unified vision of the role and mission of public health.

MISUNDERSTANDING OF THE IMPORTANCE OF MEDICAL TREATMENT COMPARED WITH POPULATION-BASED PREVENTION

Despite the widely held perception that recent advances in medical treatment have resulted in a dramatic decline in mortality, there is substantial evidence that the observed decline in mortality in the developed world during the 18th to 20th centuries was attributable largely to public health and not medical interventions (Evans, Barer, & Marmor, 1994; Lee & Estes, 1997; Levine, Feldman, & Elinson, 1983; Turnock, 1997). The most extensive research into this hypothesis was conducted by Thomas McKeown, a physician and historical demographer who, over the course of more than 20 years, has developed a convincing analysis of the reasons for mortality declines observed in England and Wales during the past three centuries (McKeown, 1971, 1976, 1978; McKeown, Record, & Turner, 1975).

McKeown concluded that declines in mortality observed during the 18th century were due to environmental changes, such as purification of water, efficient sewage disposal, and improved food, hygiene, and nutrition (McKeown, 1978). During the nineteenth century, McKeown argued, the declines in mortality were due only to a reduction in infectious diseases; chronic disease rates remained stable (McKeown et al., 1975). According to McKeown, the three major factors that contributed to the decline were (1) rising standards of living, (2) improved hygiene, and (3) improved nutrition (McKeown et al., 1975). Although the smallpox vaccination campaign was effective, McKeown attributes only 5% of the decline in mortality in the latter half of the nineteenth century to immunization. McKeown argues that declines in infectious disease rates account for about 75% of the mortality reductions observed during the 20th century (through 1971). Although immunization played a limited role, the dominant factors in the control of infectious disease were improved nutrition and hygiene.

In research on the reasons for the dramatic decline in mortality in the United States during the 20th century, John and Sonja McKinlay (1977, 1994) found that no more than 4% of the observed decline was due to medical treatment for infectious diseases. This conclusion is supported by the work of Rene Dubos (1959) and others (Cassel, 1976; Kass, 1971; Leavitt & Numbers, 1994; Lee & Estes, 1997; Magill, 1955; Powles, 1973; Weinstein, 1974). Recently, the U.S. Public Health Service (1995) estimated that of the 30 years that have been added to life expectancy since 1900, only 5 years are due to improvements in clinical medicine, while 25 years are attributable to population-based, public health programs. McKinlay and McKinlay (1994) also demonstrate that the steep decline in mortality between 1900 and 1950 slowed during the 1950s and leveled off during the 1960s. This was the precise period in which medical care expenditures skyrocketed. Increased spending for medical care does not necessarily translate into reduced mortality (Hingson, Scotch, Sorenson, & Swazey, 1981; Kim & Moody, 1992).

The work of McKeown, McKinlay and McKinlay, and others helped to reveal a shift in the 20th century in the type of diseases most responsible for mortality. The shift—known as the epidemiologic transition—was from infectious diseases to chronic diseases as the dominant cause of death in the developed countries (Omran, 1971). Whereas infectious diseases accounted for 40% of total mortality in the United States in 1900, they accounted for only 6% of mortality in 1973 (McKinlay & McKinlay, 1994). The proportion of total mortality attributable to chronic diseases (including injuries) increased from 20% to 67% during the same period.

The U.S. Department of Health and Human Services (USDHHS) estimated that approximately 75% of all premature deaths in the nation are preventable (Centers for Disease Control [CDC], 1995b; USDHHS, 1995). Of these, about 63% could have been avoided by changes in individual behavior and another 23% by changes in social and environmental conditions. Only 15% of these deaths were deemed preventable through improved access to medical care.

As McKinlay and McKinlay (1994) pointed out, the policy implications of the hypothesis that public health measures, not medical treatment, are the dominant reason for improvements in the health of the population are profound. If this perspective is accurate, then the critical strategy to achieve meaningful health reform is not the better provision of more organized, higher quality, lower cost medical services, but the societal commitment to social change. Preventing disease and illness requires changing the conditions in which people live, improving the quality of the environment, and reforming public policy. As Tesh argued, "it appears that social and political events that affect the standard of living, rather than microorganisms, are the salient determinants of health and disease" (Tesh, 1994, p. 520). Nevertheless, the current view of disease prevention continues to rely on germ theory and lifestyle theory as the explanation for illness. The most prominent public health programs aim to control infectious disease and change individual behavior. "Changing the physical environment is, from this perspective a third choice, and to attack poverty as a way to reduce disease becomes a last resort" (Tesh, 1994, p. 521).

The observed shift in causes of mortality from infectious to chronic diseases has similar implications for the improvement of the public's health. Because chronic disease is largely related to individual and societal behavior, social conditions, and social policy, public health must inherently be committed to social change. Medical care is certainly important, and recent evidence suggests that some of the modern medical interventions for atherosclerotic heart disease may explain declines in heart disease mortality during the past four decades. However, the most substantial gains in human health will be achieved only through public health—that is, the societal institution whose mission is the promotion of social change.

Even if the ultimate aim of prevention programs is to change individual behavior, the physical, social, and political environment in which people live must be the primary level of intervention. Because behavior is a product of the social conditions and social norms of the community in which a person lives (Tesh, 1994), discussing lifestyle changes without discussing the social conditions that give rise to them is misleading (Berliner, 1977). Public health practitioners cannot ignore the decades of research demonstrating that lower social class, social deprivation, and lack of social support are among the most important determinants of health (Conrad, 1987; Morris, 1982; Syme & Berkman, 1976). Substantial and sustained improvement in public health will require, first and foremost, social change.

The challenge to public health is presented clearly in a 1994 article by David Mechanic, who said, "The determinants of health risks are far too complex and forceful to succumb to ordinary efforts to inform the public and change its practices. Effective health promotion requires a deeper scrutiny of the structure of

communities and the routine activities of everyday life, as well as stronger interventions than those characteristic of much that goes on. Current efforts still function largely at the margins" (Mechanic, 1994, p. 569).

An additional reason that prevention rather than treatment of illness must form
the core of a national public health strategy is that advances in medical treatment
tend to disproportionately benefit the socioeconomically advantaged and, consequently, to increase the disparity in health status between rich and poor Americans. Dutton argues that the gap between health status of higher and lower socioeconomic classes is only partly due to differences in access to medical care
(Dutton, 1994).

> But much of the gap undoubtedly stems from a variety of nonmedical fac-
> tors, including a hazardous environment, unsafe and unrewarding work,
> poor nutrition, lack of social support, and, perhaps most important of all,
> the psychological and emotional stress of being poor and feeling powerless
> to do anything about it. . . . To be efficient as well as effective, health
> care must remedy not only the consequences of poverty, but must aid in
> efforts to change the underlying circumstances that perpetuate it. This is
> the most fundamental form of disease prevention, and perhaps ulti-
> mately the only truly effective one. (p. 479)

Foege, Amler, and White (1985) also emphasized the importance of disease prevention in closing the gap in health disparity between rich and poor.

The government's spending priorities, however, do not reflect the importance
of preventive public health measures compared with the limited effect of medical
treatment on the health status of the population (CDC, 1991, 1997; Eilbert, Barry,
Bialek, & Garufi, 1996; Eilbert et al., 1997; McGinnis, 1997; Public Health Foundation, 1994). In 1993, national health care expenditures totaled $884 billion, or
more than $3,000 per person (Gordon, Gerzoff, & Richards, 1997; USDHHS,
1996). In the same year, total public health expenditures were estimated to be
$25 billion, or slightly less than $100 per person (USDHHS, 1996). If one ex-
cludes spending for personal health care services, then the annual per capita expenditure for community-based, preventive public health programs was only $44
per person (CDC, 1995a). As a nation, then, we spend about $70 for medical treat-
ment for each $1 spent on the primary prevention of disease. Of an annual health
care budget that approaches $1 trillion, only 1% of expenditures support popula-
tion-based prevention programs (Satcher, 1996).

And although health care spending continues to skyrocket, funding for preventive public health measures is actually declining. The U.S. Public Health Service
(1995) estimated that although total U.S. health expenditures increased by more
than 210% between 1981 and 1993, the proportion of these expenditures used for
population-based public health measures declined by 25%.

The societal focus on individual-level treatment rather than population-based prevention interventions is reflected not only by the nation's spending priorities, but by the issues that dominate the national health agenda. Perhaps the two best examples of this are the inappropriate attention given to health care reform and to managed care as potential solutions to the nation's public health crisis. It is a widespread fallacy that health care reform can solve many of the nation's public health problems. An equal inaccuracy holds that managed care presents a great opportunity for public health advancement. Each of these fallacies represents a direct threat to public health practice in this country because they are sidetracking the public, policy makers, and, most importantly, public health practitioners, from the vital need to focus on social change as the vehicle to achieve societal improvement in health.

THE ILLUSION OF HEALTH CARE REFORM AS A SOLUTION TO THE PUBLIC HEALTH CRISIS

The health care reform debate in the United States is dominated by arguments over health care delivery and reimbursement methods for medical care, not by arguments about how to deliver adequate, population-based prevention programs and policies to the American people. Therefore, the debate is hardly pertinent when determining how to improve the public's health. "In spite of the evidence pointing to deficiencies in health-supporting milieus, resulting in damage that had to be remedied by health care, by the 1990s the health policy debate—in the United States and other countries—had moved to an almost exclusively economic argument about health care services, as though these considerations alone were pertinent to better health" (Milio, 1995, p. 98). Addressing the implications of the health care reform discussion initiated by President Clinton, Miller (1995) suggested the following: "The most disturbing conclusion is that current proposals are about financing, not about health care. . . . Consequently, health 'reform' is mainly about money and somewhat less about the organization of health services, and is not about broad, preventive measures that would reduce illness and injury and improve healthy functioning" (p. 356).

This country's failure to consider the real health care crisis, and its inappropriate focus on one small aspect of the problem as the solution to the whole problem, could spell doom for public health. If public and legislative debate continues to dwell on reforming the method of reimbursing physicians and hospitals, rather than on the method for ensuring the societal conditions in which people can be healthy, then the field of public health will be lost amid the complexities and conflicts of public debate.

THE ILLUSION OF MANAGED CARE AS AN OPPORTUNITY FOR PUBLIC HEALTH

Since the emergence of managed care, the field of public health has become preoccupied with it and its implications for the public's health. Managed care has dominated the agendas of major public health conferences, scientific journals, and policy debates. During the 1996 American Public Health Association (APHA) meeting, for example, 35 papers were presented on managed care (APHA, 1996). The theme for the 1998 APHA meeting is managed care and public health. The emphasis on managed care's implications for the public's health is appropriate, given the research indicating the adverse consequences of managed care on medical services and outcomes, especially for the poor, the disadvantaged, the elderly, and the chronically ill (Anders, 1996; Bickman, 1996; Brown, Clement, Hill, Retchin, & Bergeron, 1993; Clement, Retchin, Brown, & Steagall, 1994; Experton, Li, Branch, Ozminkowski, & Mellon-Lacey, 1997; Miller & Luft, 1994; Retchin & Brown, 1991; Retchin, Brown, Yeh, Chu, & Moreno, 1997; Retchin & Preston, 1991; Shaugnessy, Schenkler, & Hittle, 1994; Ware, Bayliss, Rogers, Kosinksi, & Tarlov, 1996; Webster & Feinglass, 1997; Wickizer, Lessler, & Travis, 1996).

Some public health practitioners have suggested that managed care presents tremendous opportunities for the advancement of public health goals. While efforts to integrate some aspects of public health into managed care systems certainly are important, they cannot and should not substitute for the basic effort to strengthen and preserve public health's independent role and independent infrastructure. The practitioner should not mistakenly think that managed care can be changed in a way that will allow public health to be practiced correctly. Why? Because public health and managed care are fundamentally different in their overall mission, their underlying values, and their primary goals and incentives.

Overall Mission

Managed care is simply a system of sick care delivery. But the delivery of sick care is only a small subset of public health practice. As the Institute of Medicine (1988) defined it, the mission of public health is to fulfill "society's interest in assuring conditions in which people can be healthy" (p. 7). Access to quality health care certainly is necessary to assure conditions in which people can be healthy, but it takes more than medical care to ensure that people are truly healthy.

Creating conditions in which people can be healthy requires social change: improving the infrastructure of our communities, restructuring the physical and social environments to promote healthy behaviors, and establishing social norms that support, rather than undermine, healthy behaviors. Ensuring that people are truly healthy requires the elimination of social, economic, and political barriers to an individual's ability to achieve fulfillment in his or her personal development, education, occupation, and family well-being. None of these requirements can be achieved solely through a health care system, even under ideal conditions. The best managed care could assure only the public's access to quality health care, not the quality of the public's health.

As Keck (1992) explained, there is a basic philosophical difference in the fundamental questions that managed care and public health seek to answer. While managed care asks "how do we pay for services?" public health asks "how do we maintain and restore health?" (p. 1208).

Underlying Values

The underlying values of managed care are inconsistent with those of public health. Public health is based on the principle of social justice: the assertion that society has an inherent interest in assuring a basic level of well-being for all people, regardless of their age, race, income, social status, or health status. Managed care, especially when practiced in a for-profit environment, tends to social injustice. While the system works well for people who are healthy, it is relatively unfair to the sickest and poorest individuals, who are generally those who need the most intensive intervention. The system of market justice, on which managed care is based, tends to produce inequalities in social, economic, and health status.

Managed care plans step back from the individual patient and allocate resources among their patient pool. The role of public health, however, is to step back even further and allocate public health resources among the entire population. Because of the disparities in health status, risk factors, and social and environmental conditions between different population subgroups, this means spending large amounts of money for people who are living in poverty, in the inner city, and in disadvantaged communities. This public health reality is incompatible with the mission of managed care: to reduce and control health care costs. Under managed care, people living in poverty cannot possibly receive the intensive intervention that is required.

The U.S. Department of Health and Human Services (1993), in its *Healthy People 2000* goals for the nation, called for public health efforts to "reduce health disparities among Americans" (p. 235). The managed care system will increase the disparity in health status between low- and high-income groups. In shifting the medically indigent from Medicaid and free care to managed care, the medical treatment available to people living in poverty will be limited. Although patients who have more money will be able to pay for their own health care, even if their health maintenance organization (HMO) denies coverage, the poor will have no recourse. Because managed care was developed to reduce health care spending and the groups that now require the most expensive health care are the poor, the elderly, the disabled, and the chronically, terminally, and mentally ill, it is these groups that will face a disproportionate burden of the reduction in health care spending.

Primary Goals and Incentives

The bottom line for managed care organizations is controlling medical costs for their overall patient pool, not providing the services that are in the best interests of individual patients. This is a basic, practical dilemma that cannot be overcome in a for-profit, managed care environment. Dr. Jerome Kassirer (1995b), editor of the *New England Journal of Medicine,* noted in a 1995 editorial that "although many see this as an abstract dilemma, I believe that increasingly the struggle will be more concrete and stark: physicians will be forced to choose between the best interests of their patients and their own economic survival" (p. 50). The best interests of the public's health cannot be served under a system in which quarterly earnings and shareholder value are critical concerns.

The conflict between the need to control costs and maintain corporate profit and the goal of improving the public's health is illustrated by HMOs' use of the cost savings generated by their practices. In 1994, publicly traded HMOs spent only about 75% of their patients' premiums on direct patient care (Anders, 1996). The remainder was used for executive salaries, marketing, administrative costs, retained earnings, stockholder payouts, and acquisition of other HMOs. In for-profit HMOs, the health of the public is not, and will not ever be the chief concern. Government and nonprofit health agencies and organizations are unique in having improvement of public health as their primary charge.

Managed care and public health also conflict in terms of their inherent incentives to offer expensive prevention initiatives. Attempts to encourage HMOs to enhance and expand prevention programs have generally been unsuccessful; HMOs do not appear to be interested in long-term benefits to their patients because those patients remain in a specific health plan for only a few years. Denying treatment, not expanding prevention programs, is the most effective way to increase short-term profits (Mallozzi, 1996). In contrast, prevention initiatives offer public health agencies and organizations the most effective strategies to achieve their goals of improving the societal conditions that affect health.

As long as HMOs are accountable primarily to their shareholders rather than to their patients, their providers, and their communities as a whole, the best interests of the public's health cannot be served. Investors generally want to see a return on their investments in a relatively short time period. For this reason, for-profit HMOs will always weigh short-term gains more heavily than intensive and costly preventive interventions whose payoff is in the distant future. For example, paying for intensive psychotherapy for youths with severe emotional problems might destroy an HMO's profit margin in the short term; the fact that this early intervention may prevent severe psychopathology many years in the future is of little interest to most investors. These types of interventions, however, are essential if we are to be effective in promoting public health.

The public health view is long term; social change takes many years, sometimes even decades. Programs must be administered repeatedly, consistently, and over a long period of time before the necessary changes in social conditions, norms, behavior, and policy can take place. The quarterly report framework that managed care uses for program evaluation and decision making is inappropriate for practicing public health.

Why an Emphasis on Managed Care Is Dangerous for Public Health

Because public health and managed care differ fundamentally in almost every basic premise, it is unrealistic to think that major public health achievements can be attained through the managed care system. Managed care is simply a method for the delivery and reimbursement of sick care; it cannot ever be a societal effort to create and facilitate social change. Managed care represents a threat to the survival of public health precisely because practitioners believe they can integrate public health efforts and initiatives into the managed care system. The institution that is charged with marketing social change—public health—must remain independent of managed care and must retain its focus on its fundamental mission.

Auerbach and McGuire, in a 1995 article in the *Journal of Public Health Management and Practice*, discuss the importance of maintaining a separate role for public health in human immunodeficiency virus (HIV) surveillance, education, and prevention in the era of managed care: "Surveillance programs are generally considered core public health functions that will need to be supported independent of the impact of health care reform" (p. 73). And although some argue that "under health care reform, . . . prevention messages will increasingly be provided within the context of primary care," (p. 74) Auerbach and McGuire responded by affirming the necessity for an independent role for the public health institution:

> Such an argument underestimates the extent to which individuals at highest risk are also likely to be out of care. In addition, research has shown that successful HIV prevention programs involve the community and client in the development process, are culturally competent, are specifically targeted to client subpopulations, and are grounded firmly in behavioral and social science theory. In addition, the behavior change efforts undertaken within these programs are time consuming and must

be reinforced repeatedly. Such prerequisites for success clearly exceed the capacity of most busy, primary care practices. While these practices may be able to contribute to certain aspects of individual behavior change, they are unlikely to address the community-wide attitude and norm change efforts necessary for HIV prevention. (p. 74)

Auerbach and McGuire concluded that the core public health functions necessary for HIV prevention will not and cannot flourish under health care reform unless health care reform "explicitly and separately authorizes and funds these activities and obligates the states regarding their utilization of such funds" (p. 76).

While there is pressure for public health agencies to become involved in efforts to add a more preventive focus to managed care, public health practitioners must not become so sidetracked by managed care that they lose sight of the real area in which the health of the population depends—stimulating social change for the population—not simply improving health care for the individual. To survive, public health must find, claim, and maintain its place as a societal institution outside of the managed care system. Only external to this system of health care delivery can the mission of public health be accomplished. And by sidetracking public health practitioners from the real issue at hand—the need to create and facilitate social change—the present preoccupation with finding ways to realize some marginal benefits from convincing managed care corporations to incorporate some public health programs is threatening to erode the practice of public health.

POLITICAL AND ECONOMIC FACTORS THAT DIRECTLY THREATEN PUBLIC HEALTH FUNDING

Budget Cuts

Although funding cuts for public health programs have plagued government agencies for at least two decades, unprecedented proposals to completely eliminate many of the public health functions of government emerged during the mid-1990s. During 1995 and 1996, Congressional bills were introduced to eliminate or severely weaken the ability of the Environmental Protection Agency (EPA) (S291, HR2586), the Occupational Safety and Health Administration (OSHA) (S592, HR2586), the Food and Drug Administration (FDA) (Hamdt593, S291), and the Office of the Surgeon General (HR1923) to carry out functions necessary to safeguard the health of the environment, the workplace, and the pharmaceutical supply, and to play a strong and clear leadership role in protecting the public's health (see Table 4–1). In 1995 alone, Congress considered bills that would have removed jurisdiction over tobacco products from the FDA (HR2283, HR516, S201), eliminated funding for the FDA (Hamdt593), placed a moratorium on the promulgation of regulations by all federal agencies (S219), and severely reduced Medicaid (HR3507, S1795), Medicare (HR1923), Aid for Families with Dependent Children (AFDC) and supplemental security income (SSI) (HR1157, HR4, HR1923, HR3507), food stamps (HR1135, HR3507, HR1923), school lunch programs (HR3507, HR4), and health services and other support for legal and illegal immigrants (HR1157, HR4, HR1923, HR3507) (Table 4–1).

Decreased funding for federal public health programs translates into reduced funding for state and local programs as well. Using data derived from a survey of more than 2,000 local health departments throughout the country, CDC estimated that the median per capita expenditure by local health departments in 1995 was just $20, and the mean per capita expenditure was $26 (Gordon et al., 1997). This amounts to just under a dime per day.

Federal public health agencies are not the only ones facing elimination of or severe reduction in their ability to carry out essential public health functions. Many state and local public health agencies have also faced a crisis of survival during the past few years. For example, a 1996 proposal by Governor William Weld of Massachusetts would have eliminated the state Department of Public Health as an independent entity (Kong, 1996; "Lawmaker Faults Weld Proposal To Streamline Human Services," 1996; "Public Health Successes Emerging Despite Budget Cuts, Other Stresses," 1996; Vaillancourt, 1996a, 1996b). The proposal also would have eliminated the state's role in regulation of nursing homes, hospital quality assurance, state sanitary code enforcement, lead-paint removal, and nuclear monitoring ("Public Health Successes," 1996). The bill was defeated only after a statewide lobbying effort led by the Massachusetts Public Health Association.

Block Grants

Another aspect of the push to downsize government has been the effort to eliminate public health programs that traditionally have been federal entitlements for individuals who meet specified criteria and then replacing these programs with block grants that states can administer in almost any way they choose (AMA Council on Scientific Affairs, 1997). Although these proposals are framed as a way of transferring power back to the states, they almost always result in a reduction in funding and availability of public health programs; a decrease in the provision of services; and the elimination of accountability and assurance that the services are provided as intended (AMA Council on Scientific Affairs, 1997; APHA, 1997).

For example, a 1995 Congressional proposal to restructure the Medicaid program would have eliminated Medicaid as an entitlement to individuals and replaced it with block grants to states to administer similar programs for the medically indigent (S844: Medicaid Flexibility Act of 1995). However, the block grant

Table 4–1 Legislation Introduced in the 104th Congress To Eliminate or Severely Restrict Public Health Programs and Regulatory Authority

Bill	Title	Action
HR4	Personal Responsibility Act of 1995	Cuts AFDC, SSI, school lunch programs, and social welfare benefits for legal and illegal immigrants
HR9	Administrative Procedure Reform Act of 1995	Interferes with regulatory ability of federal health agencies
HR450/S219	Regulatory Transition Act of 1995	Establishes a 1-year moratorium on the promulgation of all new federal regulations, except those necessary to address an "imminent threat" to health or safety
HR926	Regulatory Reform and Relief Act of 1995	Interferes with regulatory ability of federal health agencies
HR1022	Risk Assessment and Cost-Benefit Act of 1995	Interferes with regulatory ability of federal health agencies
HR1135	Food Stamp Simplification and Reform Act of 1995	Cuts food stamp benefits
HR1157	Welfare Transformation Act of 1995	Cuts AFDC, SSI, and aid for legal and illegal immigrants
HR2283	None	Prohibits regulation of tobacco by the U.S. Department of Health and Human Services
HR516/S201	None	Prohibits regulation of tobacco by the FDA
S291	Regulatory Reform Act of 1995	Restricts regulatory ability of the EPA and the FDA
HR1923	Restructuring a Limited Government Act	Cuts AFDC, SSI, food stamps, and Medicare; restricts aid to legal and illegal immigrants; eliminates Office of the Surgeon General
Hamdt593	None	Eliminates funding for the FDA
S592	Occupational Safety and Health Reform Act of 1995	Restricts regulatory ability of OSHA
HR3507/S1795	Personal Responsibility and Work Opportunity Act of 1996	Cuts AFDC, SSI, Medicaid, school lunch programs, food stamps, and aid to legal and illegal immigrants

proposal included significant cuts in overall funding for indigent care programs; eliminated all but an absolute minimum requirement for the basic services that states had to provide and the criteria states had to use to determine eligibility for these services; and eliminated the federal government's role in assuring that the intended services are provided equitably. Similar proposals in 1996 would have converted AFDC, food stamps, SSI, homeless assistance programs, and child service programs to a block grant funding mechanism (Table 4–2).

Ultimately, the 104th Congress passed legislation that replaced the federal AFDC, emergency assistance, and Job Opportunities and Basic Skills (JOBS) programs with a Temporary Assistance for Needy Families block grant (Personal Responsibility and Work Opportunity Reconciliation Act of 1996). An evaluation of this legislation's impact by the Tufts University Center on Hunger and Poverty concluded that in the majority of states, implementation of the new block grant program created welfare policies that worsen the economic circumstances of the poor (Center on Hunger and Poverty, 1998). In more than two-thirds of the states, the block grant mechanism resulted in welfare policies that are more likely to result in a deterioration of the economic self-sufficiency of poor families.

The consolidation of federal public health program funding into block grants to the states applies not only to entitlement programs such as AFDC, but to other public health programs as well. In 1996, Senator Nancy Kassebaum introduced legislation that would have combined 12 separate public health programs whose funding totaled $1.1 billion a year into one block grant that would be distributed to the 50 states ("Health Ranking of States Proposed," 1997).

Table 4–2 Legislation To Convert Entitlement Programs to a Block Grant Funding Mechanism, 104th Congress

Bill	Title	Action
S844	Medicaid Flexibility Act of 1995	Converts Medicaid to block grants
S842	Individual Accountability Act of 1995	Converts AFDC to block grants
S845	SSI Flexibility Act of 1995	Converts SSI to block grants
S36	Welfare to Work Act of 1995	Converts food stamp programs to block grants
HR3964	Homeless Housing Programs Consolidation and Flexibility of 1996	Converts homeless assistant programs to block grants
HR3507	Child and Family Services Block Grant Act of 1996	Converts child welfare and child protection service programs to block grants

The Influence of Special-Interest Groups and the Failure To Reform Campaign Financing

The continued influence of powerful special-interest groups, especially at the federal level, threatens the funding of many public health programs. An excellent case in point is federal funding for research on firearms-related injuries. In 1995, the National Rifle Association (NRA) lobbied Congress to eliminate all funding for the National Center for Injury Prevention and Control (NCIPC), a $46 million center that serves as the nation's leading agency dedicated to the prevention and control of intentional and unintentional injuries ("Gun Violence Remains a Public Health Risk That's Still Hard To Track," 1996; "House Cuts $2.6m for CDC Gun Study," 1996; Kassirer, 1995a; Kent, 1996). Because gun-related deaths are a significant part of injury mortality (38,500 deaths in 1994), research on firearms control is a central part of the center's mission. The NRA was successful in getting Congress to consider a bill that would have eliminated the NCIPC completely. The bill failed, but 1 year later the NRA returned with a less ambitious objective: to eliminate funding for the firearms injury research at the center, which amounted to $2.6 million in 1995. In 1996, both the House of Representatives and the Senate approved a $2.6 million cut in the NCIPC budget to eliminate firearms injury research at CDC (HR3755: Health and Human Services FY97 Appropriations Bill). Ultimately, a Congressional compromise worked out in the last days of the legislative session restored the $2.6 million to the NCIPC budget but diverted most of it to study traumatic brain injury (Kong, 1997). In addition, a clause in the appropriations bill prohibited any of the NCIPC funds from being used to advocate or promote gun control ("Gun Violence Remains a Public Health Risk That's Hard To Track," 1996; Kong, 1997).

The NRA spends $3 million to $6 million annually to influence Congressional elections and legislation (M. Gerkey, personal communication, December 1997). Of note, 75% of the 263 House members who voted to cut the NCIPC's funding accepted contributions from the NRA during the prior 3 years and only six recipients of NRA funding voted against the funding cut (Montgomery & Infield, 1996). The NRA's influence was also instrumental in House passage of a bill to repeal the ban on assault weapons (HR125: Gun Ban Repeal Act of 1995), which passed 239 to 173 but was not approved by the Senate. The NRA's influence on both bills is highlighted by the fact that 366 of the 421 members who voted on the NCIPC funding cut voted in a consistent manner on the repeal of the assault weapons ban ("How Members of Congress Voted on Issues Affecting Public Health," 1997). House Speaker Newt Gingrich stated outright in a letter to an NRA lobbyist that "as long as I am speaker of this House, no gun control legislation is going to move in committee or on the floor of this House" ("Police Take Notice," 1996).

Another example of the extent to which special-interest lobbying interferes with public health protection is the area of environmental protection and regulatory reform. Manufacturing company lobbyists have played a large role, not only in influencing the fate of environmental protection legislation, but, in some cases, actually drafting the legislation. The revision of the Clean Water Act introduced in Congress in 1995 included many provisions suggested by industry lobbyists who were allowed to work side by side with the bill's sponsors (Cushman, 1995; Jacoby, 1996). A 1995 regulatory reform bill proposed by Senator Bob Dole of Kansas contained a special provision to protect the interests of Georgia-Pacific, a wood products conglomerate. The company had worked through a Virginia law firm to persuade Dole to insert this special provision (Engelberg, 1995; Jacoby, 1996). The 1995 revision of the OSHA's enabling legislation contained language drafted by lobbyists brought in by the Labor Committee's work force protections subcommittee to help write the legislation (Jacoby, 1996).

In the 1995-1996 election year, the top three political action committees (PACs) donating to Congressional elections represented firearms, alcohol, and tobacco (McCarthy, 1997). The NRA topped the list with $1.6 million in donations, followed by the National Beer Wholesalers with $1.3 million, Philip Morris with $880,000 and R.J. Reynolds with $760,000 (McCarthy, 1997). During 1996, the alcohol industry alone contributed more than $4 million in non-PAC donations to federal candidates. Leading the list was Seagram at $1.6 million, followed by the National Beer Wholesalers ($1.4 million), Anheuser-Busch ($860,000), and Brown-Forman ($320,000; McCarthy, 1997).

Despite the continued bipartisan rhetoric about the need for campaign finance reform to reduce the influence of special interest lobbying, no meaningful campaign finance reform law has been enacted during the past 23 years (Rosenbaum, 1996). Although several campaign finance reform measures were introduced in Congress in 1996 and 1997, no significant reforms were enacted into law. And despite promises by members of both parties that 1998 would be the year that significant reforms were enacted, the U.S. Senate killed campaign finance reform legislation early in the 1998 session (Kranish, 1998).

Increasing Antiregulatory Sentiment

The practice of public health relies on a sense of public trust in government's ability to protect societal interests and a shared sense that the government has the responsibility to fund and conduct programs to accomplish this. However, recent public opinion polls have documented low levels of public trust in government and public acknowledgment of a central role and responsibility in protecting societal interests.

A May 1994 poll found that 70% of Americans were dissatisfied with the overall performance of the federal government; 70% believed that government programs are inefficient and wasteful, and 69% believed that the federal government creates more problems than it solves (Weisberg, 1996).

A May 1995 Gallup poll found that 39% of Americans feel that the federal government "has become so large and powerful it poses an immediate threat to the rights and freedoms of ordinary citizens" (Weisberg, 1996). The percentage of Americans who believe that the federal government can be trusted to "do what is right" most or all of the time declined from 76% in 1964 to a low of 14% in 1994 (Weisberg, 1996).

The public's antigovernment sentiment has been fueled by political rhetoric, heightened during and after the Republican "takeover" of Congress in 1994. House Speaker Newt Gingrich's Contract with America was based on the assertion that "Big Brother is alive and well through myriad government programs usurping personal responsibility from families and individuals" (Gillespie & Schellhas, 1994, p. 14).

The antiregulatory sentiment in Congress nearly resulted in the destruction of a significant part of the nation's public health infrastructure. During 1995 and 1996, Congressional bills were introduced that would have eliminated or severely weakened the authority of nearly every major federal health agency to protect the public's health (see Table 4–1), and there were specific proposals to eliminate the FDA (Hamdt593), the Office of the Surgeon General (HR1923), and the National Institute for Occupational Health and Safety. There also were bills to eliminate the authority of FDA (HR516/S201) or of the entire U.S. Department of Health and Human Services (HR2283) to regulate tobacco.

Perhaps more threatening than the public's lack of trust in government is the public's disinterest in the responsibility of government to promote the common good. The Progressive movement, which launched large-scale government programs to address public health issues and social problems, was based on the assertion "that social evils will not remedy themselves, and that it is wrong to sit by passively and wait for time to take care of them . . . that the people of the country should be stimulated to work energetically to bring about social progress, that the positive powers of government must be used to achieve this end" (Weisberg, 1996, p. 157).

As Weisberg argued in his 1996 book *In Defense of Government*, the values that underlie government's charge to promote social justice have not disappeared, but they need to be restored to prominence in the public, political, and media agendas: "Building a workable public activism is not a matter of starting from scratch but rather of recovering and renewing lost principles" (p. 158). What needs to be restored, according to Weisberg (1996), is the assertion of "the national government's responsibility for the welfare of the entire polity" (p. 159).

In a 1997 *American Journal of Public Health* editorial, Dr. Fitzhugh Mullan of the journal *Health Affairs* emphasized the same point, but referred specifically to the restoration of the public health movement:

> An acute hazard for the reinvention workers of our movement is that the pendulum of national life is swinging so far in the direction of propri-

etary and individual interests . . . a tougher and ultimately more central job is to retain public and communitarian principles, no small task when the rhetoric of this 'post-health-care-reform' era, both inside and outside the government, is so strongly oriented to the private sector. Yet it will be the response to this challenge—the stewardship of the public trust despite the siren calls of devolution and privatization—that will render the ultimate commentary on the leadership of federal public health at the end of the 20th century. (Mullan, 1997, p. 24)

THE LOST VISION OF PUBLIC HEALTH

In recent years, the public health community has lost a unified vision of its role and mission (Brown, 1997). The vision of public health as a form of social justice and of the mission of the public health practitioner as advocating for social justice and social change no longer guides the public health movement. To see how this has occurred, we must briefly review the historical roots of public health.

Public health has deep historical roots in what Beauchamp (1976) termed the "egalitarian tradition." Beauchamp proclaimed that "public health should be a way of doing justice, a way of asserting the value and priority of all human life" (p. 8). Turnock (1997) also explained that the underlying philosophy of public health is social justice: "In the case of public health, the goal of extending the potential benefits of the physical and behavioral sciences to all groups in the society, especially when the burden of disease and ill health within that society is unequally distributed, is largely based on principles of social justice" (pp. 15–16).

Public health was founded on three basic principles: (1) the principles of social justice; (2) the notion of an inherent public responsibility for social health and welfare; and (3) the responsibility of the public health practitioner to advocate for social justice and collective, societal action.

The first principle—social justice—is based on the view that health is not an individual privilege but a social good that should be equally available to all individuals: "While many forces influenced the development of public health, the historic dream of public health that preventable death and disability ought to be minimized is a dream of social justice" (Beauchamp, 1976, p. 6).

The second principle—public responsibility for social health and welfare—is based on the assertion that government is responsible for achieving and preserving social justice. There is a collective, societal burden to ensure equal health protection and basic standards of living for all people: "Another principle of the public health ethic is that the control of hazards cannot be achieved through voluntary mechanisms but must be undertaken by governmental or non-governmental agencies through planned, organized and collective action that is obligatory or non-voluntary in nature" (Beauchamp, 1976, p. 8). Burris (1997) explained: "While much of the most important public health work is done in the private sector and the work of the state must take a wide variety of forms beyond direct regulation, 'public health' without the dynamic leadership of government in deploying the nation's wealth against the ills arising from individual choices in the market is a contradiction in terms" (p. 1608).

The third principle—advocacy—is based on the view that the public health practitioner is, first and foremost, an advocate for social change: "Doing public health involves more than merely elaborating a new social ethic; doing public health involves the political process and the challenging of some very important and powerful interests in society. . . . While professional prestige is an important attribute in the modern day public policy process, public health is ultimately better understood as a broad social movement. . . . The political potential of public health goes beyond professionalism; at its very heart is advocacy of an explosive and radical ethic" (Beauchamp, 1976, p. 10).

The idea that public health's role is to promote social change dates back at least 150 years. Public health arose out of the establishment of healthy social conditions as a societal goal and the recognition of public institutions as responsible for achieving this social goal (Institute of Medicine, 1988). Public health is not just about studying problems and proposing solutions. It is about organizing the community to support and implement those solutions. And organizing the community requires social and political intervention. As the Institute of Medicine (1988) explained, "the history of public health has been one of identifying health problems, developing knowledge and expertise to solve problems, and rallying political and social support around the solutions" (p. 70).

Public health cannot be separated from the political process. In fact, politics is at the heart of public health. As Dr. Gro Harlem Brundtland, chief of the World Health Organization, stated, "you cannot implement it [public health] without making it a political issue" (Altman, 1998, p. C3).

Rosemary Stevens (1996) outlined these fundamental principles of public health in an *American Journal of Public Health* editorial reviewing the vision of Dr. Henry Sigerist (1891–1957), a medical historian and public health advocate: "For Sigerist, as for many of us who were socialized into public health in the 20th century, health is quite simply a social good. The role of the state is to enhance and protect that good for all members of the population; indeed, in his view, the state has a public duty to do so" (p. 1522). Further, it is the role of the public health practitioner to advocate for the necessary social reforms. For Sigerist, advocacy was a responsibility for the individual as well as for the public health institution. Sigerist "threw his own energy, commitment, and enthusiasm on the side of what he perceived to be social equity and justice" (Fee, 1996, p. 1644).

The principles of social justice, societal responsibility for public health and welfare, and advocacy for social change remain the three pillars of public health today. As expressed in a 1996 APHA policy statement, "long-standing principles of the APHA establish a commitment to the right of all people to attain and maintain good health, through population based public health services and through access to personal health care services. . . . Further, it is the responsibility of society at large, and the public health system in particular, to safeguard the public interest in achieving these objectives" (APHA, 1997, p. 511).

Public health has begun to lose sight of its historical foundation and fundamental principles. No longer united by a common vision of its mission and role, public health has come to be viewed by many in the field more as an elite profession rather than a broad, social movement. In recent years, the "advocacy of an explosive and radical ethic" is all but lost. This, more than anything else, threatens the survival of public health as an institution.

Perhaps the most poignant illustration of the loss of the vision of public health as a broad social movement and its takeover by elite professionalism is the efforts of three national public health organizations—the National Center for Tobacco-Free Kids, the American Cancer Society (ACS), and the American Heart Association (AHA)—to promote a Congressionally mediated, "global" settlement to all but a strictly defined subset of past, present, and future lawsuits by citizens, businesses, and public bodies against the tobacco industry (Califano, 1998; "Koop Opposes Immunity in Tobacco Deal," 1997; LoPucki, 1998; McGinley & Harwood, 1997; Schwartz, 1998; Shackelford, 1997; Siegel, 1996, 1997; "The Reynolds Papers," 1998; "Tobacco Talk," 1998; Torry, 1998; Weinstein & Levin, 1997). The process by which the settlement was pursued and promoted violated the core principles of public health; eschewed social justice; and co-opted a broad, social movement, wresting it from the hands of community public health practitioners across the nation and into the hands of a few powerful individuals and organizations (McGinley & Harwood, 1997; Shackelford, 1997; Siegel, 1996, 1997; Weinstein & Levin, 1997). The very organizations that claimed to represent the interests of cancer and heart disease victims were willing to trade away the legal rights of these victims. And the leadership of these organizations remained willing to consider a deal that would grant the tobacco industry immunity for its wrongdoing, even after the grassroots membership of these organizations made it clear that they opposed the concept of using the legal rights of American citizens as a bargaining chip.

A recent article in the *American Journal of Public Health* illustrated another way in which health advocates have compromised public health values. Many health advocacy groups, such as professional medical and nursing associations, the AHA, the American Lung Association, and the ACS have hired lobbyists who also represent the tobacco industry (Goldstein & Bearman, 1996). For example, in 1994 more than 300 health organizations employed one or more tobacco lobbyists (Goldstein & Bearman, 1996).

Perhaps the most egregious example is the appointment of former tobacco industry lobbyist Kim Belshe as director of the California Department of Health Services. Belshe was appointed by Governor Pete Wilson as the director of the California Department of Health Services in 1994. Belshe had been a lobbyist for the tobacco industry and had lobbied against Proposition 99, an initiative to establish a comprehensive, statewide tobacco control program funded by an increase in the state cigarette excise tax. There could hardly be a more inappropriate person to serve as director of a state health department than a former tobacco industry lobbyist who opposed one of the most important public health interventions in the state.

While some public health organizations have turned to professional lobbyists with dubious associations, many other public health groups have gone so far as to halt all advocacy in order to prevent the appearance of improper lobbying activity. The widely held perception that education is the only appropriate role for public health agencies and that advocacy is illegal or inappropriate for public health officials has arisen largely because of a widespread misunderstanding of the difference between advocacy and lobbying.

Many public health practitioners are under the impression that advocacy is synonymous with lobbying and therefore is restricted by federal law. Lobbying, however, is a very specific and legally defined term. As defined in the Internal Revenue Service Code, lobbying refers to an attempt to influence the outcome of legislation through communication with a legislator, government official, or the public (26 U.S.C.S. 4911). Generally, a communication is considered lobbying only if it (1) refers to specific legislation and (2) promotes a specific vote on that legislation (National Cancer Institute [NCI], 1993). Policy advocacy activities, such as researching, developing, planning, implementing, enforcing, and evaluating public health policy, are not lobbying, unless they involve the promotion of a specific vote on specific legislation (see Appendix 4–A).

Even when public health practitioners are convinced that their activities are legal, they often are scared into inaction by pressure from special-interest groups. A prime example is the use of federal funds to advocate for the control of tobacco use. The tobacco industry has used the Freedom of Information Act (FOIA) to intimidate tobacco control practitioners, often scaring them to inaction by forcing them to copy hundreds or even thousands of documents and accusing them of illegal activity (Levin, 1996; Mintz, 1997). For example, the Association for Non-smokers–Minnesota was hit with such a request. A spokesperson for the group explained: "They wanted people such as myself to be intimidated and fearful and confused—and at least to some extent they succeeded. Truly, we did almost nothing in the way of tobacco control for about three months" (Levin, 1996). Similar FOIA requests were made to state health departments in California, Massachusetts, Indiana, Colorado, and Washington (Levin, 1996; Mintz, 1997). According to an article in the journal *Tobacco Control*, the tobacco control section of the California Department of Health Services, which administers Proposition 99, received 59 FOIA requests from 1991 to 1993 (Aguinaga & Glantz, 1995). Although the tobacco industry's statements and actions imply that there is something wrong with the way tobacco control funds are being used, ethics board reviews have so far cleared all the groups whose activities have been challenged (Levin, 1996). Nevertheless, the tobacco industry's objective has been accomplished: Many tobacco control groups have been scared into inaction or into a state of reserved action.

CONCLUSION

The public health movement is involved in a fight not only to protect the public from the emerging epidemic of chronic disease that threatens to dominate life in the 21st century, but to save itself as a vital and integral part of the societal infrastructure. A continuing societal focus on health care reform as the solution to the nation's public health crisis, and on individual medical treatment rather than population-based prevention, threaten to obscure the need for public health. The emergence of managed care and the perception, even among public health practitioners, that public health can somehow be integrated into a managed care system threaten to erode the independent role of the public health professional. Budget cuts, block grants, special-interest group influence, and increasing antigovernment sentiment are each contributing to unprecedented cuts in funding for public health infrastructure. Finally, the failure of public health practitioners to assert their primary role as advocates for social change and the loss of a common vision for public health represent internal, yet critical, threats to the viability of the public health movement.

This is no longer a fight to protect people's health. It is now a life and death struggle for public health as a societal institution.

REFERENCES

Aguinaga, S., & Glantz, S.A. (1995). The use of public records acts to interfere with tobacco control. *Tobacco Control, 4,* 222–230.

Altman, L.K. (1998, February 3). Next W.H.O. chief will brave politics in name of science. *The New York Times,* p. C3.

AMA Council on Scientific Affairs. (1997). Federal block grants and public health: A call for physician partnership and leadership. *American Journal of Preventive Medicine, 13,* 336–342.

American Public Health Association. (1996). *Final program: Empowering the disadvantaged—Social justice in public health (124th Annual Meeting & Exposition).* Washington, DC: Author.

American Public Health Association. (1997). Policy statements adopted by the governing council of the American Public Health Association, November 20, 1996. *American Journal of Public Health, 87,* 495–518.

Anders, G. (1996). *Health against wealth: HMOs and the breakdown of medical trust.* New York: Houghton Mifflin.

Auerbach, J., & McGuire, J. (1995). The potential impact of health care reform on public health HIV-related activities. *Journal of Public Health Management and Practice, 1,* 72–77.

Beauchamp, D. (1976). Public health as social justice. *Inquiry, 13,* 3–14.

Berliner, H. (1977). Emerging ideologies in medicine. *Review of Radical Political Economics, 9,* 116–124.

Bickman, L. (1996). A continuum of care: More is not always better. *American Psychologist, 51,* 689–701.

Brown, E.R. (1997). Leadership to meet the challenges to the public's health. *American Journal of Public Health, 87,* 554–557.

Brown, R.S., Clement, D.G., Hill, J.W., Retchin, S.M., & Bergeron, J.W. (1993). Do health maintenance organizations work for Medicare? *Health Care Financing Review, 15,* 7–23.

Burris, S. (1997). The invisibility of public health: Population-level measures in a politics of market individualism. *American Journal of Public Health, 87,* 1607–1610.

Califano, J.A., Jr. (1998, January 9). Sellout to big tobacco. *The Washington Post,* p. A21.

Cassel, J. (1976). The contribution of the social environment to host resistance. *American Journal of Epidemiology, 104,* 107–123.

Center on Hunger and Poverty. (1998, February). *Are states improving the lives of poor families? A scale measure of state welfare policies.* Medford, MA: Center on Hunger and Poverty, Tufts University.

Centers for Disease Control and Prevention. (1991). *National expenditures for health promotion and disease prevention activities in the United States.* Washington, DC: U.S. Department of Health and Human Services, Centers for Disease Control and Prevention.

Centers for Disease Control and Prevention. (1995a). Expenditures for core public health functions. *Morbidity and Mortality Weekly Report, 44,* 421, 427–429.

Centers for Disease Control and Prevention. (1995b). *1994: Ten leading causes of death in the United States.* Atlanta, GA: Centers for Disease Control and Prevention, National Center for Injury Prevention and Control.

Centers for Disease Control and Prevention. (1997). Estimated expenditures for essential public health services—Selected states, fiscal year 1995. *Morbidity and Mortality Weekly Report, 46,* 150–152.

Clement, D.G., Retchin, S.M., Brown, R.S., & Steagall, M.H. (1994). Access and outcomes of elderly patients enrolled in managed care. *Journal of the American Medical Association, 271,* 1487–1492.

Conrad, P. (1987). The experience of illness: Recent and new directions. *Research in the Sociology of Health Care, 6,* 1–31.

Cushman, J., Jr. (1995, March 22). Lobbyists helped revise laws on water. *The New York Times,* p. A16.

Dubos, R. (1959). *Mirage of health.* New York: Harper & Row.

Dutton, D.B. (1994). Social class, health, and illness. In H.D. Schwartz (Ed.), *Dominant issues in medical sociology* (3rd ed., pp. 470–482). New York: McGraw-Hill.

Eilbert, K.W., Barry, M., Bialek, R., & Garufi, M. (1996). *Measuring expenditures for essential public health services.* Washington, DC: Public Health Foundation.

Eilbert, K.W., Barry, M., Bialek, R., Garufi, M., Maiese, D., Gebbie, K., & Fox, C.E. (1997). Public health expenditures: Developing estimates for improved policy making. *Journal of Public Health Management and Practice, 3,* 1–9.

Engelberg, S. (1995, April 26). Wood products company helps write a law to derail an E.P.A. inquiry. *The New York Times,* p. A18.

Evans, R.G., Barer, M., & Marmor, T.R. (Eds.). (1994). *Why are some people healthy and others not? The determinants of health of populations.* New York: Aldine DeGruyter.

Experton, B., Li, Z., Branch, L.G., Ozminkowski, R.J., & Mellon-Lacey, D.M. (1997). The impact of payor/provider type on health care use and expenditures among the frail elderly. *American Journal of Public Health, 87,* 210–216.

Fee, E. (1996). The pleasures and perils of prophetic advocacy: Henry E. Sigerist and the politics of medical reform. *American Journal of Public Health, 86,* 1637–1647.

Foege, W.H., Amler R.W., & White, C.C. (1985). Closing the gap: Report of the Carter Center health policy consultation. *Journal of the American Medical Association, 254,* 1355–1358.

Gillespie, E., & Schellhas, B. (Eds.). (1994). *Contract with America: The bold plan by Representative Newt Gingrich, Representative Dick Armey, and the House republicans to change the nation.* New York: Times Books.

Goldstein, A.O., & Bearman, N.S. (1996). State tobacco lobbyists and organizations in the United States: Crossed lines. *American Journal of Public Health, 86,* 1137–1142.

Gordon, R.L., Gerzoff, R.B., & Richards, T.B. (1997). Determinants of US local health department expenditures, 1992 through 1993. *American Journal of Public Health, 87,* 91–95.

Gun violence remains a public health risk that's still hard to track. (1996, November). In *The nation's health* (p. 24). Washington, DC: American Public Health Association.

Health ranking of states proposed. (1997, January 22). *The Boston Globe,* p. A15.

Hingson, R., Scotch, N.A., Sorenson, J., & Swazey, J.P. (1981). *In sickness and in health: Social dimensions of medical care.* St. Louis: C.V. Mosby.

House cuts $2.6m for CDC gun study: Critics, including NRA, say injury research biased toward firearms control. (1996, July 14). *The Boston Globe,* p. A19.

How members of Congress voted on issues affecting public health. (1997, February). In *The nation's health* (pp. 8–16). Washington, DC: American Public Health Association.

Institute of Medicine, Committee for the Study of the Future of Public Health. (1988). *The future of public health.* Washington, DC: National Academy Press.

Jacoby, M. (1996, Spring). A more "corrupt" Congress? *Forbes Media Critic, 3*(3), 42–46.

Kass, E.H. (1971). Infectious diseases and social change. *Journal of Infectious Diseases, 123,* 110–114.

Kassirer, J.P. (1995a). A partisan assault on science: The threat to the CDC. *New England Journal of Medicine, 333,* 793-794.

Kassirer, J.P. (1995b). Managed care and the morality of the marketplace. *New England Journal of Medicine, 332,* 50–52.

Keck, C.W. (1992). Creating a healthy public. *American Journal of Public Health, 82,* 1206–1209.

Kent, C. (1996, August 5). Fight over federal agency pits medicine vs. NRA: Funding for research on firearms injuries at issue. *American Medical News,* pp. 3, 52.

Kim, K., & Moody, P. (1992). More resources, better health? A cross-national perspective. *Social Science and Medicine, 34,* 837–842.

Kong, D. (1996, April 3). State official vows fight on downsizing. *The Boston Globe,* p. B28.

Kong, D. (1997, September 25). State loses funds to track gun injuries. *The Boston Globe,* p. B2.

Koop opposes immunity in tobacco deal. (1997, December 23). *The Los Angeles Times,* p. D12.

Kranish, M. (1998, February 27). Senate kills campaign finance bill: A 51-48 bipartisan vote falls short in bid to end a GOP-led filibuster. *The Boston Globe,* pp. A1, A8.

Lawmaker faults Weld proposal to streamline human services. (1996, February 8). *The Boston Globe,* p. B25.

Leavitt, J.W., & Numbers, R.L. (1994). Sickness and health in America: The role of public health in the prevention of disease. In H.D. Schwartz (Ed.), *Dominant issues in medical sociology* (3rd ed., pp. 529–537). New York: McGraw-Hill.

Lee, P.R., & Estes, C.L. (Eds). (1997). *The nation's health* (5th ed.). Sudbury, MA: Jones and Bartlett.

Levin, M. (1996, April 21). Legal weapon: Tobacco companies, facing increasingly strong opposition, have turned to open-records laws to fight back, inundating state offices with requests for documents. *The Los Angeles Times,* pp. D1, D4.

Levine, S., Feldman, J.J., & Elinson, J. (1983). Does medical care do any good? In D. Mechanic (Ed.), *Handbook of health, health care, and the health professions* (pp. 394–404). New York: Free Press.

LoPucki, L.M. (1998, January 20). Some settlement (op-ed column). *The Washington Post,* p. A15.

Magill, T.P. (1955). The immunologist and the evil spirits. *Journal of Immunology, 74,* 1–8.

Mallozzi, J. (1996, December). Consumer advocacy in Medicare HMOs. *States of Health, 6*(8), pp. 1–9.

McCarthy, M.J. (1997, August 18). Inside the beer industry's political machine. *The Wall Street Journal,* pp. B1, B8.

McGinley, L., & Harwood, J. (1997, August 1). Grass-roots activists try to derail tobacco settlement. *The Wall Street Journal,* p. A16.

McGinnis, J.M. (1997). What do we pay for good health? *Journal of Public Health Management and Practice, 3,* viii–ix.

McKeown, T. (1971). A historical appraisal of the medical task. In G. McLachlan & T. McKeown (Eds.), *Medical history and medical care: A symposium of perspectives* (pp. 29–55). New York: Oxford University Press.

McKeown, T. (1976). *The modern rise of population.* New York: Academic Press.

McKeown, T. (1978, April). Determinants of health. *Human Nature,* 60–67.

McKeown, T., Record, R.G., & Turner, R.D. (1975). An interpretation of the decline of mortality in England and Wales during the twentieth century. *Population Studies, 29,* 391–422.

McKinlay, J.B., & McKinlay, S.M. (1977). The questionable contribution of medical measures to the decline of mortality in the United States in the twentieth century. *Milbank Memorial Fund Quarterly/Health and Society, 55,* 405–428.

McKinlay, J.B., & McKinlay, S.M. (1994). Medical measures and the decline of mortality. In P. Conrad & R. Kern (Eds.), *The sociology of health & illness: Critical perspectives* (4th ed., pp. 10–23). New York: St. Martin's Press.

Mechanic, D. (1994). Promoting health. In H.D. Schwartz (Ed.), *Dominant issues in medical sociology* (3rd ed., pp. 569–575). New York: McGraw-Hill.

Milio, N. (1995). Health, health care reform, and the care of health. In M. Blunden & M. Dando (Eds.), *Rethinking public policy-making: Questioning assumptions, challenging beliefs* (pp. 92–107). Thousand Oaks, CA: Sage Publications.

Miller, R.H., & Luft, H.S. (1994). Managed care plan performance since 1980: A literature analysis. *Journal of the American Medical Association, 271,* 1512–1519.

Miller, S.M. (1995). Thinking strategically about society and health. In B.C. Amick, III, S. Levine, A.R. Tarlov, & D.C. Walsh (Eds.), *Society and health* (pp. 342–358). New York: Oxford University Press.

Mintz, J. (1997, April 19). 3-year-old U.S. program cuts smoking, draws fire. *The Washington Post,* p. A1.

Montgomery, L., & Infield, T. (1996, July 12). House votes to cut gun studies. The $2.6 million for the CDC was put to political use, critics said. The vote was "very important," said the NRA. *Philadelphia Inquirer,* p. A1.

Morris, J.N. (1982). Epidemiology and prevention. *Milbank Memorial Fund Quarterly/Health and Society, 60,* 1–16.

Mullan, F. (1997). Federal public health, semi-reinvented. *American Journal of Public health, 87,* 21–24.

National Cancer Institute. (1993, March 11). *Restrictions on lobbying and public policy advocacy by government contractors: The ASSIST contract.* Bethesda, MD: U.S. Department of Health and Human Services, National Institutes of Health, National Cancer Institute.

Omran, A.R. (1971). The epidemiologic transition: A theory of the epidemiology of population change. *Milbank Quarterly, 49,* 509–538.

Police take notice. (1996, September 17). *The Boston Globe,* p. A14.

Powles, J. (1973). On the limitations of modern medicine. *Science, Medicine, and Man, 1,* 1–30.

Public Health Foundation. (1994). *Measuring state expenditures for core public health functions.* Washington, DC: Author.

Public health successes emerging despite budget cuts, other stresses. (1996, September). In *The nation's health* (pp. 1, 32). Washington, DC: American Public Health Association.

Retchin, S.M., & Brown, B. (1991). Elderly patients with congestive heart failure under prepaid care. *American Journal of Medicine, 90,* 236–242.

Retchin, S.M., Brown, R.S., Yeh, S.J., Chu, D., & Moreno, L. (1997). Outcomes of stroke patients in Medicare fee for service and managed care. *Journal of the American Medical Association, 278,* 119–124.

Retchin, S.M., & Preston, J.A. (1991). The effects of cost containment on the care of elderly diabetics. *Archives of Internal Medicine, 151,* 2244–2248.

Rosenbaum, D.E. (1996, December 22). Fixing politics, more or less. *The New York Times,* pp. E1, E4 (section 4).

Satcher, D. (1996). CDC's first 50 years: Lessons learned and relearned. *American Journal of Public Health, 86,* 1705–1708.

Schwartz, J. (1998, January 22). Anti-tobacco activists may heal rift: Koop works to unite public health groups. *The Washington Post,* p. A10.

Shackelford, L. (1997, December 29). AMA leaders have betrayed doctors to protect big tobacco. *The Louisville Courier-Journal,* p. D2.

Shaughnessy, P., Schlenker, R.E., & Hittle, D.F. (1994). Home health care outcomes under capitated and fee-for-service payment. *Health Care Financing Review, 16,* 187–222.

Siegel, M. (1996, December 22). Tobacco: The $10 billion dollar debate. *The Washington Post,* p. C7.

Siegel, M. (1997, May 4). What sort of tobacco settlement? *The Washington Post,* p. C7.

Stevens, R. (1996). Editorial: Public health history and advocacy in the money-driven 1990s. *American Journal of Public Health, 86,* 1522–1523.

Syme, S.L., & Berkman, L.F. (1976). Social class, susceptibility and sickness. *American Journal of Epidemiology, 104,* 1–8.

Tesh, S.N. (1994). Hidden arguments: Political ideology and disease prevention policy. In H.D. Schwartz (Ed.), *Dominant issues in medical sociology* (3rd ed., pp. 519–529). New York: McGraw-Hill.

The Reynolds papers. (1998, January 16). *The Washington Post,* p. A20.

Tobacco talk. (1998, January 30). *The Washington Post,* p. A22.

Torry, S. (1998, February 6). Signals change on tobacco deal: White House bends on industry protection. *The Washington Post*, p. A18.

Turnock, B.J. (1997). *Public health: What it is and how it works*. Gaithersburg, MD: Aspen.

U.S. Department of Health and Human Services. (1993). *Health, United States, 1992, and healthy people 2000 review*. Hyattsville, MD: U.S. Department of Health and Human Services, Public Health Service, Centers for Disease Control and Prevention, National Center for Health Statistics.

U.S. Department of Health and Human Services. (1995). *Healthy people 2000: Midcourse review and 1995 revisions*. Washington, DC: U.S. Department of Health and Human Services, Public Health Service.

U.S. Department of Health and Human Services. (1996, May). *Health, United States, 1995* (DHHS Publication No. PHS 96–1232). Hyattsville, MD: U.S. Department of Health and Human Services, Public Health Service, Centers for Disease Control and Prevention, National Center for Health Statistics.

U.S. Public Health Service. (1995). *For a healthy nation: Returns on investment in public health*. Washington, DC: U.S. Department of Health and Human Services, Public Health Service.

Vaillancourt, M. (1996a, January 31). Eight ideas to reorganize, shrink the bureaucracy. *The Boston Globe*, p. B17.

Vaillancourt, M. (1996b, February 14). State legislators voice doubts about Weld's streamlining plan. *The Boston Globe*, p. B21.

Ware, J.E., Jr., Bayliss, M.S., Rogers, W.H., Kosinski, M., & Tarlov, A.R. (1996). Differences in 4-year health outcomes for elderly and poor, chronically ill patients treated in HMO and fee-for-service systems. Results from the Medical Outcomes Study. *Journal of the American Medical Association, 276*, 1039–1047.

Webster, J.R., & Feinglass, J. (1997). Stroke patients, "managed care," and distributive justice. *Journal of the American Medical Association, 278*, 161–162.

Weinstein, H., & Levin, M. (1997, December 15). Smoking foes split as factions oppose industry immunity. Health: As Congressional battle looms, groups struggle over how to gain passage of proposed $368.5 billion settlement. Fissure may threaten the deal, some say. *The Los Angeles Times*, p. A1.

Weinstein, L. (1974). Infectious disease: Retrospect and reminiscence. *The Journal of Infectious Diseases, 129*, 480–492.

Weisberg, J. (1996). *In defense of government: The fall and rise of public trust*. New York: Scribner.

Wickizer, T.M., Lessler, D., & Travis, D.M. (1996). Controlling inpatient psychiatric utilization through managed care. *American Journal of Psychiatry, 153*, 339–345.

Summary of Lobbying Regulations for Public Health Organizations

Although state laws may add additional restrictions, federal law prohibits for-profit and nonprofit agencies from using federal funds to lobby Congress, lobby state legislators, urge the public to contact state legislators, attempt to influence the outcome of a state or local initiative or referendum, or conduct any lobbying activities related to federal or state legislation (Alliance for Justice, 1995; Colvin & Finley, 1996; Harmon, Ladd, & Evans, 1995; National Cancer Institute [NCI], 1993). These organizations may use federal funds to lobby at the local level, to encourage the public to contact local elected officials about legislation, and to conduct a wide range of public education campaigns, as long as they do not specifically encourage the public to contact federal or state legislators about particular legislation.

Nonprofit organizations incorporated under section 501(c)(3) of the Internal Revenue Code may use non-federal funds to conduct lobbying activities, as long as they adhere to the limits on spending outlined in the Code and do not participate in a political campaign (26 U.S.C.S. 4911; Alliance for Justice, 1995; Colvin & Finley, 1996; Harmon et al., 1995). Thus, these organizations can work on federal, state, and local legislation as well as state and local ballot initiatives (Colvin & Finley, 1996). They simply cannot participate in any political campaign on behalf of or in opposition to any candidate for public office.

Nonprofit organizations incorporated under section 501(c)(4) of the Internal Revenue Code may use non-federal funds in any way they wish. However, if they participate in lobbying at the federal level, they are not eligible for federal funds (Pub. L. No. 104-65: Lobbying Disclosure Act of 1995; Alliance for Justice, 1995).

Public agencies, including state and local health departments, may not use federal funds to lobby Congress, but may lobby at the state and local levels, for example, on state and local initiatives and referenda (NCI, 1993). They may also conduct educational campaigns that address the need for federal legislation, as long as they do not urge the public to contact legislators or to support or oppose specific legislation.

REFERENCES

Alliance for Justice. (1995). *Regulation of advocacy activities of nonprofits that receive federal grants.* Washington, DC: Author.

Colvin, G.L., & Finley, L. (1996). *Seizing the initiative.* Washington, DC: Alliance for Justice.

Harmon, G.M., Ladd, J.A., & Evans, E.A. (1995). *Being a player: A guide to the IRS lobbying regulations for advocacy charities.* Washington, DC: Alliance for Justice.

National Cancer Institute. (1993, December). *5 a day for better health: NCI media campaign strategy.* Bethesda, MD: National Cancer Institute, Office of Cancer Communications.

CHAPTER 5

Marketing Public Health— A Challenge for the Public Health Practitioner

The challenge for the public health practitioner is to market the need for specific public health programs and the need for public health itself in light of the emergence of managed care; diminishing resources; tight budgets; block grants; and a growing antiregulatory, antigovernment sentiment. The demand for population-based, preventive public health programs among the public and policy makers is low because the perceived benefit (reduction in morbidity and mortality) might not be realized for many years. Programs that can demonstrate an immediate and visible impact are more attractive to policy makers and to the public. Also, the most influential political and economic sectors—business, industry, and powerful special-interest groups—are able to convince policy makers of the immediate costs of public health programs. Not only is the demand for public health programs low, but public health practitioners have not traditionally had to compete for public attention and resources. Public health practitioners have not been in the business of self-promotion. Thus, the challenge to public health professionals includes both redefining the product that public health aims to provide and stimulating demand for this product in a somewhat hostile environment. Understanding and applying marketing principles can provide public health professionals with the power and ability to compete successfully for the survival of public health programs and for public health as an institution.

——— ❧ ———

Chapter 4 showed that the practice of public health itself is threatened and that public health practitioners must compete for public attention and resources. This chapter explains the reasons that selling the need for public health institutions and public health programs to policy makers and to the public is such a profound challenge for public health practitioners.

From its inception, public health has had to overcome great obstacles to convince policy makers and the public to invest resources and intervene on behalf of society's interest in preserving health. A brief review of some highlights in public health history reveals the many significant barriers to government adoption of public health programs and institutions.

As early as the eighteenth century, public health reforms faced fierce, organized opposition. For example, despite the availability of a safe and effective vaccine against smallpox, inoculation efforts in Europe were widely criticized as interfering with God's will and spreading the disease among healthy people (McNeill, 1989). In France, the widespread resistance to inoculation did not crumble until 1774, when Louis XV died from smallpox (McNeill, 1989).

For 42 years after Dr. James Lind's 1753 paper demonstrated the effectiveness of oranges and lemons in preventing and curing scurvy, the British naval administration failed to commit the resources necessary to provide this preventive intervention to its sailors (McNeill, 1989). Even when the British Navy decided to purchase supplies of citrus juice for all sailors, it chose West Indian limes, which contained a much lower dose of vitamin C than the more expensive Mediterranean lemons. As a result, outbreaks of scurvy on British vessels occurred as late as 1875, 122 years after Lind's discovery (McNeill, 1989).

Modern public health arose as a social reform of the nineteenth century. Society began to recognize illness not only as a sign of spiritual or moral weakness, but also of poor social and environmental conditions (Amick, Levine, Tarlov, & Walsh, 1995; Institute of Medicine, 1988; McNeill, 1989; Rosen, 1958, 1972; Turnock, 1997; Winslow, 1923). "In the absence of specific etiological concepts, the social and physical conditions which accompanied urbanization were considered equally responsible for the impairment of vital bodily functions and premature death" (Institute of Medicine, 1988, p. 59). Sanitation, and therefore disease control, were then seen as a public responsibility. The control of disease shifted from simply responding to outbreaks of illness to proactively instituting preventive measures. Thus, public health arose out of the establishment of healthy social conditions as a societal goal and the recognition of public institutions as responsible for achieving this social goal (Institute of Medicine, 1988).

In 1842, Edwin Chadwick documented the high prevalence of infectious disease in England and recommended the establishment of national and local boards of health to develop, implement, and maintain a system of sewage and waste disposal (Amick et al., 1995; Chadwick, 1842/1965; Chave, 1984; Turnock, 1997). Chadwick charged the public with creating the infrastructure necessary to control and prevent the spread of infectious diseases; the public role was accepted and institutionalized in the Public Health Act of 1848. Similar reports published around 1850 by Lemuel Shattuck and John Griscom in the United States laid the foundation for the establishment of a government-directed system of public health surveillance and regulation in this country (Amick et al., 1995; Griscom, 1845/ 1970; Institute of Medicine, 1988; Rosenkrantz, 1972; Shattuck, 1850; Winslow, 1923). In 1866, New York became the first large city to establish a permanent Metropolitan Board of Health (Duffy, 1992; Institute of Medicine, 1988; McNeill, 1989; Starr, 1982).

Notably, government action to establish new sanitation systems followed more than a decade of advocacy for such changes by groups of reformers (McNeill, 1989; Turnock, 1997). England's Public Health Act of 1848 was enacted a full 6 years after Chadwick's report. New York City's Metropolitan Board of Health was established 16 years after the Shattuck and Griscom reports.

The initial outbreaks of cholera in the United States in 1832 were met with limited interventions, such as cleaning the streets, caring for the sick, and disposing of the dead (Duffy, 1992). Duffy (1992) noted that "although the cholera epidemic of 1832 shocked the country and literally panicked many citizens, insofar as public health was concerned, its impact was fleeting. . . . Cities and towns, particularly those affected by the outbreak, temporarily remedied the worst sanitary abuses, but within a year or two sanitary conditions were even worse than before. None of the health agencies that came into existence as a result of the epidemic continued to function once the danger was past" (pp. 84, 91).

A reemergence of widespread cholera outbreaks in the United States between 1849 and 1854 led public health advocates to call for sanitary reforms, but their protests were largely ignored. State and local governments did not invest in major changes in societal infrastructure until the mid-1860s, when the nation was threatened by yet another epidemic of cholera. "In almost every American city the cholera outbreaks of the mid-nineteenth century occasioned sanitary surveys and reports. And in almost every case these reports recommended the building of water and sewer systems, the institution of street-cleaning and garbage-collection programs, the creation of strong health departments with extensive authority, and the passage of a whole series of sanitary measures" (Duffy, 1992, p. 100). Nevertheless, "the various sanitary reports in this period were largely ignored" (Duffy, 1992, p. 100).

Ultimately, it took the threat of a reemergence of a cholera epidemic in England to precipitate Parliamentary action in 1848 (McNeill, 1989) and the threat of a third wave of approaching cholera to prompt the establishment of a formal and permanent Metropolitan Board of Health in New York City in 1866 (Duffy, 1992; McNeill, 1989; Rosenberg, 1962; Starr, 1982), almost 25 years after Chadwick's report and 15 years after similar reports by Shattuck and Griscom.

One reason for delayed implementation of sanitary reforms was that the early cholera epidemics largely affected the poor and were perceived as a scourge on their filthy living conditions. As Duffy (1992) pointed out, "in New Orleans, where civic leaders insisted that only strangers and the intemperate poor fell prey to pestilential disorders, the city's experience with cholera merely reinforced their belief" (p. 84). Further, the large capital expenditures required to build water and sewage systems would increase taxes for the wealthy. Duffy explained that "the upper classes in general had no desire to tax themselves for the welfare of the poor" (p. 100).

The necessary reforms were finally adopted only when the impending cholera outbreaks threatened to affect all segments of society. During the urbanization and industrialization of the nineteenth century, infectious diseases began to ravage the entire population, rich and poor alike. In New York City, for example, an 1865 field survey found more than 1,200 cases of smallpox and more than 2,000 cases of typhus in a single tenement district (Institute of Medicine, 1988; Winslow, 1923). Moreover, persons of all social classes were susceptible to these contagious diseases. "Increasingly, it dawned upon the rich that they could not ignore the plight of the poor; the proximity of gold coast and slum was too close" (Institute of Medicine, 1988, p. 59). Whereas disease had previously been viewed as a problem of the underclass, the poor, and the morally flawed, contagion throughout communities of rich and poor alike fostered the view of disease as a societal, not a personal, problem. "Poverty and disease could no longer be treated simply as individual failings" (Institute of Medicine, 1988, p. 59). The implication of this change in the disease paradigm was profound: Disease was a societal problem, thus prevention and control were societal responsibilities. Social reform gave rise to the establishment of public health agencies (Institute of Medicine, 1988). And because unhealthy social and environmental conditions threatened not only the poor but the entire community, public health came to be seen as a public responsibility (McNeill, 1989; Rosenkrantz, 1972).

Other governments were even slower to respond to the need for sanitary reforms. For example, Hamburg, Germany, held back the necessary expenditures to establish a clean water supply until 1892 when a widespread cholera epidemic affected all social classes in the city (McNeill, 1989).

The public in general, and government in particular, were relatively apathetic to the welfare of the poor. Public health advocates countered this sentiment in order to secure funding for many of their programs. "Health and social reformers inveighed against the prevailing social injustices and unsanitary conditions of the times, but the propertied classes had little concern for the welfare of the poor, and without their support little could be done" (Duffy, 1992, p. 118).

The delay in implementing sanitary reforms also was due, in part, to political opposition, especially the firmly held principle of individual freedom and control over one's property (McNeill, 1989). Installation of water and sewer pipes required intrusion onto private property as well as huge capital expenditures. The challenge to public health reformers at the time was not one of finding effective solutions, but of convincing policy makers to adopt these solutions. As McNeill (1989) explained, "the problem as it presented itself to sanitary reformers of the 1830s and 1840s was less one of technique than of organization . . . a libertarian prejudice against regulation, infringing the individual's right to do what he chose with his own property was deeply rooted" (p. 239). Duffy (1992) argued that government did not respond more aggressively to the first wave of cholera because it was hesitant to infringe on "individual liberty and private property rights" (p. 84).

Public health measures were perceived as treading not only on individual rights but also on the rights and opportunities of business owners. The development of water and sewer systems was very costly. Other public health measures, such as quarantines, were perceived as interfering with free enterprise and harmful to business and economic development. For example, in 1866 the city of Memphis rejected its Board of Health's recommendations for preventing a cholera epidemic (Duffy, 1992). "The dominant commercial interests in Memphis reflected the prevailing view in the urban South that the only functions of government were to protect property and preserve the existing social order. That quarantines hindered trade and that sanitary programs cost money only reinforced this assumption" (p. 115).

Paul Starr, in *The Social Transformation of American Medicine*, reinforced Duffy's point:

> The economic boundaries of public health were determined partly by constraints of cost—not simply the direct cost of public health programs to taxpayers, but the indirect cost of such measures to business and to society at large. In the first half of the nineteenth century, some authorities attributed epidemics to contagion and recommended quarantines—an economically damaging measure because of the disruption of commerce. Others ascribed epidemics to miasmas and advised general cleanups of the environment. The environmental approach may have been favored by commercial interest because it was less disruptive than the closing of markets. But wholesale cleanups and quarantines were both costly responses to disease. (Starr, 1982, p. 189)

Public health measures often have been perceived as interfering not with individual or business rights, but with individual behavior. As the Institute of Medicine (1988) explained, "repeatedly, the role of the government in regulating individual behavior has been challenged" (p. 71). Soon after it was formed, Britain's Board of Health was disbanded because Chadwick, its director, "claimed a wide scope for state intervention in an age when laissez-faire was the doctrine of the day" (Chave, 1984, p. 7).

A fourth reason for the delay in implementing sanitary reforms was that the public seemed interested in public health only during an outbreak—there was little interest in instituting preventive measures. For example, Duffy (1992) explained that despite the widespread second wave of cholera in the United States in the mid-nineteenth century, recommendations of public health reformers were ignored because citizens quickly lost interest after the epidemic disappeared: "Carrying out these recommendations would have required relatively huge capital expenditures and large increases in annual government budgets, but once cholera had disappeared, the average citizen had little interest in public health" (p. 100).

The routine nature of endemic infectious diseases also might explain why government officials did not respond with greater urgency (Duffy, 1971; Leavitt, 1982; Rosenberg, 1962). "The endemic disorders responsible for the high morbidity and mortality rates were all too familiar, and without the stimulus provided by a strange and highly fatal pestilence, the average citizen had little interest in—and even less inclination to spend money for—public health" (Duffy, 1992, p. 179). During the late 1800s, tuberculosis, diphtheria, scarlet fever, and typhoid were the chief killers, but newspapers and the public paid little attention (Duffy, 1992). Instead, "the press and the public worried about Asiatic cholera, which was of no consequence after 1873, and smallpox, which was relatively minor compared to the other epidemic disorders" (p. 179). Why the lack of public concern? According to Duffy, all of these endemic disorders "were familiar ones" (p. 179).

Leavitt (1982), discussing the history of Milwaukee's public health system, made a similar point:

> The frightening and dramatic quality of the unexpected provided the first impetus to health reform. . . . When smallpox or cholera threatened Milwaukee, citizens reacted vigorously. Not only were these diseases infrequent visitors, and therefore possibly preventable, they also carried ghastly symptoms and produced perilous outcomes. . . . Because of the fear generated at times of acute distress, epidemics frequently increased the power and authority of the health department. Conversely, chronic diseases, which killed more people than the epidemics, did not easily win the attention of citizen groups or health officials. (pp. 241, 242)

Leavitt (1982) explained: "The Milwaukee experience abounds with other examples that support the contention that unusual and acute disasters encouraged health reforms more than did the typical endemic problems. Tuberculosis, the city's major killer, received almost no attention until the turn of the twentieth century, in part because it was familiar, its symptoms lacked drama, and the disease took many years to kill its victims" (p. 243).

Even during colonial times, disease was viewed as a burden on society only when it represented something that was not well understood, something mysterious, or something unfamiliar—all conditions that evoke societal fear. As Duffy (1992) noted, malaria was by far the greatest threat to health and life in colonial times, but the epidemics that aroused the most attention during this period were smallpox and yellow fever. Although malaria was far more significant in terms of its public health burden on society, smallpox and yellow fever were less predictable, less well understood, more mysterious, and brought about quicker, more visible, and more graphic death:

> They appeared mysteriously, swept through the community with deadly force, struck down old and young alike, and brought a ghastly death to many of their victims. . . . The constant references in colonial letters, diaries, journals, newspapers, and official records to the two great killer diseases, smallpox and yellow fever, speak more for their dramatic nature than for their actual impact upon colonial health. People have always feared strange and unknown dangers far more than familiar ones, and this holds true for diseases. (Duffy, 1992, p. 23)

A final reason for the delay in implementing public health reforms was organized opposition from the medical profession, which historically has viewed many public health programs as intrusions on its autonomy. As Starr (1982) explained, "extending the boundaries of public health to incorporate more of medicine seemed necessary and desirable to some public health officials, but as one might imagine, private practitioners regarded such extensions as a usurpation. Doctors fought against public treatment of the sick, requirements for reporting cases of tuberculosis and venereal disease, and attempts by public health authorities to establish health centers to coordinate preventive and curative medical services" (p. 181).

Perhaps the most striking example of medical opposition to public health measures was the medical profession's opposition to the proposal for a series of rural health centers in New York State in the 1920s. "When the bill came before the state legislature, it had the backing of public health, social welfare, labor, and farming groups, but was opposed by the medical profession. The doctors' opposition, according to C.-E.A. Winslow's account, proved fatal" (Starr, 1982, p. 196).

Starr (1982) summarized public health's perpetual struggle against social forces that oppose government intervention into personal or societal interests: "Much of the history of public health is a record of struggles over the limits of its mandate. On one frontier, public health authorities have met opposition from religious groups and others with moral objections to state intervention on behalf of the officially sponsored conceptions of health and hygiene. On another frontier, public health has met opposition from business and commerce, anxious to protect their economic interests" (pp. 180–181).

The lessons of public health history have three important implications in terms of the marketing environment that public health practitioners face. First, the nature of the public health product puts it in an unfavorable state of demand by the public and by policy makers. Second, the environment in which public health must be marketed is hostile. Third, the type of effort required to market public health involves skills that many public health practitioners have not developed and that are rarely taught to public health students. The reasons that marketing public health is a formidable challenge for the public health practitioner are explored in the following sections.

AN UNFAVORABLE STATE OF DEMAND FOR PUBLIC HEALTH PROGRAMS

As was just described, the public and policy makers have not demanded public health programs and policies and public health as an institution. The great public health reforms of the nineteenth century, for example, took many years of persistent advocacy by public health practitioners before they were adopted. From the foregoing discussion, several major reasons for the low level of public and political demand for public health interventions can be identified. The common denominator is that the benefits of public health programs are remote in time and remote in the mind of the consumer. In contrast, the benefits of medical interventions are usually immediate, both in time and in the mind of the patient. This point is illustrated by comparing characteristics of the benefits of medical interventions and public health programs.

The benefits of medical treatment are usually immediate. A patient with appendicitis, for example, entered the hospital in severe pain and with her life in jeopardy. Within hours of surgery, the patient's condition was stabilized and her pain was relieved. On the other hand, the very nature of prevention implies that benefits will not be seen for a long time after intervention, sometimes for many years. For example, cities that invested in new water and sewer systems did not benefit for many years. Although improved sanitation might prevent an epidemic from occurring in the future, it cannot alleviate the epidemic conditions that already exist. Similarly, the benefits of programs that prevent smoking among adolescents, decrease fat intake, or increase physical activity might not be seen until many years later.

Because of the immediate benefits of medical treatment and interventions to control communicable diseases, it is easy to convince policy makers of the need for medical treatment and for infectious disease control programs. When Ebola virus attacks, people die within days and the immediate survival of a community is imminently threatened. It is easy to see the benefit of intervening to treat victims of Ebola infection. When an epidemic of smoking affects youth in a community, there is no immediate threat to survival or even to health. The benefits of intervention are not as readily apparent, not as immediate, and not nearly as compelling.

The benefits of public health interventions are remote in time as well as in the mind of the consumer, while the connection between a medical intervention and its benefits is much more apparent to the observer. For example, the benefits of instituting sanitary reforms were not visible when New York City's Metropolitan

Board of Health was established in 1866 although it resulted in far better control of the subsequent cholera outbreak. In the public's perception, there simply were fewer victims after the implementation of the reforms.

The remote connection between public health programs and their benefits makes it more difficult to market public health programs to policy makers. Few, if any, policy makers question whether treatment of heart attack victims has a positive impact on their health and survival or whether treatment of victims of infectious diseases is beneficial. Even without scientific demonstration of a positive impact of treatment, a strong and unquestioned link between treatment and outcome is present, leading, for example, to the expenditure of billions of health care dollars on increasing the quantity, but not the quality, of the last years of life. In contrast, the relation between public health interventions and effects is often questioned seriously, even when scientific evidence clearly demonstrates a significant effect of the public health program on both longevity and quality of life. Despite a wealth of evidence that public assistance helps alleviate poverty and make life more tolerable for the impoverished, policy makers continue to question this link, even suggesting that public assistance causes the poverty. Mikhail, Swint, Casperson, and Spitz (1997) noted that "curative services often have been judged by their perceived value, while preventive services have been held to a more rigorous standard of documentation" (p. 37).

Because the results of public health programs often are invisible, it is much more difficult to develop vocal constituencies around public health issues than around medical treatment issues. As Turnock (1997) explained "prevention efforts often lack a clear constituency because success results in unseen consequences. Because these consequences are unseen, people are less likely to develop an attachment for or to support the efforts preventing them. Advocates for mental health services, care for individuals with developmental disabilities, organ transplants, and end-stage renal disease often make their presence felt. But few state capitols have seen candlelight demonstrations by thousands of people who did not get diphtheria" (p. 20).

A major reason for the obscurity of the impact of public health programs, especially those that address chronic disease, is that the outcomes are neither visible nor graphic. The effect of medical treatment (or its absence), however, is highly visible and pervasive in our culture, especially through the media. Movies such as *Outbreak* and *Twelve Monkeys* show the immediate and vividly disturbing consequences of infection with "killer" viruses. Television portrays the immediate impact of treatment in medical emergencies weekly on *ER* and *Chicago Hope*. Television news stories show vivid images of malnourished children in Africa, prompting an outpouring of concern and money for medical aid. No equally compelling images exist for most public health problems and interventions.

Harvard University researcher Graham Colditz explained: "One of the things we can't get away from is that if you're in a clinic treating patients with cancer, you can count the number treated and the successes. But if you have 10,000 people who increase their physical activity and 10 fewer of them get colon cancer in 10 years, well, those people are not identifiable. That's particularly frustrating when you're trying to lobby for dollars for prevention" (as cited in Lauerman, 1997, p. 14).

Mikhail and colleagues (1997) made the distinction between "identified" lives and "statistical" lives and argued that society favors treatment programs over prevention programs because they address the needs of identifiable individuals. "The clear social preference is to provide health care resources to respond to specific and immediate needs of identified individuals. By its very nature, prevention generally deals with amorphous populations; curative care deals with identified personalized lives and thus seems to carry a greater societal ethical imperative for committing resources in response to specific health care needs" (p. 38).

The nature of the demand for public health compared with medical intervention also is different in terms of its urgency. Physicians do not typically go out into the community trying to stimulate demand for medical treatment: When people become sick, they demand medical treatment. This is not the case with public health. The presence of public health problems does not itself imply an immediate demand for intervention. Usually, the demand for public health attention is dormant until a crisis arises. The nature of demand for public health interventions during the nineteenth century largely followed such a pattern. While temporary public health programs were established with each of the three waves of the cholera epidemic, demand dissipated when the outbreaks subsided.

Medical interventions often involve technological problems and solutions, while public health problems usually require social, economic, and political solutions. Americans tend to view technological challenges as a true test of the nation's strength. Atwood, Colditz, and Kawachi (1997) compared U.S. investment in sequencing the human genome with the limited effort in controlling tobacco use: "Tobacco is responsible for 30% of all cancer deaths, while 5% to 10% can be linked to inherited genetic causes. Yet the tobacco control budget of the National Cancer Institute (NCI) amounted to $60 million in 1996, as compared with the multibillion-dollar research project under way to sequence the human genome" (Atwood et al., 1997, p. 1604).

A HOSTILE ENVIRONMENT FOR MARKETING PUBLIC HEALTH PROGRAMS

Because public health interventions often interfere with individual rights or behavior, or the conduct and livelihood of business, marketing public health programs often is done in a hostile environment. By their very nature, public health programs tend to interfere with personal behaviors and might well be interpreted as interfering with individual rights. As John Duffy (1992) noted in *The Sanitarians: A History of American Public Health,* "unfortunately, sanitary and health regulations inevitably infringe on individual rights, a situation compounded by the general American distrust of all laws and regulations. . . . The zealous guarding of individual rights creates major problems for health officials in a democracy" (p. 3).

For this reason, public health measures often run up against fierce opposition by many stakeholders, including the public. Regulations against public smoking are criticized on the grounds that individuals have the right to decide when and where to smoke and that infringing on this freedom will lead to regulating other aspects of personal behavior, including eating, drinking, and exercising. In such an environment, public health advocates aiming to reduce tobacco-related mortality are considered zealots seeking prohibition.

Not only do population-based, preventive, public health programs tend to intrude into the lives of individuals, they also often interfere with the autonomy of business and the perceived integrity of the free enterprise system. Public health programs often are seen as intruding into the free market system and placing undue economic burdens on business owners. The debate over public health regulations often is framed in terms of health versus wealth, implying that public health programs are, by definition, economically harmful.

In contrast, medical treatment programs are viewed as providing the individual with personal freedoms and individual rights. Efforts to limit the provision of medical care are attacked as being unfair encroachments on the health care system. Even when medical treatment does affect personal freedom, society often sanctions the treatment on the grounds that it safeguards the right of other individuals. For example, several states have enacted laws that require pregnant women who are infected with the human immunodeficiency virus (HIV) to be treated with AZT. Although this interferes far more with individual freedom than do most public health programs, society still views forced treatment as a mechanism to ensure the rights of others—in this case, the unborn child.

The appropriateness of medical treatment interventions also tends to be unquestioned from an economic perspective. Even when their potential cost-effectiveness is not clear, treatment interventions generally are acceptable (Mikhail et al., 1997). Treatment programs are rarely challenged on the grounds that they will adversely affect the nation's economy in spite of the tremendous burden placed on the national economy by the increasing costs of medical treatment.

In addition to interfering with individual rights and business autonomy, public health programs often run up against firmly held social and economic norms. Because the central goal of effective public health interventions is to change social and economic conditions or policies, these interventions must in some way challenge existing norms. In contrast, medical treatment programs tend to support the established economic norms of the health care system. The more specialists, specialized equipment, and specialized procedures there are, the more deeply entrenched the health care industry becomes as an economic force in society. On the other hand, poorly funded public health agencies have been accused of promoting programs simply to ensure their continued personal livelihood. "Implications for life-style and resource allocation inherent in the modern definition of public health are often in conflict with prevailing social policy or perceived feasibility in an age of growing awareness of scarcity and debate regarding the limits of government" (Ellencweig & Yoshpe, 1984, p. 75).

The presence of opposition groups that fight public health measures that they perceive will harm their economic livelihood make for a hostile environment for marketing public health. In contrast, no established industry opposes medical treatment programs because they perceive them as threats to economic viability. For example, there is no anti–liver transplant industry opposing the extreme medical interventions required to treat liver disease. However, as soon as one proposes regulations on the advertising or sale of alcohol to prevent the need for some liver transplants, one runs into well-funded and well-organized opposition from the alcoholic beverage industry.

Often, public health programs run up against industries whose financial interests would be directly affected by the implementation of the program. Public health interventions to reduce alcohol and tobacco use, for example, can be successful only if they reduce alcohol and tobacco sales and therefore the profits of these industries. In contrast, there are no major special-interest groups whose primary purpose is to oppose medical treatment programs. There is no pro-hypertension industry, for example, that opposes treatment of hypertension. However, if public health officials were to propose a federal program to prevent hypertension in the population by regulating the sodium content of foods, a large and powerful food industry would be waiting for them at the Capitol steps. As Ellencweig and Yoshpe (1984) explained, "emphasis upon preventive medicine and environment threatens most prevailing systems of medical care organization and entrenched industrial and professional lobbies" (p. 75).

LIMITED CAPACITY OF PUBLIC HEALTH PRACTITIONERS TO COMPETE FOR PUBLIC ATTENTION AND RESOURCES

Because public health practitioners generally are not trained in marketing, communications, political science, and public relations, it might be difficult for them to compete in the battle to secure scarce resources to fund their programs. To gain attention and resources, public health practitioners must be able to work with lawmakers in the legislative process, build constituencies and coalitions, and form collaborative relations with other organizations. And to generate public understanding, appreciation, and support, they must employ public relations techniques and marketing and communications principles. The lack of training of public health practitioners in these areas makes the marketing challenge particularly difficult.

Fred Kroger, director of the Centers for Disease Control and Prevention's Office of Health Communications, summarized:

> When colleagues at the state and local levels try to sell city councils, their boards of supervisors, or their state legislators on the merits of public health, folks are not buying. Some in public health have even admitted publicly that public health has done a singularly poor job of marketing. This failure to effectively market public health became more painfully evident when the Clinton administration's initial proposals on health care reform surfaced. Public health found itself all but absent from the planning process, and consequently from the plans themselves. (Kroger, McKenna, Shepherd, Howze, & Knight, 1997, p. 273)

In addition, public health practitioners generally have not played the same kind of prominent leadership and advocacy roles for themselves, their programs, and their institutions that they have played for the health of their constituents. At the 1996 annual meeting of the American Public Health Association, public health leaders emphasized that "in a time when public health faces some of its greatest challenges, leadership and advocacy will be the most important tools for safeguarding the nation's health" ("Record Attendance Marks 124th Annual Meeting," 1996, p. 1). Outgoing president, Dr. Richard E. Brown, stated that "as managed care continues to grow, we must have strong advocacy skills to keep public health providers in networks and provide for preventive services. We have a responsibility to be public health leaders. . . . Critical resources for public health can be assured only if our agencies and associations strengthen their political advocacy. Public health leadership is our most powerful instrument to create a healthier society" ("Record Attendance," 1996, pp. 1, 3). Executive director Katherine McCarter told the delegates: "We are meeting here today during a time of great change, a time of challenges and a time of opportunities. Our challenge as public health officials is to educate and inform our elected officials. Our challenge and our opportunity is to define and redefine our role as public health professionals" ("Record Attendance," 1996, p. 1).

To promote the continued survival and growth of public health as an institution, public health practitioners must take more prominent leadership and advocacy roles, guided by improved knowledge of and competence in political advocacy.

CONCLUSION

Stimulating demand for public health programs is a formidable challenge for the public health practitioner because public health programs (1) tend to have delayed benefits that are not easily recognized and are not visible, (2) are perceived as intruding into individual autonomy and the free enterprise system or as conflicting with established social and economic norms, and (3) face heavy opposition by powerful special-interest groups.

Fortunately, the strategic application of marketing principles can be a powerful tool in redefining and repositioning public health as a product that is in demand by the public and by policy makers. Chapter 6 demonstrates that marketing public health is both a challenge and an opportunity for the public health practitioner.

REFERENCES

Amick, B.C., III, Levine, S., Tarlov, A.R., & Walsh, D.C. (1995). Introduction. In B.C. Amick, III, S. Levine, A.R. Tarlov, & D.C. Walsh (Eds.), *Society and health* (pp. 3–17). New York: Oxford University Press.

Atwood, K., Colditz, G.A., & Kawachi, I. (1997). From public health science to prevention policy: Placing science in its social and political contexts. *American Journal of Public Health, 87,* 1603–1606.

Chadwick, E. (1842/1965). *Report on the sanitary condition of the labouring population of Great Britain.* Edinburgh, Scotland: Edinburgh University Press.

Chave, S.P.W. (1984). The origins and development of public health. In W.W. Holland, R. Detels, & G. Knox (Eds.), *Oxford textbook of public health: Vol. 1. History, determinants, scope, and strategies.* New York: Oxford University Press.

Duffy, J. (1971). Social impact of disease in the late 19th century. *Bulletin of the New York Academy of Medicine, 47,* 797–811.

Duffy, J. (1992). *The sanitarians: A history of American public health.* Urbana, IL: University of Illinois Press.

Ellencweig, A., & Yoshpe, R. (1984). Definition of public health. *Public Health Review, 12,* 65–78.

Griscom, J.H. (1845/1970). *The sanitary condition of the laboring population of New York.* New York: Arno.

Institute of Medicine, Committee for the Study of the Future of Public Health. (1988). *The future of public health.* Washington, DC: National Academy Press.

Kroger, F., McKenna, J.W., Shepherd, M., Howze, E.H., & Knight, D.S. (1997). Marketing public health: The CDC experience. In M.E. Goldberg, M. Fishbein, & S.E. Middlestadt (Eds.), *Social marketing: Theoretical and practical perspectives* (pp. 267–290). Mahwah, NJ: Lawrence Erlbaum Associates.

Lauerman, J.F. (1997). Combating cancer: The power of prevention has scarcely been tapped. *Harvard Magazine, 99,* 11–14.

Leavitt, J.W. (1982). *The healthiest city. Milwaukee and the politics of health reform.* Princeton, NJ: Princeton University Press.

McNeill, W.H. (1989). *Plagues and peoples.* New York: Anchor Books.

Mikhail, O.I., Swint, J.M., Casperson, P.R., & Spitz, M.R. (1997). Health care's double standard: The prevention dilemma. *Journal of Public Health Management and Practice, 3,* 37–42.

Record attendance marks 124th annual meeting: Leadership, advocacy will be most important tools in meeting coming challenges, speakers say. (1996, December). In *The nation's health* (pp. 1, 3). Washington, DC: American Public Health Association.

Rosen, G. (1958). *A history of public health*. New York: MD Publications.

Rosen, G. (1972). The evolution of social medicine. In H.E. Freeman, S. Levine, & L.G. Reeder (Eds.), *Handbook of medical sociology* (2nd ed., pp. 30–60). Englewood Cliffs, NJ: Prentice-Hall.

Rosenberg, C.E. (1962). *The cholera years: The United States in 1832, 1849, and 1866*. Chicago: University of Chicago Press.

Rosenkrantz, B.G. (1972). *Public health and the state*. Cambridge, MA: Harvard University Press.

Shattuck, L. (1850). *Report of the Sanitary Commission of Massachusetts, 1850*. Boston: Dutton & Wentworth: State Printers.

Starr, P. (1982). *The social transformation of American medicine*. New York: Basic Books.

Turnock, B.J. (1997). *Public health: What it is and how it works*. Gaithersburg, MD: Aspen.

Winslow, C-E.A. (1923). *The evolution and significance of the modern public health campaign*. New Haven, CT: Yale University Press.

CHAPTER 6

Marketing Public Health— An Opportunity for the Public Health Practitioner

Public health practitioners must market population-based, preventive public health programs in the absence of significant demand among the public and policy makers for these programs. They must also market the need for public health itself in hostile and competitive political and social environments. The strategic use of marketing principles can help public health practitioners effectively confront these challenges. The key is to abandon the traditional approach of deciding what they want the public and policy makers to buy and then attempting to sell this product to an audience that has little demand for it. Instead, public health practitioners must first identify the needs and desires of the audience and then redefine, package, position, and frame the product in such a way that it satisfies an existing demand among the target audience. The public health practitioner must be able to offer programs with a benefit that the audience appreciates and demands, to back up this offer, and to communicate an image of public health programs or the public health institution that reinforces core values of the target audience.

—————— ❧ ——————

Chapter 5 demonstrated that public health practitioners must sell the need for specific public health programs and for public health itself to a public and to policy makers for whom the demand is low. Fortunately, the strategic application of basic marketing principles can provide the public health practitioner with a powerful tool to promote public health programs and policies and to establish public health as a highly regarded societal institution.

This chapter discusses the two major steps in marketing a public health program or policy: (1) identifying the needs, wants, and core values of the target audience to define the product as beneficial to that audience; and (2) packaging and positioning the program or policy so that it reinforces the core values of the target audience.

DEFINING THE PRODUCT: THE IMPORTANCE OF FORMATIVE RESEARCH IN MARKETING PUBLIC HEALTH POLICIES AND PROGRAMS

The first marketing principle that the public health practitioner must apply is the importance of identifying and understanding the needs and wants of the target audience and defining the product so that it offers a benefit that is desired by the target audience. Two major audiences for promoting a public health program or policy are policy makers and the public. Too often, public health practitioners determine the benefits that policy makers and the public ought to want and then attempt to sell these benefits even when there is low, or no, demand. Often, for example, practitioners try to sell a program or a policy based solely on the benefit of improving the health of individual members of society.

However, as described in Chapter 5, the intrinsic presence of disease among the population was not the policy makers' motivation for adopting major public health programs, policies, and reforms over the past two centuries. It was fear of the political and economic consequences of losing control over the spread of disease. The prospect of disease is dreaded not because it signifies that individuals are sick or suffering, but because it represents a threat to a society's freedom, independence, autonomy, and control. Just as freedom, independence, autonomy, and control form the individual's core values and underscore the value he or she places on health, the policy maker holds these same values, which explains his or her desire to exert some control over the spread of disease in society (see Appendix 6–A).

Therefore, in defining the public health product in a campaign to promote a public health program or policy, the practitioner may need to go beyond simply offering health as the benefit to society. The public health practitioner must redefine the product and its benefits. The product is not health for society's members, but something more basic, more compelling, and more at the core of the American policy makers' values system. The product is the preservation of freedom, independence, autonomy, and control for society.

While public health practitioners traditionally have based their public health campaigns solely on what they think should be important—health—their opponents have used marketing principles to define their campaign themes. They determine what the consumer (the public or policy makers) wants and then design, package, and position the product so that it satisfies the need. Often, this leads to campaigns based on themes that have little to do with health. The marketing research process is used not only in consumer product campaigns to influence individual behavior, but it also is used in political campaigns to promote or oppose a specific legislative policy or program.

An example of the use of marketing research to defeat a public health campaign was the insurance industry's effort to defeat President Clinton's proposed health care reform initiative in 1994. The Coalition for Health Insurance Choices, an insurance industry front, conducted a carefully crafted media and grassroots lobbying campaign based on extensive research (Stauber & Rampton, 1995). Stauber and Rampton (1995) described how the coalition used formative research to identify campaign themes that would resonate with voters: "Instead of forming a single coalition, health reform opponents used opinion polling to develop a point-by-point list of vulnerabilities in the Clinton administration proposal and organized over 20 separate coalitions to hammer away at each point" (p. 96). Campaign organizer Blair Childs emphasized the importance of formative research: "In naming your coalition . . . use words that you've identified in your research. There are certain words that . . . have a general positive reaction. That's where focus group and survey work can be very beneficial. 'Fairness,' 'balance,' 'choice,' 'coalition,' and 'alliance' are all words that resonate very positively" (Stauber & Rampton, 1995, pp. 96, 97).

Using careful, formative research, the coalition framed Clinton's health reform proposal in a way that conflicted with the core values of American voters, generating subsequent opposition to the proposal. The coalition identified a fear among Americans that government-sponsored health care would "bankrupt the country, reduce the quality of care, and lead to jail terms for people who wanted to stick with their family doctor" (Stauber & Rampton, 1995, p. 97). Clinton's proposal was framed as the archetypal example of government-sponsored health care, which would take away all individual choice, put health care into a helpless bureaucracy, hurt small businesses, and eliminate America's position as the international leader in quality of medical care. These messages appealed to the American core values of independence, autonomy, self-determination, free choice, free enterprise, capitalism, economic stability, and the democratic principle. With these core values at the heart of its arguments, it is no surprise that the insurance coalition's campaign was so effective.

A now-legendary television spot vividly illustrated to the public how the Clinton plan would affect them personally. In it, a middle-class couple named Harry and Louise lamented "the complexity of Clinton's plan and the menace of a new 'billion-dollar bureaucracy.' . . . 'Harry and Louise' symbolized everything that went wrong with the great health care struggle of 1994" (Stauber & Rampton, 1995, p. 97). Harry and Louise became a symbol for the entire campaign and effectively suggested that the Clinton plan represented the opposite of everything for which America is supposed to stand. A pro-health-care reform campaign that relied primarily on the arguments that millions of Americans lacked health insurance, that the costs of health care were increasing, and that the insurance and pharmaceutical industries were acting irresponsibly (White House Domestic Policy Council, 1993) simply could not stand up against a campaign for the hearts and minds of the American people.

Another excellent example of the use of marketing research to defeat a public health campaign is the tobacco industry's successful effort to defeat a proposed Montana ballot initiative to raise the state cigarette excise tax in 1990. The tobacco industry did not restrict itself to the health-oriented aspects of the proposed cigarette tax in fighting this initiative. Nor did it design its campaign based on the public health community's definition and packaging of the product (Moon, Males, & Nelson, 1993). Instead, the tobacco industry conducted marketing research to identify the basic needs and desires of the Montana voters, messages that would and would not appeal to the voters, and the core values influencing their voting intentions. The industry then redefined the product and reframed the discussion over the product's benefits and costs such that voting against the initiative would be perceived as fulfilling the identified needs and desires and as reinforcing the most influential core values of Montana voters. Specifically, freedom, security, and fairness were targeted by tobacco interests as campaign messages to sway voters from supporting the tax increase.

First, the tobacco industry argued that the ballot initiative would interfere with the core value of security by causing cigarette smuggling problems: Gang members would bootleg cigarettes from nearby states with lower taxes. Second, the industry showed how the proposal conflicted with the core values of fairness and equality: Poor families would be harder hit by the cigarette tax than wealthier families. Third, the industry explained that the initiative would take control away from the voters: Bureaucrats would take the taxpayers' money and use it however they saw fit. Fourth, the proposed cigarette tax interfered with the core values of freedom and autonomy: The proposal represented an effort on the part of special-interest groups to override the concerns of the people of Montana and to manipulate voters into establishing programs favored by these special-interest groups. At the most basic level, the tobacco industry was not selling opposition to the initiative; it was selling freedom and independence, fairness, security, control over one's life, individual rights, and the democratic ideal.

In contrast, the public health coalition in Montana did not conduct extensive marketing research studies. Because of the lack of adequate resources, only one poll was conducted during the campaign. The coalition defined and positioned the initiative based on its health content alone and on speculation about the health benefits that would be most important to the voters: reducing the number of smokers, preventing children from starting to smoke, reducing exposure to secondhand smoke, and establishing better prenatal care programs for poor families.

A third example of how opponents of public health policies use marketing principles to fight reform comes from the environmental health movement. Stauber and Rampton (1995) explained how corporations that pollute the environment also use marketing principles to prevent significant policy reforms that could hurt their profits. Many corporations hire sophisticated public relations, marketing, and advertising firms to determine what the public thinks about them and about environmental policy issues. In this way, they learn how to frame environmental policy issues so that citizens perceive increased environmental regulation as conflicting with their core values. Joanna Underwood, president of one environmental research firm, explained the importance of talking to people to find out how they think: "Companies must have some vehicle for knowing what the intelligent public thinks about their products and processes. If they want to understand sophisticated outside views of environmental issues affecting their companies, they would do well to have someone in the room" (Stauber & Rampton, 1995, pp. 127, 128). Too often, public health practitioners attempt to design policy campaigns without having anyone else "in the room."

The key strategy of corporate polluters, according to Stauber and Rampton (1995), is to frame environmental issues so that the blame is shifted from corporations to the individual. In other words, these corporations rely on the core American value of rugged individualism, convincing people that individual actions are at the root of environmental problems. "In place of systemic analysis and systemic solutions to social problems, they offer an individualistic and deeply hypocritical analysis in which 'all of us' are to blame for our collective 'irresponsibility.' If we would all just pick up after ourselves . . . the problems would go away" (Stauber & Rampton, 1995, p. 132).

About 200 companies fund an organization called Keep America Beautiful, the "industry's most organized proponent of the belief that individual irresponsibility is at the root of the pollution" (Stauber & Rampton, 1995, p. 133). Although these companies produce products that are estimated to account for about a third of the material in U.S. landfills, Keep America Beautiful's message to consumers is that they are responsible for the trash problem in this country. Although Keep America Beautiful has used more than half a billion dollars of donated advertising time and space to encourage guilty consumers to "put litter in its place," the organization's leadership "opposes a national bottle bill that would place a deposit on glass and metal drink containers" (Stauber & Rampton, 1995, p. 133). These companies are strategically applying basic marketing principles to reframe the issue of environmental pollution so that responsibility for the problem shifts from the corporation to the individual.

Just as the industries that oppose public health programs and policies use marketing principles to convince the public that these policies are detrimental, public health practitioners must begin to use marketing principles to *promote* them. The key is to redefine the public health product and its benefits in a way that appeals to the most compelling core values of the target audience. To do this, the public health practitioner must first abandon the traditional approach of deciding for himself or herself what product he or she wants the target audience to buy and then attempting to sell this product to an audience that has little demand for it. Instead, the public health practitioner must begin to use formative research to determine what the public wants and to identify the arguments, messages, themes, and values that are highly salient and influential among these target groups. Case studies that demonstrate how practitioners can accomplish this are reviewed in Chapters 7 and 8, and the process is detailed in Chapters 11 and 12.

PACKAGING AND POSITIONING THE PRODUCT: FRAMING PUBLIC HEALTH PROGRAMS AND POLICIES

We have just explained that the first step in marketing a public health program or policy is to define the product such that it offers benefits that will satisfy the needs and desires of the public, and that formative research is an essential tool to identify these basic needs and desires. The second step is to package and position the program or policy so that it communicates these benefits in a way that reinforces the core values of the public—both general citizens and policy makers. The public health practitioner must provide support for the promised benefits and must communicate a compelling image for the product. The process of packaging and positioning a public health program or policy so that it reinforces the public's core values is called framing.

In the remainder of this chapter, we explain the process of framing public health programs and policies in order to tap into core values of policy makers and the public. We illustrate how opposition marketers (e.g., the tobacco industry) frame public health programs in a way that leads the public to perceive the program as conflicting with basic core values. We then demonstrate how issues can be reframed in such a way that the desired public health policy or program is actually perceived as reinforcing these same core values.

Framing—Definition and Examples

A *frame* is a way of packaging and positioning an issue to convey a certain meaning (Chapman & Lupton, 1994; Entman, 1993; Iyengar, 1991; Kaniss, 1991; Ryan, 1991; Schon & Rein, 1994; Wallack & Dorfman, 1996; Wallack, Dorfman, Jernigan, & Themba, 1993). Framing has been described as the emphasis placed around particular issues "that seeks to define 'what this issue is really about'" (Chapman & Lupton, 1994, p. 12) and as "the process by which someone packages a group of facts to create a story" (Wallack et al., 1993, p. 68). Schon and Rein (1994) defined frames as "the broadly shared beliefs, values, and perspectives familiar to the members of a societal culture and likely to endure in that culture over long periods of time, on which individuals and institutions draw in order to give meaning, sense, and normative direction to their thinking and action in policy matters" (p. xiii).

In 1922, political pundit and author Walter Lippmann wrote that people see the world through certain frameworks and that these frameworks affect what a person sees. Lippmann wrote, "We do not first see, and then define, we define first and then see" (Steel, 1981, p. 181). Steel (1981) expanded on the point: "We define, not at random, but according to 'stereotypes' demanded by our culture. The stereotypes, while limiting, are essential. . . . But if stereotypes determine not only how we see but what we see, clearly our opinions are only partial truths. What we assume to be 'facts' are often really judgments" (p. 181).

The concept of framing was formally introduced as early as 1954 (Tannen, 1993). Gregory Bateson theorized that "no communicative move, verbal or nonverbal, could be understood without reference to a metacommunicative message, or metamessage, about what is going on—that is, what frame of interpretation applies to the move" (Tannen, 1993, p. 3). Tversky and Kahneman (1982) showed that minor changes in the way decision problems are framed may influence people's decisions: "Systematic reversals of preference are observed when a decision problem is framed in different ways" (p. 3). The concept of framing has important implications for individuals' opinions and attitudes. On the most basic level, the framing of questions influences responses to attitude surveys and public opinion polls (Krosnick & Alwin, 1988).

On a broader level, the framing of an issue forms "the basis by which public policy decisions are made" (Wallack et al., 1993, p. 68; see also Nelkin, 1987). Framing not only defines the issue, it also suggests the solution: "If we alter the definition of problems, then the response also changes" (Wallack et al., 1993, p. 82; see also Ryan, 1991; Watzlawick, Weakland, & Fisch, 1974). As Wagenaar and Streff pointed out, "how questions are worded is related to how policy advocates and opponents shape and present policy options to legislators and other opinion leaders, as well as to the general public" (Wagenaar & Streff, 1990, p. 203).

The effect of framing has been demonstrated in studies of public opinion on alcohol policies (Wagenaar & Streff, 1990), mandatory seat belt laws (Slovic, Fischhoff, & Lichtenstein, 1982), affirmative action (Fine, 1992), environmental policy (Vaughan & Seifert, 1992), and welfare policy (Smith, 1987). Message framing has been shown to influence not only public opinion, but individual behavior as well (Meyerowitz & Chaiken, 1987; Rothman, Salovey, Antone, Keough, & Martin, 1993; Vookles & Carr, 1993; Wilson, Purdon, & Wallston, 1988; Wilson, Wallston, & King, 1990).

Ryan (1991), one of the developers of framing theory and its applications in public policy advocacy, argued that a frame is defined by a core value or principle that underlies it. Ryan further characterized frames by their core positions, meta-phors, images, catch phrases, attribution of responsibility for the problem, and the solution implied by the frame.

For example, one frame used by the tobacco industry in debates over citywide smoking restrictions in restaurants is the "level playing field" frame (Table 6–1). The core position of this frame is that restricting smoking in restaurants in one city creates an unlevel playing field—customers will shift their business to restaurants in nearby cities that allow smoking, resulting in a loss of business for restaurants in the affected city. The metaphor suggested by this frame is that of an unlevel playing field that favors one team over another. The core values or principles to which this frame appeals are fairness, equality, justice, and economic opportunity. It is simply unfair for the government to create an advantage for restaurants in one city over those in another city.

The Importance of Framing in Public Policy Debates

In their case studies of antismoking legislation in six states, Jacobson, Wasserman, and Raube (1993) found that the tobacco industry "attempted to shift the nature of the debate from the credibility of the scientific evidence to personal freedoms" (p. 800). Moreover, they observed that "antismoking forces fare better

---

Table 6–1 The Level Playing Field Frame Used by the Tobacco Industry in Fighting Local Smoke-free Restaurant Ordinances

Frame	Level Playing Field
Core position	Restricting smoking in restaurants in one city creates a selective advantage for restaurants in nearby cities.
Metaphor	An unlevel playing field in a sports event, favoring one team over another
Images	An unlevel playing field in a sports event
Catch phrases	"Level playing field"; "unfair advantage"; "discrimination"
Attribution of responsibility for problem	The government, which is creating a selective advantage for some businesses
Implied solution	Maintain a level playing field by banning smoking in all restaurants nationwide, or do nothing
Core values	Fairness Equality Justice Economic opportunity

when public health issues dominate and that the tobacco industry benefits when personal freedoms arguments are predominant. . . . [L]egislative outcomes favored antismoking advocates during the time that public health dominated the debate. Once the debate shifted to personal freedoms, statewide antismoking legislation stalled" (p. 801).

As Jacobson and colleagues (1993) described it, the tobacco industry

> shifted its opposition to smoking restrictions to a broadly conceived argument equating smoking behavior with other personal liberties, such as freedom of speech and protection against racial discrimination. This argument involves three interconnected concepts: first, governmental interference—that smoking restrictions should be determined by private economic arrangements, not by governmental fiat; second, smokers' rights—that smokers have certain rights and autonomy in pursuing personal social behavior; and third—nondiscrimination—that smokers cannot be discriminated against for their smoking behavior, particularly in employment, for smoking during nonworking hours. (p. 802)

In the late 1980s the tobacco industry shifted its strategy from a focus on challenging the scientific evidence about the health effects of tobacco to a focus on discussing non–health-related frames: civil liberties, government interference, individual rights, and discrimination. This was not a lucky guess but the result of public opinion research showing that these frames resonated well with American voters. For example, in 1988 a Tobacco Institute poll appraised the strength of various core values as well as alternative campaign messages and arguments. This poll assessed the extent of antiregulatory sentiment among American voters to determine whether an antigovernment interference theme might be effective in generating opposition to tobacco policy proposals (Roper Center at University of Connecticut, 1989). In addition to assessing voter attitudes concerning specific tobacco policies, the poll also asked questions about government regulation of food, federal restrictions on the number of commercial flights that can be scheduled out of airports, and Environmental Protection Agency (EPA) regulation of the use, transportation, and disposal of toxic chemicals (Roper Center at University of Connecticut, 1989; Exhibit 6–1).

The tobacco industry's strategy has been quite successful because of the extent to which the core values of its messages are an inherent part of American thinking:

> The concept and symbolic importance of individual freedoms are deeply ingrained in American myth, culture, and law. Antismoking advocates may have underestimated how powerfully the idea of personal autonomy for life-style choices resonates among legislators, especially

Exhibit 6–1 Sample Questions from a 1988 Tobacco Institute Public Opinion Poll

1. The U.S. Agriculture Department currently inspects food processing plants to make sure that they are sanitary. Do you think that these inspections should be made more strict than they are now, made less strict than they are now, or should they be left about as they are now?
2. The Federal Aviation Administration now places restrictions on the number of commercial flights that can be scheduled in and out of major airports. Do you think that these restrictions should be made more strict than they are now, made less strict than they are now, or should they be left about as they are now?
3. The Environmental Protection Agency now requires companies using toxic chemicals to follow certain procedures in the use, transportation, and disposal of those chemicals. Do you think that those procedures should be made more strict than they are now, made less strict than they are now, or should they be left about as they are now?

Source: Data from Roper Center at University of Connecticut, 1989.

when used creatively to obscure the tobacco industry's goals. As the tobacco industry has correctly calculated, the individual liberties arguments are seductive when framed as unfair restrictions on private social behavior, even in the presence of compelling scientific evidence on the adverse health effects from smoking. (Jacobson et al., 1993, p. 807)

The findings of Jacobson and colleagues (1993) suggest that although health is an important core value, personal freedoms, civil liberties, and individual rights may be even more compelling values for the public. When the debate is framed in a way such that antismoking legislation is seen as conflicting with these values, antismoking advocates are unlikely to be successful. Moreover, to succeed, antismoking advocates must directly confront the opposition frames. They must develop their own frames that appeal to the same compelling core values being tapped into by the opposition. The development of these frames should be guided by market research, not by mere conjecture.

Wallack and associates (1993) have argued that, in a sense, debates over public health policy issues represent a battle for framing the issue in the eyes of the public. It is not necessarily the relative merits of various arguments for and against a proposal that most influence its legislative fate. Rather, it is the relative success of proponents and opponents in framing the overall terms of the debate. For example, in tobacco control, "the battle for framing is evident in how the tobacco industry uses symbols and images to promote itself as a good corporate citizen, defender of the First

Amendment, protector of free choice, and friend of the family farmer. The industry paints antitobacco people, on the other hand, as zealots, health fascists, paternalists, and government interventionists" (Wallack et al., 1993, p. 71). As Jacobson and associates (1993) argued, "how the issue of smoking restrictions is framed is an important component of the legislative debate and outcome" (p. 806).

Similarly, Schon and Rein (1994) explained that in a policy controversy, "two or more parties contend with one another over the definition of a problematic policy situation and vie for control of the policy-making process. Their struggles over the naming and framing of a policy situation are symbolic contests over the social meaning of an issue domain, where meaning implies not only what is at issue but what is to be done" (pp. 28, 29).

The public's perception of how an issue relates to its needs, wants, and values most influences public opinion. The way in which a debate is framed has important implications for how the public relates the issue to its needs and core values. The battle over public health programs and policy initiatives, then, can be viewed not only as a battle over specific facts and arguments, but as a battle over the framing of the overall issue; not solely as a battle over policy, but as a battle over the packaging of that policy into symbols, images, and themes.

In their discussion of "the framing of debate," Chapman and Lupton (1994) emphasized the need to understand "how issues need to be reframed in order to steer public and political support in the desired directions" (p. 18). The authors stated that "political battles are seldom won only on the elegance of logic or by those who can best assemble rational arguments. These are mere strategies within a wider battle front. The real issue is which are the overall framings of debates that best succeed in capturing public opinion and political will" (p. 125).

Similarly, Schon and Rein (1994) saw policy controversies as "disputes in which the contending parties hold conflicting frames. Such disputes are resistant to resolution by appeal to facts or reasoned argumentation because the parties' conflicting frames determine what counts as a fact and what arguments are taken to be relevant and compelling" (p. 23).

Kaniss (1991), too, emphasized the importance of the "symbolic framing of the proposal," concluding that "the way in which new initiatives are presented and framed for the media is particularly important" (pp. 182, 183). She stressed that symbols play a critical role in the framing of policies and showed how the battle for the symbolic framing of a policy issue in a way that best appeals to the media is the central battle over a public health policy.

Framing can be viewed as the packaging and positioning of a public health policy or program so that it appeals to deeply ingrained, widely shared principles held by the target audience. Framing is an integral part of developing a strategy to market public health programs and policies.

Developing Public Health Frames

In developing frames, public health practitioners must identify how to define, position, and package an issue in ways that (1) present a unified, coherent core position; (2) evoke desired visual images; (3) employ recognizable "catch phrases"; (4) suggest appropriate metaphors; (5) attribute responsibility for the problem to society, rather than merely to the individual; and (6) imply as a solution the program or policy being marketed by the practitioner (Exhibit 6–2). All of these individual objectives must work together effectively to reinforce the deeply ingrained, widely held principles and values of the target audience.

For example, consider the framing of a local ordinance to protect the health of restaurant workers by eliminating smoking in restaurants. To market such a policy, one might develop four frames based on widely held core values: freedom, independence, control, and fairness. Instead of defining the product of an anti-smoking ordinance campaign as a law to protect the health of nonsmokers and offering health for restaurant customers as a benefit, the product and benefits can be redefined as the freedom to work in an environment free of health hazards, the right to make a living without being involuntarily exposed to carcinogens, creating a level playing field for all workers by affording restaurant workers the same protection that is provided to almost all other workers, helping business by preventing huge liability risks for damages caused by secondhand smoke, preventing discrimination against blue-collar workers by extending to all workers the protection that almost all white-collar workers have from secondhand smoke, and protecting the livelihood of workers in small restaurants by ending the suffering they endure from exposure to a hazardous working environment (Table 6–2).

Similarly, instead of framing an initiative to increase the cigarette tax simply as a measure to reduce cigarette consumption and improve health, supporting the

---

Exhibit 6–2 Key Objectives in Development of Framing Strategy for Public Health Programs and Policies

1. Present unified, coherent core position on the policy or program that is consistent with the core values of target audience.
2. Evoke visual images that appeal to the core values.
3. Develop catch phrases (verbal images) that appeal to the core values.
4. Suggest appropriate metaphors that evoke themes and images that appeal to the core values.
5. Attribute responsibility for the public health problem to society (including government), not merely to individuals.
6. Imply as a solution the program or policy being marketed.

Table 6–2 Core Values and Messages That Appeal to These Values for Several Public Health Policies

Public Health Policy	Core Value	Message
Eliminate smoking in restaurants	Freedom/Free enterprise	What could possibly be a more basic freedom to Americans than the freedom to make a living and support one's children without having to be exposed to dangerous working conditions? What is a more basic civil liberty than the right to work in a safe environment? Forcing employees to breathe in carcinogens in order to make a living is a violation of the free enterprise principle.
	Independence/ Economic opportunity	Liability risks posed by allowing employees to be exposed to secondhand smoke (workers' compensation, disability, etc.) could hurt business owners. Illnesses and deaths will cause a loss of jobs, productivity, and sales.
	Control	How can workers pursue a livelihood and support children if they are too sick to work or suffer (can't breathe) at work?
	Fairness/Equality	Excluding restaurant workers from health protection that all other workers take for granted is not fair; it represents discrimination against a certain class of workers; this is a class issue. Excluding restaurant workers from protection is hardly a level playing field.
Increase cigarette tax	Freedom	Voting for the tax is a way to assert freedom from tobacco industry influence. Rejecting the tax is just playing into the hands of the industry and letting it dictate state policies.
	Independence	Without a higher tax, parents cannot effectively keep children from smoking, cannot effectively fight the tobacco industry's pressure on their children to smoke.
	Control	Voting for the tax allows you, not the tobacco industry, to decide the fate of your children's health.

continues

Table 6–2 continued

Public Health Policy	Core Value	Message
	Democracy	Voting for the tax preserves the democratic ideal by keeping government in the hands of the people, not in the hands of a powerful, greedy, special-interest group that has intruded into our state.
Adopt stricter environmental regulations	Control	Regulations will allow society to retain control over the unknown consequences of environmental destruction.
	Economic opportunity	Regulations will help preserve livelihoods and economic opportunity by protecting tourism; rejecting the regulations will lead to economic devastation of the community.
Adopt needle exchange program	Freedom	The program will allow society to remain free of the scourge of acquired immuno-deficiency syndrome (AIDS); without it, AIDS may spread from the drug-using population to the general population.
	Control	If AIDS spreads to the general population, the epidemic may soon be out of control.
Adopt mandatory seat belt law	Fairness	It is not fair for taxpayers to have to pay medical bills for people seriously injured because they were irresponsible and failed to wear seat belts.
	Economic livelihood	The medical costs of accidents involving individuals not wearing seat belts are wreaking havoc on the budget and the economy and increasing taxes for everyone. The law will create savings that will translate into lower taxes and increased economic livelihood.
Adopt tuberculosis (TB) screening and treatment program in drug treatment clinics	Freedom	The program will prevent the epidemic scourge of TB that threatens to affect all of us, as TB spreads from drug users into the general population.
	Control	The program will allow society to retain control over the unknown consequences of the spread of multidrug-resistant TB into the general population. The consequences are unknown, but could be devastating to society.

initiative could be framed as a way for voters to remain free of the tobacco industry's influence, raise their children independent of the pressure being placed on their children to smoke, maintain control of the health of their communities, and preserve the principles of democracy (see Table 6–2).

Programs to adopt such measures as stricter environmental regulations, needle exchange programs, mandatory seat belt laws, and screening and treatment programs also could be framed to appeal to the core values of freedom, independence, economic opportunity, autonomy, control, fairness, and equality (see Table 6–2).

Reframing Public Health Issues

In addition to developing their own frames, public health practitioners must also learn to confront directly the frames developed by opponents of their proposed policies and programs.

How can public health advocates confront opposition framing? Two approaches are possible. Take, for example, the level playing field frame used by the tobacco industry in fighting local smoking regulations (see Table 6–1). First, advocates can simply ignore the opposition frame and emphasize that this is a health issue. The success of this approach depends on policy makers perceiving the policy's reinforcement of the value they place on health as more compelling than the policy's conflict with the value they place on fairness and equality. As Jacobson and colleagues (1993) noted, this approach may be successful, but only if advocates are able to make the public health frame the dominant one.

An alternative approach is to reframe the issue so that supporting the policy reinforces rather than conflicts with the core values being tapped by the opposition frame. In other words, public health advocates must develop a new frame that shows policy makers how a local restaurant smoking ordinance is necessary to preserve fairness and equality for the city's residents.

One way the issue could be reframed is to demonstrate how the exclusion of restaurant workers from the protection from secondhand smoke that we afford most other workers is unfair (Table 6–3). The real unlevel playing field is the singling out of restaurant workers as the one occupational group not deserving of basic public health protections that most other workers take for granted and consider to be their right.

A second way to reframe the issue might be to show how the failure to protect citizens in the city would perpetuate an unlevel playing field by denying citizens in that city a basic right guaranteed to the citizens of more than 200 cities throughout the country—the right to work in an environment free of hazards (Table 6–3).

In both frames, the core values are the same: fairness and equality. However, in the opposition frame, voting for the ordinance would conflict with these values, while in the proponent frame, voting for the ordinance would reinforce these values. (See Appendix 6–B.)

Table 6–3 The Level Playing Field Frame: Reframing for Use by Public Health Advocates in Promoting Local Smoke-free Restaurant Ordinances

Frame	Level Playing Field— Reframe 1	Level Playing Field— Reframe 2
Core position	Singling out restaurant workers as the one occupational group not deserving basic health protection afforded to nearly all other workers creates an unlevel playing field for these workers.	Failing to protect citizens in this city from secondhand smoke when more than 200 cities nationwide have already afforded these protections to their workers creates an unlevel playing field for our residents.
Metaphor	An unlevel playing field in a sports event, favoring one team over another	An unlevel playing field in a sports event, favoring one team over another
Images	An unlevel playing field in a sports event	An unlevel playing field in a sports event
Catch phrases	"Level playing field"; "unfair"; "disadvantage"; "discrimination"	"Level playing field"; "unfair"; "disadvantage"; "discrimination"
Attribution of responsibility for problem	Government, which is selectively protecting workers in typical offices, but excluding restaurant workers from protection	Government, which is selectively excluding our city's residents from protection that many residents in other cities have
Implied solution	Extend smoke-free working environment protections to all workers	Extend smoke-free working environment protections to workers in our city
Core values	Fairness Equality Justice Economic opportunity	Fairness Equality Justice Economic opportunity

Another excellent example of the technique of redefining public health issues so that the desired program reinforces rather than opposes core values was provided by former Surgeon General Joycelyn Elders. In 1994, public health practitioners in Baltimore proposed a program to offer Norplant—a system of long-term contraception that involves the surgical insertion of a slow-release hormone delivery device under the skin of the upper arm—to teenage girls at a city health department clinic. The plan was condemned on the grounds that it would interfere with the autonomy and freedom of the young women and restrict their reproductive rights. In response, Dr. Elders redefined the Norplant program as a method to *free* young women from the enslaving grip of unwanted pregnancies: "If you're poor and ignorant, with a child, you're a slave. Meaning that you're never going to get out of it. These women are in bondage to a kind of slavery that the Thirteenth Amendment just didn't deal with" (Gaylin & Jennings, 1996, p. 16). As Gaylin and Jennings (1996) explained, Surgeon General Elders framed the use of Norplant as "a liberating factor from the veritable 'slavery' of teenage pregnancy" (p. 16).

Beauchamp (1976) discussed how public health practitioners can use the core value of justice to redefine public health problems in ways that will gain public support and motivate the public and policy makers to collective action: "In building these collective redefinitions of health problems, however, public health must take care to do more than merely shed light on specific public health problems. . . . This means that the function of each different redefinition of a specific problem must be to raise the common and recurrent issue of justice by exposing the aggressive and powerful structures implicated in all instances of preventable death and disability, and further to point to the necessity for collective measures to confront and resist these structures" (p. 10).

The process of reframing public health programs and policies effectively can be aided by considering the nature of societal core values. In particular, two characteristics of these core values are most salient. First, as discussed in Chapter 3, the deeply ingrained core value of freedom represents both the absence of interference from others (negative liberty) and the presence of control over one's life and destiny (positive liberty). Special-interest groups that oppose public health programs tend to emphasize their infringement on negative liberty. Public health practitioners can often reframe the debate by pointing out how the program or policy will actually enhance positive liberties. Thus, while a law that limits individuals' ability to drink and drive may be perceived as interfering with personal freedom, public health practitioners can market such a law by pointing out that it actually preserves individual autonomy by protecting society's members from being killed by drunk drivers and therefore preserves their ability to control their lives.

Second, core values such as freedom, independence, autonomy, and even justice have tended to be interpreted with an individualistic perspective. Civil rights laws, for example, usually have been interpreted as protecting the rights of individuals. But Gaylin and Jennings (1996) argued that "nothing inherent in civil rights laws . . . requires that they be interpreted in individualistic terms; their meaning could easily be construed in terms of nondiscrimination or equality" (p. 53). In other words, public health practitioners may be able to reframe public health programs and policies in a way that highlights how they will promote a communitarian or societal advancement of civil rights. For example, a law that eliminates smoking in bars could be promoted as a necessary measure to en-

sure equality of occupational safety protections for all workers. A smoke-free ordinance is simply an expression of a societal interpretation of civil rights.

Gaylin and Jennings (1996) suggested that in America, civil rights have become
"a framework for individual claims against others," but that they could just as
easily become "a framework for social solidarity" and a means of "building a
moral community of equal citizens" (p. 53). Etzioni (1993) even claimed that a
communitarian perspective of rights is not only consistent with, but is necessary
for, the preservation of individual liberty: "Neither human existence nor individual liberty can be sustained for long outside the interdependent and overlap-
ping communities to which all of us belong. . . . The exclusive pursuit of private
interest erodes the network of social environments on which we all depend and is
destructive to our shared experiment in democratic self-government. For these
reasons, we hold that the rights of individuals cannot long be preserved without a
Communitarian perspective" (pp. 253, 254).

Sunstein (1997) wrote that the government effort to change social norms is often necessary to advance individual autonomy:

> In fact, there are many reasons why a legal system might seek to alter
> norms, meanings, and roles. The most important reason is that the resulting
> reforms might enhance autonomy. . . . Obstacles to autonomy and to good
> lives can also come from bad roles, norms, and meaning. . . . In some cases,
> existing norms undermine people's autonomy, by discouraging them
> from being exposed to diverse conceptions of the good and from giving
> critical scrutiny to their own conceptions, in such a way as to make it
> impossible for them to be, in any sense, masters of the narratives of their
> own lives. (pp. 37, 55, 59)

Thus, in reframing public health programs and policies, public health practitioners can confront antiregulatory sentiment by positioning these reforms as necessary to eliminate obstacles to individual freedom and autonomy. "It should be
clear that social norms, meanings, and roles may undermine individual autonomy.
Above all, this is because norms can compromise autonomy itself, by stigmatizing
it. . . . In such cases, autonomy cannot exist without collective assistance; people
are able to produce the norms, meanings, and roles that they reflectively endorse
only with governmental involvement. Something must be done collectively if the
situation is to be changed" (Sunstein, 1997, p. 62).

In general, public health practitioners can confront the antiregulatory sentiment
in the nation by reframing public health issues to show that government action is
necessary precisely to preserve the societal interest in individual freedom and autonomy. As Sunstein (1997) wrote,

> more broadly, a democratic government should sometimes take private
> preferences as an object of deliberation, evaluation, and even control—

an inevitable task in light of the need to define initial entitlements—and precisely in the interest of welfare and autonomy. . . . The interest in liberty or autonomy does not call for government inaction, even if that were an intelligible category. Indeed, in many or perhaps all of the cases, regulation removes a kind of coercion. . . . The view that freedom requires an opportunity to choose among alternatives finds a natural supplement in the view that people should not face unjustifiable constraints on the free development of their preferences and beliefs. . . . Liberalism does not forbid citizens, operating through democratic channels, from enacting their considered judgments into law, or from counteracting, through the provision of opportunities and information, preferences and beliefs that have adjusted to an unjust status quo. Ironically, a system that forecloses these routes—and that claims to do so in the name of liberalism or democracy—will defeat many of the aspirations that gave both liberalism and democracy their original appeal, and that continue to fuel them in so many parts of the world. (pp. 20, 30, 31)

Perhaps the best example of reframing social policy so as to reinforce the core values of freedom and autonomy is the description offered by Sunstein (1997) of the rationale for government programs to address poverty:

Poverty itself is perhaps the most severe obstacle to the free development of preferences and beliefs. Programs that attempt to respond to the deprivation faced by poor people—most obviously by eliminating poverty, but also through broad public education and regulatory efforts designed to make cultural resources generally available regardless of wealth—are fully justified in this light. They should hardly be seen as objectionable paternalism or as unsupportable redistribution. Indeed, antipoverty efforts are tightly linked with traditional efforts to promote security and independence in the interest of creating the conditions for full and equal citizenship. (p. 28)

The strategic use of issue framing to redefine the public health product and package and position it so that it supports the most compelling core values of the public and policy makers can play an important role in helping public health practitioners deal with the unique marketing challenge they face. Evidence suggests that issue-framing strategies derived from marketing and public opinion research can help promote support for public health policies. For example, a 1988 survey funded by the Coalition for a Healthy California explored the effectiveness of various issue-framing strategies for a state cigarette tax initiative and was used in developing the campaign that led to the passage of Proposition 99 (Marr, 1990; Traynor & Glantz, 1996). A 1991 survey funded by the Massachusetts division of the American Cancer Society played a key role in developing the campaign that led to the passage of a cigarette tax initiative in 1992 (Marttila & Kiley, Inc., 1991). Similar marketing research helped a public health coalition in Arizona promote the passage of a cigarette tax initiative in 1994 (Ross, 1996). The role of marketing principles in these campaigns is discussed in detail in the case studies in Chapter 7.

Despite the promise of issue framing in marketing public health programs and policies, more research must be done in this area. Chapman and Lupton (1994) suggested four specific questions to address in such research:

> (1) Are there important differences in the framings favored by those working in public health, and those that hold most public and political appeal?; (2) Are there methodologies that are sufficiently sensitive to be reliably used in pretesting different framings used in advocacy?; (3) What examples are there, where dominant framings that run against the interests of public health appear to have been successfully reversed?; (4) Are there principles that characterize such reversals, which can be applied in practical ways in future debates? (p. 12)

CONCLUSION

To advocate successfully for public health policies and programs and to promote the survival of public health as a societal institution, public health practitioners must adopt two basic marketing principles.

1. The first step in developing campaigns to promote a public health policy or program is *not* to decide how to convince the public or policy makers to support the program, but to use market research to identify the basic needs, desires, and core values of the target audience.
2. When referring to public health, practitioners must define the product they are selling based on the results of formative research. Public health practitioners must acknowledge that they cannot always effectively sell public health programs. They must begin to sell basic values such as freedom, independence, control, and the democratic way. Public health must be positioned, packaged, and framed in such a way that it will be perceived as fulfilling the needs, desires, and values of the target audience. And then the message must be reinforced.

In the new view of public health presented in this chapter, epidemiologic research and formative research combine to form a basic foundation. Epidemiologic research helps identify the most effective programs and policies to solve public health problems. Then, based on the findings of formative research, the most important needs, desires, and values of the target audience (policy makers and/or the public) can be identified. Next, the public health practitioner must define the product so that it will offer as a benefit the fulfillment of these desires and needs. Finally, the practitioner can package, position, and frame the product in an effort to demonstrate to the audience how it will indeed fulfill these desires and needs (Figure 6–1).

This model differs from traditional models of public health practice because it includes two intermediate steps not generally included in other models. Most

---

A. Program evaluation research
1. Identify effective public health programs and policies.
2. Identify the specific target audience for each desired program and policy (the target).

B. Formative research (understanding the target audience)
1. Identify and prioritize basic needs, desires, and values of target audience.
2. Identify attributes of the public health program or policy that satisfy or fulfill these needs, desires, and values.
3. Test potential themes, arguments, phrases, and images to see how well they resonate with core values of target audience.
4. Test potential themes, arguments, phrases, and images of opposition.
5. Test ways of counterarguing or opposing the frames presented by the opposition.

C. Strategic marketing for public health
1. Redefine the product so that it offers as a benefit fulfillment of important needs and desires (the product).
2. Package and position the product as a way to fulfill important needs and desires (the promise).
3. Show how the alternative policy or program conflicts with fulfillment of underlying needs and desires.
4. Frame the communications in a way that reinforces, and does not conflict with, audience's core values.
5. Develop support for the promise: Demonstrate to and convince audience that the product does and will fulfill their specific needs and desires (the support).

D. Planning, Implementing, and Evaluating the Public Health Campaign

Figure 6–1 A New Marketing Strategy for Public Health: Confronting Threats to the Survival of Public Health

models begin with step A and jump immediately to the final step D, running the campaign. In our model, before the actual planning, implementation, and evaluation of the public health campaign, we add two steps: formative research (understanding the consumer's needs, desires, and values) and strategic marketing for public health (using the results of formative research to effectively define, package, position, and frame the public health program or policy being promoted).

The next two chapters present case studies to illustrate the most important points of the first part of the book. Chapter 7 presents a case study of the use of marketing principles to market a public health policy: the adoption of cigarette excise tax increases with earmarking of revenue for antitobacco programs. Chapter 8 presents a case study of the use of framing principles to market a major public health institution: the Centers for Disease Control and Prevention.

REFERENCES

Beauchamp, D. (1976). Public health as social justice. *Inquiry, 13,* 3–14.

Chapman, S., & Lupton, D. (1994). *The fight for public health: Principles and practice of media advocacy.* London: BMJ Publishing Group.

Entman R. (1993). Framing: Toward clarification of a fractured paradigm. *Journal of Communication, 43,* 51–58.

Etzioni, A. (1993). *The spirit of community: Rights, responsibilities, and the communitarian agenda.* New York: Crown.

Fine, T.S. (1992). The impact of issue framing on public opinion toward affirmative action programs. *The Social Science Journal, 29,* 323–334.

Gaylin, W., & Jennings, B. (1996). *The perversion of autonomy: The proper uses of coercion and constraints in a liberal society.* New York: The Free Press.

Iyengar, S. (1991). *Is anyone responsible? How television frames political issues.* Chicago: University of Chicago Press.

Jacobson, P.D., Wasserman, J., & Raube, K. (1993). The politics of antismoking legislation. *Journal of Health Politics, Policy and Law, 18,* 787–819.

Kaniss, P. (1991). *Making local news.* Chicago: University of Chicago Press.

Krosnick, J., & Alwin, D. (1988). A test of the form-resistant correlation hypothesis: Ratings, rankings and the measurement of values. *Public Opinion Quarterly, 52,* 526–538.

Marr, M. (1990, April). *Proposition 99: The California tobacco tax initiative, a case study.* Berkeley, CA: Western Consortium for Public Health.

Marttila & Kiley, Inc. (1991). *A survey of voter attitudes in Massachusetts: Benchmark survey.* Boston: Author.

Meyerowitz, B.E., & Chaiken, S. (1987). The effect of message framing on breast self-examination attitudes, intentions, and behavior. *Journal of Personality and Social Psychology, 52,* 500–510.

Moon, R.W., Males, M.A., & Nelson, D.E. (1993). The 1990 Montana initiative to increase cigarette taxes: Lessons for other states and localities. *Journal of Public Health Policy, 14,* 19–33.

Nelkin, D. (1987). *Selling science: How the press covers science and technology.* New York: Freeman.

Roper Center at University of Connecticut. (1989). *Public opinion online.* Tobacco Institute sponsored survey conducted by Hamilton, Frederick, and Schneiders, November 23–December 6, 1988.

Ross, M. (1996). *Tobacco tax campaigns: A case study of two states.* Washington, DC: Advocacy Institute.

Rothman, A.J., Salovey, P., Antone, C., Keough, K., & Martin, C.D. (1993). The influence of message framing on intentions to perform health behaviors. *Journal of Experimental and Social Psychology, 29,* 408–433.

Ryan, C. (1991). *Prime time activism: Media strategies for grassroots organizing.* Boston: South End Press.

Schon, D.A., & Rein, M. (1994). *Frame reflection: Toward the resolution of intractable policy controversies.* New York: Basic Books.

Slovic, P., Fischhoff, B., & Lichtenstein, S. (1982). Response mode, framing, and information-processing effects in risk assessment. In R.M. Hogarth (Ed.), *Question framing and response consistency* (pp. 21–36). San Francisco: Jossey-Bass.

Smith, T. (1987). That which we call welfare by any other name would smell sweeter: An analysis of the impact of question wording on response patterns. *Public Opinion Quarterly, 51,* 75–83.

Stauber, J., & Rampton, S. (1995). *Toxic sludge is good for you! Lies, damn lies and the public relations industry.* Monroe, ME: Common Courage Press.

Steel, R. (1981). *Walter Lippmann and the American century.* New York: Vintage Books.

Sunstein, C.R. (1997). *Free markets and social justice.* New York: Oxford University Press.

Tannen, D. (Ed.). (1993). *Framing in discourse.* New York: Oxford University Press.

Traynor, M.P., & Glantz, S.A. (1996). California's tobacco tax initiative: The development and passage of Proposition 99. *Journal of Health Politics, Policy and Law, 21*(3), 543–585.

Tversky, A. & Kahneman, D. (1982). The framing of decisions and the psychology of choice. In R.M. Hogarth (Ed.), *Question framing and response consistency* (pp. 3–20). San Francisco: Jossey-Bass.

Vaughan, E., & Seifert, M. (1992). Variability in the framing of risk issues. *Journal of Social Issues, 48,* 119–135.

Vookles, J., & Carr, J. (1993). The effects of message framing manipulations on AIDS preventive behavior. *AIDS Weekly,* 16.

Wagenaar, A.C., & Streff, F.M. (1990). Public opinion on alcohol policies. *Journal of Public Health Policy, 11,* 189–205.

Wallack, L., & Dorfman, L. (1996). Media advocacy: A strategy for advancing policy and promoting health. *Health Education Quarterly, 23,* 293–317.

Wallack, L., Dorfman, L., Jernigan, D., & Themba, M. (1993). *Media advocacy and public health: Power for prevention.* Newbury Park, CA: Sage Publications.

Watzlawick, P., Weakland, J., & Fisch, R. (1974). *Change: Principles of problem formation and problem resolution.* New York: Norton.

White House Domestic Policy Council. (1993). *Health security: The President's report to the American people.* New York: Touchstone.

Wilson, D.K., Purdon, S.E., & Wallston, K.A. (1988). Compliance to health recommendations: A theoretical overview of message framing. *Health Education Research: Theory and Practice, 3,* 161–171.

Wilson, D.K., Wallston, K.A., & King, J.E. (1990). Effect of contract framing, motivation to quit, and self-efficacy on smoking reduction. *Journal of Applied Social Psychology, 20,* 531–547.

Exploring the Core Values of Policy Makers: Lessons from Public Health History

To see how the public health practitioner can use the principles of marketing to promote the institution of public health, we must return to the importance of identifying and understanding the needs and wants of the target audience. In this case, we must identify what it is that policy makers need and want to support specific health programs and policies and to fund public health agencies.

What does public health mean to the policy maker? Why is it that policy makers want to protect the health of their constituents? What are the values associated with having healthy individuals in society that lead policy makers to allocate funds for public health protection?

Perhaps the best way to find out what public health means to policy makers is to study the conditions under which the institution of public health was created. What were the conditions that have led to the funding of major public health interventions during the past two centuries? To answer this question, we must turn to our review of major highlights in public health history that was presented in Chapter 5.

If one looks at the major events that have led to the adoption and funding of public health programs and institutions throughout history, one finds that a governmental concern over the health of the public has rarely been the driving force. Instead, it has generally been one factor or the combination of two factors that has led to government action: (1) the perception of broad, societal susceptibility to a disease and (2) the perception of societal lack of control over the spread and consequences of a disease.

The perception that all persons—rich and poor alike—were susceptible to a disease has been a powerful stimulus for organized government action. Often, public policy–making bodies ignored diseases when they affected only the poorer classes, and acted only when a disease penetrated into the higher classes of society.

As was described in Chapter 5, it was because unhealthy social and environmental conditions threatened not only the poor but also the entire community that public health first came to be seen as a public responsibility. Government action to establish new sanitation systems followed more than a decade of advocacy for such changes by groups of reformers. It took the "lively fear" that cholera provoked among policy makers themselves to overcome entrenched opposition to public health action. The visible and widespread threat of cholera was the "catalyst" to action (McNeill, 1989). "To do nothing was no longer sufficient; old debates and stubborn clashes had to be quickly resolved by public bodies acting literally under fear of death" (McNeill, 1989, pp. 239, 240).

It has always been more difficult to motivate policy makers to allocate funds to improve social conditions in impoverished areas than in areas inhabited by the wealthy and politically powerful. As Duffy (1992) noted, referring to the late 1800s, "generally, accumulated piles of garbage and refuse characterized most urban areas. The one exception was the neighborhoods occupied by the well-to-do, which usually received special attention from the city authorities" (p. 175).

However, the penetration of disease across the boundaries of social class changed policy makers' views. The rapid changes in transportation that occurred in the nineteenth century helped bring infectious disease within the confines of all neighborhoods, regardless of socioeconomic level:

> One of the obvious lessons of this period, drawn from experiences with contagious diseases, was that no community was an island. With yellow fever striking the southern coastal states and spreading up the Mississippi Valley, and with recurrent outbreaks of smallpox and Asiatic cholera plaguing the entire country, state officials took it upon themselves to proclaim statewide quarantines. The sanitary movement also demonstrated the interdependence of communities. Water pollution, for example, affected not only the community responsible for the pollution but also other communities dependent upon the polluted water source. (Duffy, 1992, p. 148)

Policy makers acted because it was no longer possible to ignore the afflictions of the poor. Diseases whose spread was initiated among the poor would sooner or later affect the upper classes as well: "In earlier centuries, disease was more readily identified as only the plight of the impoverished and immoral. The plague had been regarded as a disease of the poor; the wealthy could retreat to country estates and, in essence, quarantine themselves. In the urbanized nineteenth century, it became obvious that the wealthy could not escape contact with the poor" (Institute of Medicine, 1988, p. 59).

The broadened susceptibility to disease also changed the way policy makers came to view the reasons for disease. When it was only the poor who were affected, disease could be attributed to poor personal hygiene. But as soon as the wealthy were affected as well, disease had to be seen as a societal problem. "Almost all families lost children to diphtheria, smallpox, or other infectious diseases.

Because of the deplorable social and environmental conditions and the constant threat of disease spread, diseases came to be considered an indicator of a societal problem as well as a personal problem" (Institute of Medicine, 1988, p. 59).

Even when government action did occur in response to hazards within impoverished communities, the stimulus for action was the fear that the hazard could spread outside poor neighborhoods and affect everyone in the community. As Starr (1982) writes about the evolution of public health in the nineteenth century, "earlier in the century, cholera and yellow fever epidemics and concern about the squalid living conditions of the 'dangerous classes' had stimulated the organization of citizens' sanitary or hygiene associations to clean up the cities" (p. 184). It was not the suffering of the poor that precipitated action, but the fact that they were perceived as being dangerous to others.

The perception that a disease is out of the control of societal effort, that it represents a threat to the economic and political fabric of society, and that it is unfamiliar, mysterious, unexplained, or graphically destructive of human life has also been a powerful stimulus for government action. Policy makers have not tended to take action when they perceived a disease as controlled, familiar, or explained, even if it was taking a huge toll on human life. But a new disease that is unfamiliar, mysterious, or out of society's control brings prompt government action to control it even if its mortality toll is relatively low.

Throughout public health history, the fear of the unknown, the ghastly, and the mysterious—not the actual public health impact of a disease—has determined the speed and extent of organized government action against the disease. It was these characteristics of cholera, for example, that prompted many of the sanitary reforms of the mid-nineteenth century. As McNeill (1989) explained,

> the speed with which cholera killed was profoundly alarming, since perfectly healthy people could never feel safe from sudden death when the infection was anywhere near. In addition, the symptoms were peculiarly horrible: radical dehydration meant that a victim shrank into a wizened caricature of his former self within a few hours, while ruptured capillaries discolored the skin, turning it black and blue. The effect was to make mortality uniquely visible: patterns of bodily decay were exacerbated and accelerated, as in a time-lapse motion picture, to remind all who saw it of death's ugly horror and utter inevitability. (p. 231)

Not only did cholera produce graphic demonstrations of the impact of a disease on human victims, but it also represented a threat to society's sense of control over its own existence and viability. McNeill (1989) spoke of "the unique psychological impact of the approach of such a killer. . . . Cholera seemed capable of penetrating any quarantine, of bypassing any man-made obstacle: it chose its victims erratically" (p. 231).

Society also tended to take action against public health hazards when it perceived those hazards as a threat to its economic stability. As Duffy (1992) explained, the institutionalization of public health in many American cities occurred only when policy makers realized that having an unhealthy population was a threat to the economic viability of the population as a whole: "In Memphis and other southern cities, it would be some years before enlightened businessmen finally realized that a healthy population was necessary for a healthy economy" (p. 115). As Leavitt (1982) explained, competition between cities for economic progress was often the stimulus for investment in the public health infrastructure: "Local pride and inter-city competition provided an economic dimension of support for health campaigns to clean the streets and to eradicate epidemic diseases. Milwaukeeans believed that Chicago and Minneapolis–St. Paul threatened their own economic progress and, trying to surpass their rivals, became intolerant of serious sanitation problems. A prosperous Milwaukee could not rise from the piles of rotting garbage that supposedly caused high death rates" (p. 247).

And as Dr. James Howard Means, former president of the American College of Physicians, wrote in 1953,

> when he is sick the individual creates a social vacuum which affects others than his immediate family. . . . The cost of his illness must be paid for somehow. . . . Illness of the individual, therefore, like fire, flood, or other destructive processes, is always an economic loss to the community. . . . Ill health subordinates other values, both on the part of the patient and of those immediately affected by his illness. Illness may even be said to be a political loss through the deterioration it causes in the sense of public responsibility. . . . Communities with many cases of chronic illness suffer economically, socially, and politically. (pp. 4, 5)

The factors that influence government funding of public health programs and institutions are little different today. For example, it was the threat of the uncontrolled and indiscriminate spread of acquired immunodeficiency syndrome (AIDS) that led to increased government funding of AIDS prevention programs in 1985, several years after the disease was first identified among homosexual men in San Francisco. It was not until AIDS affected a celebrity—Rock Hudson—in 1985, that the issue finally reached the media agenda, the public agenda, and the public policy agenda. When AIDS was perceived as being confined to the general homosexual population, it was viewed neither as a national newsworthy public health problem, nor as a funding priority. As Randy Shilts (1987) explained in *And the Band Played On,* "there was something about Hudson's diagnosis that seemed to strike an archetypal chord in the American consciousness. For decades, Hudson had been among the handful of screen actors who personified wholesome American masculinity; now, in one stroke, he was revealed as both gay and suffering from the affliction of pariahs" (pp. 578, 579). Hudson's announcement is viewed as "the single most important event in the history of the epidemic" (Shilts, 1987, p. 579). Even after Hudson's announcement and subsequent death, funding for AIDS prevention continued to be determined largely by its affecting celebrities. Odets (1995) noted that American society "more or less ignores AIDS between sporadic public concern about celebrities who contract it" (p. 24).

Reports of AIDS among heterosexuals also helped unleash the funding that, if released several years earlier, could have done much to prevent the epidemic from reaching the level it did. As Shilts (1987) explained,

> the outpouring of official attention to the handful of heterosexual AIDS cases in early 1985 proved a crucial event in determining the direction of the AIDS debate in the next two years. It instructed health officials and AIDS researchers, who had had such a difficult time seizing government and media interest in the epidemic, that nothing captured the attention of editors and news directors like the talk of widespread heterosexual transmission of AIDS. Such talk could be guaranteed air time and news space, which, in the AIDS business, quickly translated into funds and resources. (p. 513)

Indeed, funding for AIDS prevention, education, and research programs at the Centers for Disease Control and Prevention (CDC) increased from just $2 million in 1982, $6.2 million in 1983, and $13.8 million in 1984 to $33.3 million in 1985, $62.1 million in 1986, and $136.1 million in 1987.

As Duffy (1992) noted, "the appearance of a few cases of Legionnaire's disease or bubonic plague in the twentieth century has been enough to cause newspaper headlines and bring demands for action by the federal government. . . . By contrast, the thousands of deaths caused by smoking or drunken driving are familiar and hence acceptable. We may deplore them, but they arouse no fear or consternation among us" (pp. 23, 24).

From a societal perspective, disease is viewed as a burden not so much because of the individual suffering or loss that it causes, but because it impinges upon, ultimately, the freedom of other individuals and societal institutions. For example, disease places a burden on society because it imposes significant costs: for medical care, lost productivity, increased health insurance premiums, increased taxes, and strained public budgets. The government tends to respond to the threat of disease not when individual suffering reaches a certain level, but when the magnitude of the perceived threat to the freedom and autonomy of the rest of society's members reaches a level that demands public attention.

Disease has important societal meanings that go beyond the value society places on the absence of diseased individuals. In a sense, society as a whole has an "illness experience," a way in which it experiences, perceives, interprets, and reacts to the presence of disease. And similar to the experience of individuals, it is not the existence of diseased individuals itself, but the threats to the freedom, independence, autonomy, and control of the members of society at large that most accurately characterize the salience of the experience to society.

REFERENCES

Duffy, J. (1992). *The sanitarians: A history of American public health.* Urbana, IL: University of Illinois Press.

Institute of Medicine, Committee for the Study of the Future of Public Health. (1988). *The future of public health.* Washington, DC: National Academy Press.

Leavitt, J.W. (1982). *The healthiest city: Milwaukee and the politics of health reform.* Princeton, NJ: Princeton University Press.

McNeill, W.H. (1989). *Plagues and peoples.* New York: Anchor Books.

Means, J.H. (1953). *Doctors, people, and government.* Boston: Little, Brown.

Odets, W. (1995). *In the shadow of the epidemic: Being HIV-negative in the age of AIDS.* Durham, NC: Duke University Press.

Shilts, R. (1987). *And the band played on: Politics, people, and the AIDS epidemic.* New York: St. Martin's Press.

Starr, P. (1982). *The social transformation of American medicine.* New York: Basic Books.

An Example of Reframing a Public Health Policy Issue: Antismoking Ordinances

In 1995, the Ontario legislature considered a law to eliminate smoking in restaurants. The Ontario Restaurant Association (ORA) lobbied against the proposal, arguing that it would harm businesses there; result in job losses for workers; and create hardship and suffering for restaurant owners, employees, and their families.

In an April 5, 1995, letter to the Ontario Campaign for Action on Tobacco, the ORA outlined its position. In response, Michael Siegel prepared a letter that was sent to Ontario government officials, attempting to reframe the issues. Excerpts from the two statements follow.

ORA:

> The ORA believes that it is important to understand that any negative impact, if it is experienced by 1 restaurant or 1,000 restaurants, is a very serious situation to a restaurant owner, and depending on the degree and length of the negative impact, a foodservice operator could be forced to go out of business.

Response:

> We believe that it is important to understand that any adverse health effects of secondhand smoke, if they are experienced by 1 restaurant worker or 1000 restaurant workers, are a very serious situation for a restaurant owner, and depending on the degree and duration of the health effects, a restaurant worker could be forced to suffer, to have to stop working, or even to die.

ORA:

> I do not believe that we can make light of a situation in which a negative impact on business is experienced, as it is both very serious and fright-

ening for business owners who have placed their savings into their business and rely on their business for their livelihood. Nor can we ignore the fact that businesses employ people who will also be forced out of employment, if a severe negative impact is experienced as a result of a smoking by-law.

Response:

I do not believe that we can make light of a situation in which devastating health effects on restaurant workers are experienced, as it is both very serious and frightening for restaurant workers who have placed their careers into the food service business and rely on their work for their livelihood. Nor can we ignore the fact that businesses employ people who will be forced out of employment if they become sick due to a severe negative impact of secondhand smoke.

ORA:

No one knows the true impact of smoking bans on foodservice establishments in Ontario, except for foodservice operators who have the most direct contact with their customers and therefore know what percentage smoke.

Response:

No one knows the true impact of smoking in restaurants on foodservice workers in Ontario, except for the workers themselves, who have the most direct contact with secondhand smoke in their workplace, and therefore know the devastating impact that secondhand smoke has on their health and their lives.

SECTION III

Marketing Public Health— Case Studies

This section presents two case studies. The first case study illustrates the strategic application of marketing principles to advance a public health policy: increasing state cigarette excise taxes to support comprehensive, statewide, antitobacco programs. The second case study illustrates the role of issue framing in promoting funding for a major public health institution: the Centers for Disease Control and Prevention.

CHAPTER 7

Marketing Public Health Programs and Policies— A Case Study

The following case study illustrates the importance of the strategic use of marketing principles to public health coalitions. From 1988 to 1994, health coalitions in five states drafted ballot propositions calling for an increase in the state tobacco excise tax. The proposed increases, ranging from 25 to 50 cents per pack, faced similar attacks by the tobacco industry. However, the success of the initiatives varied. While the 1988 proposition in California passed with 58% support, others, such as Colorado's 1994 initiative, garnered only 38% support by election day. An analysis of these five battles over a tobacco tax initiative sheds light on the importance of an effective marketing campaign in a successful public health initiative. In particular, the success of public health coalitions formed to promote the tax increases was directly related to their ability to identify the needs and wants of their target audience, define the product, control the debate, reframe issues, and craft arguments that would appeal to the core values of voters.

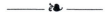

Effective marketing strategies are crucial to public health initiatives opposed by politically connected and well-financed industries such as the tobacco industry. Tobacco use, the chief cause of preventable death in America, provides a clear target for the public health community. Until recently, tobacco companies have maintained a tight grip on the legislative agendas of both Congress and individual states. Recognizing the need for government intervention in tobacco control efforts and the lack of legislative action, health advocates have turned to state proposition campaigns in which decisions regarding the establishment of tobacco control programs are left directly to the voters. These ballot initiatives have called for tobacco tax increases, particularly cigarette taxes, with a portion of the tax revenue going toward statewide tobacco control programs. From 1988 to 1994, health coalitions in five states conducted successful petition drives that enabled such initiatives to be placed on the ballot and voted on by the public. Of these five, the ballot initiatives passed in three states: California (1988), Massachusetts (1992), and Arizona (1994). Similar propositions in Montana (1990) and Colorado (1994) failed. What follows is an analysis of the marketing strategies used in each campaign and their relationship to the success or failure of each public health campaign.

The importance of an effective marketing strategy by public health advocates is amplified by the dearth of financial resources available to promote the proposition in the face of high-cost tobacco industry campaigns against tax increases (Table 7–1).

Over the years, the tobacco industry has mastered a strategy designed to move the debate about tobacco taxes away from health relevance and toward an issue of government bureaucracy and tax fairness. These issues appeal to American voters who have come to be wary of government programs and compassionate toward groups who claim unfair tax burdens. The challenge for health advocates is to go beyond simply educating voters about the health benefits of a cigarette tax. They must recognize that health is not the only issue in the minds of voters and must prepare to conduct formative research in order to develop a campaign strategy that reflects voter attitudes and values rather than merely the intuition of the public health community.

CALIFORNIA

The passage of Proposition 99 in California resulted in a 25-cent-per-pack cigarette tax increase with 20% of the new revenue going toward education programs intended to reduce tobacco use (Bal, Kizer, Felten, Mozar, & Niemeyer, 1990; Marr, 1990; Traynor & Glantz, 1996). California's tax initiative campaign repre-

---

Table 7–1 Total Campaign Spending in Five Cigarette Tax Initiative Campaigns

State	Tobacco Industry	Health Coalition
California	$21.4 million	$1.6 million
Massachusetts	$7.3 million	$800,000
Arizona	$6.0 million	$2.0 million
Montana	$1.5 million	$40,000
Colorado	$5.0 million	$300,000

Source: Data from Koh, 1996, Moon et al., 1993, Ross, 1996, and Traynor and Glantz, 1996.

sented a major step for health advocates: It was one of the first public health campaigns to recognize the role of marketing and strategically apply marketing principles to obtain voter support. The success of this campaign came only after carefully crafting the initiative in response to public opinion polls.

The Coalition for a Healthy California, which consisted of the California Medical Association (CMA), the Planning and Conservation League (PCL), California
Association of Hospital and Health Systems (CAHHS), the American Lung Association (ALA), American Cancer Society (ACS), and the American Heart Association (AHA), spearheaded the Proposition 99 campaign (Marr, 1990; Traynor &
Glantz, 1996). In January 1987, the coalition sponsored its first poll to determine
the level of public support for a tobacco tax and to determine how the public
wanted the revenue distributed (Charlton Research, Inc., 1987). The results were
extremely promising with 73% of voters supporting a 25- to 35-cent-per-pack
cigarette tax increase. The initial polls also examined the reasons voters would
support or oppose a cigarette tax increase. The most popular arguments in support
of a tax increase (almost two-thirds support) included (a) tobacco use costs society
billions of dollars, (b) the tax would discourage smoking among young people,
and (c) tobacco use is the single most preventable cause of death in America. This
early polling enabled the coalition to develop a campaign using arguments that
resonated with voters. In addition, the poll helped identify weaknesses in the initiative. The strongest argument against the tax, with 46% of respondents stating
that they were less likely to vote for it after hearing the argument, was that "increasing cigarette taxes would mean another government bureaucracy and more
bureaucrats spending more of our money" (Charlton Research, Inc., 1987).

The poll also indicated that funding education programs to prevent drug and
tobacco use was the most popular destination for the tax revenue (72% support)
followed by health research for tobacco-related disease (60%) (Traynor & Glantz,
1996). After seeing how popular these programs were with voters, the Coalition
for a Healthy California made sure that the initiative clearly stated that 25% of the
new tax revenue would go to such programs.

In the meantime, the tobacco industry conducted its own polls, from which it soon
realized that its only hope for success was to move the debate away from smoking and
frame the issue as a matter of regressive taxes and increased government bureaucracy. Other arguments that resonated well with the voters included (a) the tax would
lead to higher crime due to cigarette bootlegging and (b) the tax was being promoted
by special interests, like physicians, who wanted to pad their pockets. With this in
mind, Californians against Unfair Tax Increases (CAUTI) was formed. Funded almost entirely by the tobacco industry, CAUTI was a citizens' group that served as a
front to allow the tobacco industry to attack the initiative from behind the scenes.

Early tobacco industry advertising focused on attacking the "greedy intentions"
of the initiative's sponsors. However, the strategy soon focused on crime and

bootlegging. Billboards across the state reinforced the notion that higher cigarette taxes would lead to gang-directed smuggling of cheaper tobacco from other states. Despite the lack of any reasonable evidence to suggest that this was at all likely, the tobacco companies had put into question the core value of security in the minds of Californians. Polls conducted by Mervin Field suggested that these fears were having an effect at the polls. Support for Proposition 99 fell from 73% to 58%, with an increase in the number of undecided voters (Marr, 1990). The industry, realizing the impact of this theme, continued framing the tax initiative in this way in television and radio advertisements.

A series of fortunate events for the coalition led to the unraveling of the crime issue. California's attorney general, John Van de Kamp, called a press conference, at which he criticized the increased crime allegations brought forth by the tobacco industry. In addition, a police officer who played an undercover cop in a "No on 99" ad had signed an affidavit at the request of a local television station claiming that he was a police officer and not an actor. It was later brought to the coalition's attention that the "undercover cop" acted in a movie in which his character killed two secret service agents (Traynor & Glantz, 1996). Thus, he had lied, or at least been deceitful, in his affidavit. This information was quickly distributed to media outlets and received widespread attention. The tactics of the tobacco industry had been publicly exposed. The industry's use of lies and deceit in the Proposition 99 campaign did not sit well with the voters.

This public relations debacle forced the industry to drop the crime ads with just 3 weeks left until election day. While the crime theme had at one point been effective, the industry had now lost some credibility and instead focused on the regressive nature of cigarette taxes and "smokers' rights." However, the damage was done, and support for Prop 99 stabilized for the rest of the campaign. On November 8, Proposition 99 passed with 57.8% of the vote.

Even though the leadership of the California campaign chose to frame the tax proposal primarily as a health issue, some of their most effective advertising appealed to voters' other core values, such as independence and autonomy. For example, one television ad featured actor Jack Klugman asking voters who they believed about the tax initiative: the tobacco industry or health groups. This ad touched the surface of the inner desire of voters to make their own decisions and not allow themselves to become puppets of the tobacco industry.

Campaign activists recognized that the David versus Goliath struggle between health and Big Tobacco could serve as a rallying cry for voters. Americans love an underdog. In addition, the David/Goliath argument is consistently used by the tobacco industry. In this case, however, David is the taxpayer while Goliath represents the government. Using this frame in addition to the health argument strengthened the position of health advocates and forged a more appealing bond with the voter while taking campaign angles away from the industry.

Ultimately, it was sustained formative research and effective issue framing and reframing that led to the success of Proposition 99. Had the coalition not conducted public opinion polls during the campaign, it would not have detected the precipitous drop in voter support for the tax and it would not have identified the crime frame as the reason for this loss of support. The coalition would not have been able to reframe this issue by exposing how the tobacco industry was using lies and deceitful manipulation. The tobacco industry was the real "criminal" here. And the citizens of California were the true underdogs: the victims of tobacco industry deceit and manipulation.

The coalition framed the tax issue in a way that turned the core values of freedom, independence, autonomy, and security into powerful incentives to vote for Proposition 99. The platform on which the industry was standing was pulled right out from under it and now supported public health frames.

MONTANA

The decline in cigarette consumption after Proposition 99 was implemented in California received national attention and prompted states such as Montana to attempt to pass similar tobacco tax initiatives. In 1990, after gathering enough signatures to put Initiative 115 on the ballot, proponents had only $40,000 to finance the campaign (Moon, Males, & Nelson, 1993). An analysis of Montana's campaign underscores the relationship between effective marketing and success at the polls.

In contrast to the health coalition in California, the Montana coalition conducted only one public opinion survey and only after the initiative language had been finalized (Howard/Johnson Associates, 1990; Moon et al., 1993). The August 1990 poll indicated that 77% of voters had already decided how they were voting (Howard/Johnson Associates, 1990). While these voters supported the initiative by a 50% to 45% margin, the fact that nearly 80% of voters had already decided how they would vote in November illustrates that the poll was conducted too late. Because the initiative language had already been finalized, it could not be changed so as to garner greater public support. Such a small margin of support offered little chance that the initiative campaign could withstand the tobacco industry's million dollar ad campaign in September and October. In November, Initiative 115 was voted down 59% to 41%.

As stated in Initiative 115, "revenue raised as a result of the tax would be allocated between the state's long-range building program fund and a newly-established Montana tobacco education and preventive health care fund." The August 1990 poll revealed that 62% agreed that "with Montana's economy as bad as it is, now is not the time for any form of new taxes" (Howard/Johnson Associates, 1990). In addition, 52% agreed that "a consumption tax is a bad idea because it taxes those who can least afford it." If the poll had been conducted earlier, the initiative could have allocated a portion of the revenue toward programs that addressed these concerns. For example, a portion of the revenues could have been earmarked for an economy stimulation package.

In contrast to the late start in market research by the public health coalition, the tobacco industry conducted telephone tracking surveys as early as January 1990 to test possible campaign themes. Realizing the impact that a message of increased taxes and bureaucracy had on the voters, the industry developed its primary strategy: Frame the issue as "more tax and bureaucracy." The tobacco industry–funded "citizens' group" opposing Initiative 115 took the name "Committee Against More Tax and Bureaucracy" and focused on this theme continually until election day with the ever-present slogan, "Put the ax to more tax and bureaucracy, vote against I-115." The tobacco industry ads successfully framed the initiative as one that would further aggravate the economic stability and security of Montana citizens.

While opponents of Initiative 115 ran ads questioning where the money would go, the public health community ran ads that reminded voters that the initiative was a health issue. "It's not about taxes . . . it's about saving lives," one ad mentions. Regardless of whether it was or wasn't a health issue, the ability of tobacco interests to frame the initiative as a tax issue made these ads ineffective. During the California campaign a CAUTI staff member remarked, "We truly didn't believe it was a health initiative, and even if it was, even if we hadn't thought about it that way, we couldn't argue [with] a health initiative. I mean, you argue with a health initiative, you lose. And so we felt what we needed to do was attack the weak points. I mean in any political campaign or any battle you go after the weak spots in the campaign" (Traynor & Glantz, 1996, p. 561).

As the focus of the initiative became less about health and more about taxes, much of the press viewed Initiative 115 as a flawed measure despite good intentions. This perception could have been altered had I-115 proponents been more aggressive in reframing rather than ignoring the tobacco industry themes. Instead of telling voters not to "be fooled by smoke and mirror tactics" and then barraging them with health statistics, the public health coalition should have molded their argument around the economic issues that were persuading voters. In particular, opponents consistently brought up the prudence of a new tax of which no part was targeted toward alleviating the expected $100 million state deficit. The health coalition could have defused this issue by suggesting that at least part of the deficit was due to the economic drain placed on society by tobacco products.

The public health coalition's August 1990 poll provided at least some feedback on the popularity of a variety of arguments for and against the initiative. However, additional polls could have provided some assessment of what was causing support for I-115 to fall from 50% to 41% during the campaign. The lack of additional polling also prevented a testing ground for new arguments that the coalition might use to defend against the industry's attacks. In contrast to the coalition in California, the Montana health coalition did not successfully reframe the key tobacco industry arguments.

For public health advocates to run successful political campaigns, marketing must play an integral role from start to finish. A political campaign must rapidly adjust its message and constantly evaluate the effectiveness of the message sent. Public health advocates in Massachusetts would recognize this in 1992 to wage an effective tobacco tax campaign.

MASSACHUSETTS

Much of the credit for the success of the Massachusetts tobacco tax campaign (Question 1) lies with the ACS. In April 1991, the ACS hired the political consulting firm of Marttila & Kiley, Inc., to conduct a statewide poll to obtain information regarding public support for a tobacco tax increase. The results were promising, with 68% in favor of a 25-cent-per-pack cigarette tax increase (Marttila & Kiley, Inc., 1991a, 1991b).

The value of the poll went further than simply demonstrating widespread support for the tax increase. Of those who were not in favor of a 25-cent increase, only 6% changed their minds to favor a tax increase of 20 cents per pack. However, 14% of voters who supported a 25-cent increase would not support an increase of 30 cents. This information demonstrates that an initiative calling for a 25-cent increase was the maximum tobacco tax increase that could receive widespread support. Lowering the tax increase to 20 cents would not result in a gain of much support, and increasing the tax by 30 cents would lose considerable support. In addition, the poll asked voters to choose where they would most like to direct revenue from a tobacco tax increase. Seventy percent of those polled supported using the tax revenue to fund programs to prevent tobacco use. Unlike the Montana initiative, this information could be used before the drafting of the initiative to ensure a tax proposal that would satisfy the goals of public health advocates with a strong level of popular support. Because the Massachusetts state constitution prohibits allocating particular tax revenues for specific purposes, the authors of the initiative could not be as specific as California in designating how the new revenue would be spent. Instead, the initiative called for the establishment of a "Health Protection Fund" from the tax revenue "subject to appropriation by the legislature" (Heiser & Begay, 1997, p. 969; see also Koh, 1996). But the initiative language clearly suggested that the Health Protection Fund moneys were to be used for tobacco prevention and education programs.

Just as California and Montana had done in previous polls, Massachusetts tested the popularity of a variety of arguments for and against the initiative (Marttila & Kiley, Inc., 1991a, 1991b). While this research was extremely valuable in identifying arguments that would be most effective with voters, perhaps the most important result of the poll was identifying who the public trusted. Potential voters were presented with a list of groups that included health and tobacco organizations. For each group they were asked "would you trust what they have to say almost completely, a great deal, only somewhat, hardly at all, or not sure?" Seventy-seven percent trusted the ACS a great deal or almost completely, the most of any group in the poll. In contrast, only 7% trusted the tobacco industry a great deal. This information provided the newly formed Massachusetts Coalition for a Healthy Future with its chief strategic goal: to frame the campaign as a fight between good and evil, that is, the ACS and the medical community versus the tobacco industry. Polling and focus group research had revealed that ACS's credibility as a sponsor of Question 1—especially when compared with the tobacco industry's lack of credibility—was the most effective argument in support of the initiative (Marttila & Kiley, Inc., 1992a).

Unfortunately, two focus group sessions in early September 1992 revealed that the public was unaware that Question 1 was sponsored by the ACS. Instead, most had assumed that it was being promoted by a state agency. Another poll, conducted on October 1, revealed that voters were three times more likely to think the state or political system (20%) was the chief sponsor of Question 1, rather than the ACS (7%; Marttila & Kiley, Inc., 1992a).

Had the Massachusetts coalition not conducted this formative research, it would never have known that the public was not aware that ACS was behind Question 1, even though such awareness could have a huge impact on public support. Thanks to its research efforts, the coalition was able to step up the visibility of the ACS and to frame the battle over Question 1 as one between the ACS and the tobacco industry. By election day, the coalition had distributed more than 750,000 brochures with the headline, "Help the American Cancer Society fight the tobacco industry."

On November 2 and November 3 (election day), the coalition took out full-page ads in *The Boston Globe* that simply stated "Help the American Cancer Society Defeat Big Tobacco. Vote Yes on 1" (Figure 7–1). Marttila & Kiley, Inc., designed this ad not based on intuition, but based on careful formative research. They knew the ad would appeal to voters because they had asked them in advance.

In addition to providing the coalition with its primary issue frame, the formative research also showed health groups how they could effectively reframe tobacco industry arguments. The focus groups conducted by Marttila & Kiley, Inc. for the coalition revealed that while voters were receptive to the basic antitax message of Question 1's opponents, they were extremely skeptical when they realized that the opposition was funded almost entirely by the tobacco industry. In fact, the major Massachusetts citizen antitax group, Citizens for Limited Taxation, did not oppose the initiative. In addition, voters readily accepted that the industry's motives against Question 1 were to protect its profits rather than any true concern for citizens' financial burdens.

Help the American Cancer Society Defeat Big Tobacco.

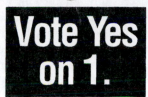

Vote Yes on 1.

Question #1 is sponsored by the American Cancer Society and 200 other health organizations.

The American Cancer Society put Question #1 on the ballot to reduce smoking and save lives. More than 200 other health and medical groups across the state have joined the Cancer Society as co-sponsors of Question #1.

The tobacco industry has spent more than $6.5 million in Massachusetts to kill Question #1.

The campaign against Question #1 has been funded entirely by these seven out-of-state tobacco companies:

R.J. Reynolds Tobacco Co.   The Tobacco Institute
Philip Morris Co.   Smokeless Tobacco Council
Lorillard Tobacco Co.   Brown & Williamson
The American Tobacco Co.   Tobacco Corp.

The tobacco industry is desperate to defeat Question #1 because they know it will reduce smoking rates in Massachusetts—which means fewer customers and less profits for the big cigarette manufacturers.

Cigarette smoking is the leading cause of preventable death in Massachusetts today.

Cigarettes kill more people in Massachusetts every year than car accidents, fires, murders, suicides, alcohol abuse, cocaine, heroin, and AIDS *combined*. And each year they cost Massachusetts taxpayers $1.5 billion in medical expenses and lost productivity.

Raising the cigarette tax is a proven way to reduce smoking.

When California voted for a 25¢ increase in the cigarette tax, people stopped smoking at twice the national average. Independent analysts project that Massachusetts would see a similar drop in smoking if Question #1 passes—as many as 80,000 fewer smokers in the first year alone.

Question #1 is aimed at reducing smoking among kids.

Question #1 is especially intended to discourage young kinds from taking up smoking. More than 90% of all smokers begin their habit as teenagers. Today, about one out of every three high school students smokes. Studies show that adolescents are the most sensitive to a cigarette tax increase—as the price goes up, fewer kids smoke.

Former U.S. Surgeon General C. Everett Koop supports Question #1

"I strongly endorse Question #1. Raising the excise tax on cigarettes is one of the most direct and effective ways to reduce smoking rates—especially among adolescents. The tobacco industry knows this, which is why they are spending millions of dollars in Massachusetts to defeat Question #1."

Question #1 has also been endorsed by:

The Boston Globe   Boston Business Journal
Springfield Union News   WBZ-TV Channel 4
Worcester Telegram & Gazette   WCVB-TV Channel 5
Quincy Patriot Ledger   WHDH-TV Channel 7

Paid for by the Massachusetts Coalition for a Healthy Future, Blake Cady, M.D., Chairman

Figure 7–1 Advertisement for Cigarette Tax Initiative—Massachusetts, 1992. *Source:* Copyright © American Cancer Society.

While opponents of Question 1 rehashed their argument of unfairness toward smokers, particularly poor smokers, the coalition lashed back and focused on "the unfairness of the $45 billion tobacco industry, their addiction of children, and their efforts to buy the election. The coalition maintained that cancer was far more disproportionately afflicting the poor and minority groups while burdening taxpayers with huge costs" (Koh, 1996, p. 222). This line of attack took the core value of fairness away from the industry and used it as an important argument in favor of Question 1. The coalition successfully reframed the tobacco tax initiative as one that would reinforce, rather than conflict with, the core value of fairness.

From October 1 until election day, the public health coalition conducted four tracking polls in an effort to receive constant feedback on the effectiveness of campaign strategies and the susceptibilities of their opponents (Marttila & Kiley, Inc., 1992a, 1992b, 1992c, 1992d, 1993). This was a benefit unavailable to activists in the failed Montana campaign. The first tracking poll identified that despite strong public support for Question 1, there was potential for significant loss in the weeks ahead (Marttila & Kiley, Inc., 1992a). After voters heard a list of strong arguments against the tax, support for Question 1 declined from 68% to 55%. This made it clear that an aggressive media campaign would be required to pull out a victory. If not for the unexpected realization from poll results that support was "soft," the coalition would not have taken such an aggressive campaign marketing approach and Question 1 probably would have failed.

Two weeks later a second tracking poll showed that support had dropped from 68% to 59% (Marttila & Kiley, Inc., 1992b). During the same period, awareness of the opposition's television advertising increased from 15% to 40%. Of those who had seen opposition ads, support was 51% compared with 65% for those who had not seen the advertising. In addition, the campaign was still not effective in educating the public about the primary sponsor of Question 1. A majority of voters did not know that the ACS was the primary group behind the initiative. Without making this fact known to voters, the campaign could not capitalize on the David versus Goliath struggle between ACS and Big Tobacco. In addition, only 41% of voters agreed that "raising the cigarette excise tax is an effective way to reduce smoking" (Marttila & Kiley, Inc., 1992b). In response to this information, the campaign developed a television ad that clearly highlighted the ACS sponsorship of Question 1 and the success that Proposition 99 had on reducing smoking in California.

A third tracking poll on October 26 showed support for Question 1 stabilizing at 60% (Marttila & Kiley, Inc., 1992c). While voter awareness of opposition television advertising had risen from 40% to 61%, the appearance of pro-Question 1 ads, which 42% had seen, was effectively neutralizing the opposition. The fourth and final tracking poll indicated that support had fallen to 56% (Marttila & Kiley,

Inc., 1992d), prompting a last-minute, paid newspaper advertising blitz that focused on the theme of protecting children from the tobacco companies and their products and discussed the success of the California tobacco control program. In addition, Blue Cross/Blue Shield placed a highly effective ad that focused on the economics of smoking: "The real point about Question #1 isn't what it will cost smokers. It's what it will save the rest of us" (Figure 7–2).

It was clear to all participants that the public supported less cigarette consumption, especially by children. The question was whether Question 1 would be effectively framed as an issue of public health or as one of increased and unfair taxes. The coalition's intensive marketing research enabled it to continually monitor the impact of its campaign strategy and of the opposition's campaign as well, allowing the coalition to retain control of the framing of the issue. The ability of the ACS to do this is best exemplified by the tobacco industry's 11th-hour strategy change. Although the industry had focused its entire campaign on an antitax message, just before the election ads began to portray Question 1 supporters as intolerant, using images of Martin Luther King to depict smokers as a targeted group in danger of losing its rights. This late-in-the-game maneuver shows how anxious the industry was to frame the debate under its own terms without the public health coalition redirecting it. Demonstrating the strong ability of the coalition to fight back and redirect opponents' arguments, Dr. Blake Cady, the coalition chairperson, responded publicly: "How dare the tobacco industry pretend to be a defender of tolerance. What could be more intolerant than the tyranny of an industry that hooks kids before they can make a reasonable choice" (Phillips, 1992, p. 13).

The primary spokesperson for the Committee against Unfair Taxes for most of the campaign was a former chair of the Massachusetts Legislature's Joint Committee on Taxation, Jack Flood. While Flood at first represented a legitimate authority against Question 1, his credibility quickly eroded and he was far less visible by the end of the campaign. "Declining public opinion of Mr. Flood was epitomized by a *Boston Globe* political cartoon depicting him as a monkey dancing to the tune of the tobacco industry's organ grinder" (Koh, 1996, p. 223). Would the public allow themselves to vote against the tax increase and become puppets of the industry as well? The issues that had gripped the press and were driving the campaign did not even remotely relate to health. In this case, Question 1 became an issue of autonomy. Voters may not be able to relate to a patient with lung cancer, but everyone can relate to a time in their life when they felt as if they were losing control. The threat of tobacco influencing individual decisions on behavior resonated with the public. The issue was not what tobacco would do to your body but how it would control your life.

The coalition made sure the public knew that the tobacco industry was behind the "No on Question 1" campaign with weekly updates publicizing the large

Throat Cancer Operation
$16,000

Electronic Voice Generator
$2,000

Esophageal Speech Training
$3,500

Pack of Cigarettes
$2.25

Lung Cancer Removal
$19,000

Radiation Treatments
$15,000

Chemotherapy
$5,000

Lung Transplant
$20,000

The Real Point About Question #1 Isn't What It Will Cost Smokers. It's What It Will Save The Rest Of Us.

By now, everyone knows the medical facts on smoking. So let's talk medical figures. Tobacco related illnesses cost all of us in Massachusetts over $1.5 billion in medical costs and lost productivity last year alone. Costs everyone pays for in higher health plan rates. Question #1 will increase the excise tax on cigarettes by 25 cents a pack. The point isn't to raise money. It's to reduce smoking, especially by our teenagers, a new target of the tobacco industry. It will work. When California voters approved a similar bill, smoking there fell 17%. We strongly urge you to join us in voting yes on Question #1. Because if we don't do it now, we'll all pay for it later.

Vote Yes On Question #1   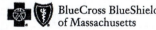 BlueCross BlueShield of Massachusetts

Paid for by Blue Cross and Blue Shield of Massachusetts, Inc.,
William C. Van Faasen, President, Joseph C. Avellono, M.D., Executive Vice President
® Registered Mark of The Blue Cross and Blue Shield Association. © 1992 Blue Cross and Blue Shield of Massachusetts, Inc.

Figure 7–2 Advertisement for Cigarette Tax Increase—Massachusetts, 1992. *Source:* Copyright © BlueCross BlueShield.

amounts of tobacco money being poured into media efforts across the state. Placing the spotlight on the industry allowed the health coalition to present Question 1 as a health issue rather than spend its time defending industry attacks that confuse the issue. When opponents of Question 1 did attack, the coalition not only defended themselves quickly and effectively but used the opportunity to attack the industry on a similar point. As early as July 1992, the ACS had already prepared question-and-answer sheets for key members of the coalition to use when defending their principles against the inevitable attack by the tobacco industry.

A TALE OF TWO STATES: COLORADO AND ARIZONA

Perhaps partly due to the success of the Massachusetts campaign, tobacco taxes truly became a national issue. President Clinton hoped to impose a $1- to $2-per-pack federal excise tax to pay for a national health insurance plan. In addition, in 1994 Arizona and Colorado saw battle over ballot propositions for 40- and 50-cent-per-pack cigarette tax increases, respectively, with revenue going toward tobacco control programs. With both states undergoing tax fights in a similar political climate, these battles provided an excellent opportunity for analysis because Arizona's campaign was successful, while Colorado's attempt failed.

Before evaluating the marketing strategies in each state, it is only fair to point out the disparity in financial resources available to the respective health coalitions. The coalition in Arizona, led by the Arizona Hospital Association, had $2 million at its disposal (Ross, 1996). In contrast, Colorado, which lacked any participation from the Colorado Hospital Association, could only muster $400,000 (Ross, 1996). While this large difference in financial support goes a long way toward explaining the results of the two campaigns, an analysis of the marketing strategies is helpful nevertheless.

Just as in California and Massachusetts, both states conducted polls before drafting any initiative (Ridder/Braden, Inc., 1993; Ross, 1996; Strategies West Research, 1993). A public opinion poll conducted in 1992, well before the initiative was even proposed, revealed strong support for a cigarette tax increase among Arizona voters (Ross, 1996). Further research revealed that 70% of Arizona voters would vote in favor of a tax up to 50 cents per pack. The poll also indicated strong voter support for allocating the tax for specific programs. Seventy-five percent favored using the money to educate children and teens about smoking, and 74% supported using the tax increase to fund health care for the poor and uninsured. However, 63% said they would oppose the measure if the legislature were allowed to spend the money on programs other than those specified by voters.

A similar poll conducted in March 1993 by the Colorado campaign showed comparable levels of support for a cigarette tax increase of 50 cents per pack, with 72% of voters in favor of a tax increase (Strategies West Research, 1993). In addition, the top three choices for spending tobacco tax revenue were to support health care for children (25%), health care for the poor (28%), and education programs on the dangers of tobacco (18%).

With this information in hand more than 18 months before election day, both groups were able to draft tax initiatives that reflected voter attitude by calling for a 40- to 50-cent increase and specifically allocating revenue to the programs that voters most supported. Under state law, for Colorado to specifically allocate revenue, the initiative had to be drafted as a constitutional amendment. Unfortunately, the fact that the initiative would amend the state's constitution became a source of debate later in the campaign and could not be defended effectively from attacks by opponents.

From the beginning, the health coalition in Arizona took a very proactive stance during the campaign. Once the initiative was qualified for the November ballot as Proposition 200, supporters brought in campaign veterans from other states that had recently fought for tobacco tax increases and asked them to brief Arizona reporters on the tactics the tobacco industry would use to fight Proposition 200. The coalition in Arizona was so concerned with controlling the debate from the beginning that they made sure to air the first television ad discussing the tax increase. While the ad was not very successful in its attempt to discredit the tobacco industry without first establishing its own credibility, it demonstrated the Arizona coalition's efforts to control the debate from the onset.

In contrast, the tobacco industry controlled the tax debate in Colorado (Dreyfuss, 1996). In January 1994, the tobacco industry claimed that it found evidence that state and local government health officials were engaging in illegal political activities, such as campaigning for the tax initiative on government time. These allegations persisted straight through election day. While no major violations were ever identified, the press coverage was more about government scandal than about the benefits of the tax initiative. By August 1994, support for the tobacco tax had fallen to 60% (Ross, 1996). The 10% drop before tobacco industry advertising even got under way showed little promise for the success of the campaign.

Arizona was outspent by the tobacco industry by only a 3 to 1 margin, enabling its coalition to remain competitive with tobacco industry advertising. Although the Arizona coalition used the health theme to sell the tax, the coalition also crafted ads designed to appeal to other core values of the Arizona voters, such as autonomy. One very successful ad depicted a man urging voters to support Proposition 200. The man had a laryngectomy due to smoking-induced cancer and now smoked through a voice box. The ad may have been in line with the campaign message on health, but something deeper may have caught the voters' attention. This man's voice was taken from him because he smoked. Would voters allow their children's voices to be taken from them by the tobacco industry? It was not just an issue of health. It also was about parental sovereignty in safeguarding their children. Would parents cede control of their children to the industry?

A poll taken in mid-October showed that support for Proposition 200 had fallen from over 60% to 44% in 3 weeks (Ross, 1996). While some strong arguments had been made for the initiative, voters reacted to allegations by the industry that there would be no accountability for how the tax revenue was spent. The political climate in 1994 was strongly antigovernment; incumbents lost heavily and the ensuing turnover in Congress gave control to Republicans for the first time in 40 years (Gillespie & Schellhas, 1994). Considering the conservative, antitax sentiment of the time, suggestions of wasted tax revenue had an effect on the voters. The campaign quickly responded with a flurry of ads that refuted the claims of the industry and clearly demonstrated how the initiative guaranteed accountability. It is important to note again that, without continuous polling, coalition members would not have realized the need to redirect their strategy away from health issues. Polling close to election day gave the coalition the information they needed to concentrate on last-minute techniques such as contesting effective arguments put forth by the tobacco industry. The coalition's effort was rewarded: On November 8, Proposition 200 passed by a 51% to 49% margin.

The tobacco industry, which had already placed the health coalition in Colorado on the defensive by suggesting improper lobbying by government workers, strengthened its position further by framing the cigarette tax as an issue of fairness. One newspaper ad depicted a hand squeezing blood from a rock: "They've squeezed smokers one too many times. . . . Don't you think they've picked on smokers enough?" A radio ad remarked, "Is it fair to target a single group for a $132 million tax increase? Is it fair to make smokers pay for problems that are everyone's responsibility?" (Lipsher, 1994). Smokers rather than children were being viewed as the victims. The industry instructed the public to think about how unfair a tax burden Amendment 1 would place on smokers. As tobacco industry spokesman Frank Hays commented, "There's a real feeling out there among voters that enough is enough. We've kicked smokers out in the snow, we've ostracized them from co-workers and friends. I think maybe nonsmokers are tired of kicking the dog. There is a fairness question" (Sanko, 1994, p. 5A).

By election day, the industry's arguments were strongly ingrained and the tax was soundly defeated 62% to 38%. The coalition in Colorado did not have the resources to conduct tracking polls that would go beyond measuring public support of the tax. Polling would have provided valuable feedback on the effectiveness of campaign messages from both sides of the proposition, allowing the coalition to respond with targeted advertising. No reframing of the debate was possible in Colorado.

SUMMARY

Raising the price of cigarettes through tobacco taxes is one of the most effective ways of reducing cigarette consumption, especially among children. As these recent tobacco tax campaigns indicate, a political environment differs greatly from an academic setting, to which many health professionals are accustomed. While results sell theories to scientists, images sell ideas to the public. To date, the public health community has been outmaneuvered by an industry that has spent many years pinpointing the best method of selling its product to citizens. While the public health community tends to market a proposal based on how it subjectively views the issue, the tobacco companies market opposition to these proposals based on carefully measured public attitudes, beliefs, and values.

The case studies clearly indicate that the success of a campaign is directly related to the amount of marketing research conducted in a campaign and the actions taken as a result of this research (Table 7–2). The dynamics of the political arena represent a stark contrast from the public health classroom. Relying on intuition and health statistics is no substitute for relying on marketing research that allows

Table 7–2 Characteristics of Successful and Failed Cigarette Tax Initiative Campaigns: The Role of Marketing Research

	Passed			Failed	
	California	Massachusetts	Arizona	Montana	Colorado
Ratio of campaign expenditures, tobacco industry: health coalition	13:1	9:1	3:1	37:1	17:1
Number of polls conducted by health coalition	2	6	4	1	2
Polling conducted before drafting initiative	Yes	Yes	Yes	Yes	No
Polls tested ways to frame issue	Yes	Yes	Yes	Yes	Yes
Polls assessed opponents' arguments	Yes	Yes	Yes	Yes	Yes
Conducted tracking polls	No	Yes	Yes	No	No
Health advocates controlled debate	Yes	Yes	Yes	No	No
Health advocates reframed issue	Yes	Yes	Yes	No	No

practitioners to generate an image that resonates with the deepest core values of a target audience.

While all of the campaigns described here relied on a health frame to sell the issue, it is clear that some of the most effective marketing was also directed at other core values, which may have been more salient and more influential on voter behavior. In the future, health professionals must seize the marketing tools used by the tobacco companies and use these tools against them. Public health practitioners must incorporate the strategic application of basic marketing principles into their public health campaigns if they are to have any chance of defeating such strong and experienced opponents.

First and foremost, public health coalitions need to take control of the debate by framing the issue. They must decide how they want the issue to be perceived by voters and then carry out a media campaign that reflects this strategy. Regardless of the final outcome of the initiatives described earlier, the tobacco industry made significant inroads in the level of support for the tobacco tax by consistently moving the issue away from health and toward alternate frames, most notably those of increased taxes, fairness, government bureaucracy, special-interest legislation, and accountable management of revenue.

When these alternative themes are presented, they must be confronted quickly. The most effective way of doing this involves reframing the issue so that opponents are taking the defensive on the arguments they pose. As mentioned earlier, Massachusetts demonstrated a large degree of success in reframing Question 1. When the industry called the tax intolerant, the coalition responded by attacking the intolerance of the marketing of cigarettes to children before they have a chance to make an educated decision about smoking. Complaints about the regressive nature of the tax were met with statistics demonstrating the regressive nature of lung cancer. When the industry referred to Question 1 as just another tax, the coalition responded with information on how "taxed" society is by the health care costs of treating sick smokers.

To convey an effective frame to the public, formative research plays an essential role. It must begin before finalizing the initiative and continue throughout the campaign, up until election day. Initial research efforts should focus on gauging public support for a measure, and then testing the effectiveness of possible arguments for and against the proposition. Later polls must assess the impact of opponents' arguments and the success of coalition arguments, and must consistently probe for changes in voter attitudes that warrant altering the campaign message. These polls provide the information necessary to make a campaign flexible and responsive to its desired market: the voters. Public polling is the testing ground for campaign themes, arguments, and issue frames. There simply is no substitute for sound marketing research to promote a public health policy.

The most important difference in successful versus failed cigarette tax initiative campaigns is the integration of marketing principles into the public health campaign. In most of the failed campaigns, the coalition had little success in recognizing the values that appealed to individuals—and influencing their behavior by appealing to these values. The case studies demonstrate the consistent and almost complete reliance on health to sell the issue in all of the failed campaigns. But health cannot stand alone as a selling point. It must be accompanied by an appeal to more central values, such as fairness, autonomy, and independence. What characterizes the successful tax campaigns is the realization that these core values are not off limits to public health. In fact, all were used effectively to market important public health initiatives.

CONCLUSION

These case studies demonstrate the success of integrating basic marketing principles into a public health campaign. Identifying and understanding important core values of the voters—such as fairness, autonomy, and independence—and evaluating alternative arguments to tap into these values must play a central role in developing a public health campaign message and in revising that message during the campaign. Ultimately, the issue at stake in the voting booth must not be simply improved health, but a reaffirmation of the values that Americans hold dearly: freedom, independence, autonomy, and fairness. The strategic use of marketing principles offers the public health practitioner a powerful tool to make this happen.

REFERENCES

Bal, D.G., Kizer, K.W., Felten, P.G., Mozar, H.N., & Niemeyer, D. (1990). Reducing tobacco consumption in California: Development of a statewide anti–tobacco use campaign. *Journal of the American Medical Association, 264,* 1570–1574.

Charlton Research, Inc. (1987). *California tobacco tax poll.* San Francisco: Author.

Dreyfuss, R. (1996). The campaign against the states. Tobacco's current strategy: Use state politicians to pre-empt local smoking controls. Attacking "big government" works. *Mother Jones,* p. 55.

Gillespie, E., & Schellhas, B. (Eds.). (1994). *Contract with America: The bold plan by Representative Newt Gingrich, Representative Dick Armey, and the House Republicans to change the nation.* New York: Times Books.

Heiser, P.F., & Begay, M.E. (1997). The campaign to raise the tobacco tax in Massachusetts. *American Journal of Public Health, 87,* 968–973.

Howard/Johnson Associates. (1990). *Results of market research regarding attitudes of Montana voters towards Initiative 115.* Helena, MT: Howard/Johnson Associates.

Koh, H.D. (1996). An analysis of the successful 1992 Massachusetts tobacco tax initiative. *Tobacco Control, 5,* 220–225.

Lipsher, S. (1994, September 10). Ads to blast cigarette tax lobby's $3.3 million fund worries measure's supporters. *The Denver Post,* p. A1.

Marr, M. (1990, April). Proposition 99: *The California tobacco tax initiative, a case study.* Berkeley, CA: Western Consortium for Public Health.

Marttila & Kiley, Inc. (1991a). *A survey of voter attitudes in Massachusetts: Benchmark survey.* Boston: Author.

Marttila & Kiley, Inc. (1991b). *Executive summary: A study of attitudes among voters in Massachusetts.* Boston: Author.

Marttila & Kiley, Inc. (1992a). *A survey of voter attitudes in Massachusetts: Track #1.* Boston: Author.

Marttila & Kiley, Inc. (1992b). *A survey of voter attitudes in Massachusetts: Track #2.* Boston: Author.

Marttila & Kiley, Inc. (1992c). *A survey of voter attitudes in Massachusetts: Track #3.* Boston: Author.

Marttila & Kiley, Inc. (1992d). *A survey of voter attitudes in Massachusetts: Track #4.* Boston: Author.

Marttila & Kiley, Inc. (1993). *Raising the tobacco tax: The campaign for Question One in Massachusetts (Prepared for the American Cancer Society, Massachusetts Division).* Boston: Author.

Moon, R.W., Males, M.A., & Nelson, D.E. (1993). The 1990 Montana initiative to increase cigarette taxes: Lessons for other states and localities. *Journal of Public Health Policy, 14,* 19–33.

Phillips, F. (1992, October 24). Tobacco industry ads tout tolerance. *The Boston Globe,* pp. 13, 17.

Ridder/Braden, Inc. (1993). *Tobacco tax initiative survey.* Denver, CO: Author.

Ross, M. (1996). *Tobacco tax campaigns: A case study of two states.* Washington, DC: Advocacy Institute.

Sanko, J. (1994, October 19). 50 cents tobacco tax hike losing steam: Poll shows backing of only 42% of registered voters, compared to 70% in 1992. *Rocky Mountain News,* p. 5A.

Strategies West Research. (1993, March 18). *Tobacco tax initiative survey.* Denver, CO: Author.

Traynor, M.P., & Glantz, S.A. (1996). California's tobacco tax initiative: The development and passage of Proposition 99. *Journal of Health Politics, Policy and Law, 21*(3), 543–585.

CHAPTER 8

Marketing Public Health as an Institution—A Case Study

Public health practitioners must market not only changes in health behavior, adoption of public health policies, and funding of specific public health programs, they also must market public health itself as a fundamental societal institution. With the threats of managed care, budget cuts, block grants, and other factors discussed in Chapter 4, public health practitioners often must compete to obtain funding for their agencies, independent of promoting specific policies or the adoption and funding of specific programs.

Perhaps the grandest example of the need to market public health as an institution is the annual Congressional debate over the level of funding for the nation's chief public health agency—the Centers for Disease Control and Prevention (CDC). This marketing effort is conducted not only by the CDC itself, but by national public health organizations, such as American Public Health Association (APHA), and by a broad coalition of nearly 100 national organizations (the CDC Coalition) established in 1987 by APHA to support the CDC and promote funding of its activities and programs.

Examination of the Congressional debate over CDC funding in the 104th Congress (1995–1996) helps to illustrate the use of framing principles discussed in Chapter 6 in marketing the institution of public health. The framing of CDC as an essential public health institution during the 104th Congress was extremely effective. While nearly every other federal public health agency suffered budget cuts during this period of revolt against government, CDC's budget was increased. The way in which public health and CDC's role in preserving public health were defined and framed may be instructive for public health practitioners in future efforts to promote their own agencies' funding.

———— ❧ ————

The period of the 104th Congress was one of revolt against big government. The Republicans, after gaining control of Congress for the first time in 40 years, pledged to downsize government; decrease government spending and regulation; consolidate or eliminate government programs and call on personal responsibility to solve societal problems; and make government simpler and more accountable. During the 104th Congress, and especially during the 1995 session, there were unprecedented attempts to limit the regulatory authority of government agencies, to cut funding for most government agencies, and even to eliminate agencies completely. (See Chapter 4 for a more detailed discussion.)

Despite this antigovernment, budget-slashing rhetoric, and although nearly every other federal public health agency suffered budget cuts during this period, Congress increased CDC's budget considerably in both 1995 and 1996. This disparity between the antigovernment sentiment in Congress and the success of CDC in maintaining and even increasing its funding presents a great opportunity to examine the role of defining and framing public health and public health institutions in the effort to secure funding for these institutions. As we will show, it was the way in which public health in general, and CDC in particular, were framed during the 104th Congress that explains CDC's budget success during this period.

Perhaps the best way to illustrate the framing of the debate over CDC funding is to examine the floor debate that occurred in Congress. The excerpts from the *Congressional Record* in Appendix 8–A at the end of this chapter are representative of the overall CDC funding debate in the 104th Congress.

During the 104th Congress, the leadership of the executive and legislative branches was concerned with the effort to balance the budget or reduce the federal budget deficit, to downsize government, and to decrease the federal payroll and bureaucracy. President Clinton, however, refused to sign budget resolutions passed by the Republican-controlled Congress that he felt went too far in eliminating essential government services. A prolonged budget impasse resulted, and the federal government was shut down for several weeks. Also of note, 1996 marked the 50th anniversary of the Centers for Disease Control and Prevention. It is in this context that the following excerpts of statements made in the *Congressional Record* are presented. These excerpts are taken from floor debates in the U.S. House of Representatives and the U.S. Senate in 1995 and 1996 concerning funding for CDC and the National Institutes of Health (NIH) (see Appendix 8–A).

Our most striking observation about the framing of CDC during the 104th Congress is not the way CDC was framed, but the way it was not framed. The CDC did not decide for itself what product it believed was important for Congress to buy. The CDC did not, for example, list and prioritize its programs in terms of their public health impact (e.g., the number of lives saved) and promote these programs by trying to convince Congress of the need to save as many lives as possible. Had this been the case, CDC's rationale for funding would have relied mainly on the importance of its programs to prevent chronic diseases—especially those related to tobacco use (420,000 deaths per year), alcohol (100,000 deaths per year), motor vehicle accidents (42,000 deaths per year), and firearms (40,000 deaths per year). Framing CDC's importance in this way would have engendered fierce opposition from powerful special-interest lobbies, including the tobacco industry, the alcohol industry, and the National Rifle Association (NRA). These groups would have called on Congress to preserve the principles of freedom, individual rights, autonomy, free enterprise, economic opportunity, equality, and capitalism by rejecting excessive government interference in these areas.

Instead, advocates for CDC funding relied on a framing of public health and the agency's role, which reinforced rather than conflicted with these widely held values. Ultimately, the argument for CDC funding was based not on an appeal to Congress's desire to improve health, but on an appeal to the value Congress places on the core American values of freedom; independence; autonomy; and control over one's life, one's liberty, and one's pursuit of happiness.

Specifically, it was the threat of newly emerging, mysterious, deadly, and potentially uncontrolled infectious disease epidemics like the Ebola virus outbreak that ensured continued across-the-board funding for CDC and sheltered the agency from the budget slashing that affected almost every other federal agency during the same legislative session.

Using the threat of an Ebola virus epidemic to frame the need for funding CDC was effective. Because Ebola virus infection is new, mysterious, deadly, and contagious, it represents a severe threat to the public's perception of freedom, independence, autonomy, and control over their lives. Because the virus can infect anyone, its threat is felt by everyone, and the fear of loss of control over one's life is salient, strong, and universal. Ebola virus kills its victims in a horrific way: the virus attacks the internal organs, causing them to slowly bleed until they cannot function. Thus, the very mention of the virus evokes graphic visual images that reinforce the complete loss of control over one's own body and its basic functions. And many catch phrases widely associated with Ebola virus (e.g., killer virus, hemorrhagic fever, outbreak, deadly, horror, victims, the hot zone) work in concert with the visual images to attack the most basic core values held by the public.

The sense of potential danger from Ebola virus was created, in part, by what Daniel McGee (1996) called *signification*, which he defined as "a cultural process by which meanings are assigned to signs; although these meanings appear to be stable and 'natural,' they actually can only be fully understood within the social context in which signification occurs" (p. 1095). McGee (1996) suggested that "emerging infections have become an 'epidemic of meanings or signification' as well as being a set of pathogens with the potential to cause epidemics" (p. 1095). McGee (1996) described the process by which these meanings create a sense of public threat as follows: "The very term 'emerging' becomes threatening, conjuring up an image of some menacing threat rising out of the steaming primordial ooze to ravage the peaceful denizens of Western civilization. The mass media in turn signify risk by creating horrific images of infectious diseases violating the boundaries of people's bodies, and these bodies issuing forth dangerous, filthy, infectious substances such as vomit, blood, and pus that threaten to contaminate bystanders" (p. 1097).

McGee (1996) concluded: "Because research funds and public health measures are shifted toward some diseases and away from others by both media attention and the 'emerging infections' scientific paradigm, the relationships between science and the mass media, as well as the relationships between public health priorities and infectious disease research, need critical examination" (p. 1097).

John Graham, director of the Center for Risk Analysis at the Harvard School of Public Health, has concluded that the health threats that policy makers and the public react to are "mysterious, unfamiliar, hard to explain, ones that we perceive are imposed upon us without our knowledge or consent—and that affect, frankly, upper-middle-class white people. If things hit those buttons, then the media gets very interested in them, politicians get very interested, and you can get an enormous amount of attention. Other risks may be factors of 10 and 100 times bigger, but if they don't hit those hot buttons, apathy may ensue" (Henig, 1997, p. 165).

The appeal of the threat of Ebola virus infection to the deepest and most vivid aspects of human fear is demonstrated by the many popular books and movies devoted to the topic (Exhibit 8–1). In *Virus Hunter,* Dr. C.J. Peters, chief of the CDC's Special Pathogens Branch and Mark Olshaker wrote that these books played a role in Congressional funding of CDC initiatives to control emerging infectious diseases: "One of the greatest boosts [to our funding] has been the public success of popular books and journalistic accounts [of emerging infectious diseases]" (Peters & Olshaker, 1997, p. x).

These excerpts from the *Congressional Record* illustrate the widespread use and effectiveness of the "killer virus" frame in defining, positioning, and packaging the product and benefits that CDC can offer to the public in a way that appeals to the widely held core values of freedom, independence, autonomy, and control. For the most part, these statements were not simply appeals for the protection of health. They were appeals for safeguarding the very security of the nation and the survival and freedom of its people. One did not hear similar appeals using the worldwide epidemic of tobacco use, which kills millions of people each year. The debate was dominated by appeals to protection from a virus that has never been reported in humans in this country. But the threat of this virus symbolized much more than Ebola virus infection. It symbolized everything that is profoundly basic to American values, everything that goes to the fundamental reason that public health exists in the first place.

This framing of the debate over the CDC and NIH budgets in 1995 and 1996 was extremely effective. While many federal agencies saw considerable declines in funding during this period of government downsizing, both CDC and NIH saw budget increases during this period (Figure 8–1).

Exhibit 8–1 Books and Movies about the Threat of Ebola Virus and Other Emerging "Killer Virus" Infections

---

Books

Virus X: Tracking the New Killer Plagues Out of the Present and into the Future. Frank Ryan. Boston: Little, Brown and Company, 1997.

A Dancing Matrix: Voyages along the Viral Frontier. Robin Marantz Henig. New York: A.A. Knopf, 1993.

The Hot Zone: A Terrifying True Story. Richard Preston. New York: Random House, 1994.

Virus Hunter: Thirty Years of Battling Hot Viruses around the World. C.J. Peters and Mark Olshaker. New York: Anchor Books, 1997.

Ebola: A Documentary Novel of Its First Explosion in Zaire by a Doctor Who Was There. William T. Close. New York: Ivy Books, 1995.

Emerging Viruses. Ed. Stephen S. Morse. New York: Oxford University Press, 1993.

The Coming Plague: Newly Emerging Diseases in a World Out of Balance. Laurie Garrett. New York: Farrar, Straus, and Giroux, 1994.

Deadly Feasts: Tracking the Secrets of a Terrifying New Plague. Richard Rhodes. New York: Simon & Schuster, 1997.

Virus Ground Zero: Stalking the Killer Viruses with the Centers for Disease Control. Ed Regis. New York: Pocket Books, 1996.

Level 4: Virus Hunters of the CDC. J.B. McCormick and S. Fisher-Hoch. Atlanta, GA: Turner Publishing, 1995.

The Plague Tales. Ann Benson. New York: Delacorte Press, 1997.

Biohazard: The Hot Zone and Beyond—Mankind's Battle Against Deadly Disease. Peter Brookesmith. London: Barnes & Noble, Inc., 1997.

The Third Pandemic: A Novel. Pierre Oulette. New York: Pocket Books, 1996.

Carriers. Patrick Lynch. New York: Villard, 1995.

Movies
Outbreak
Twelve Monkeys

Of all the federal health agencies shown in Figure 8–1, only CDC and NIH received a budget increase between fiscal year 1995 and fiscal year 1996. All of the other agencies, including the Food and Drug Administration (FDA), the Environmental Protection Agency (EPA), the Occupational Safety and Health Administration (OSHA), the Substance Abuse and Mental Health Services Administration (SAMHSA), the Agency for Health Care Policy Research (AHCPR), the Office of the Assistant Secretary for Health (OASH), the Office of the Inspector General (OIG), the Office of Consumer Research (OCR), the Office of Civil Rights (OCR), and the Administration on Aging saw budget cuts in fiscal year

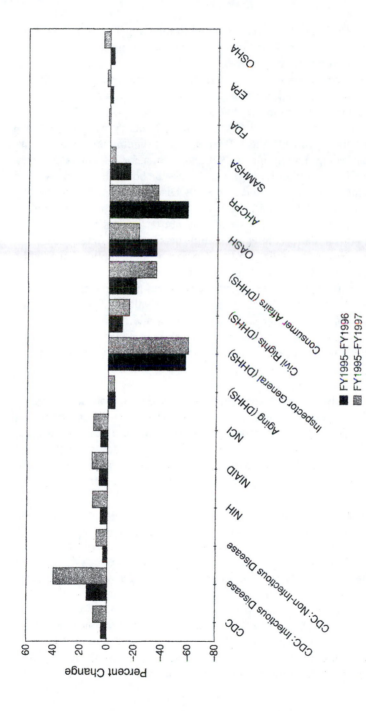

Figure 8–1 Percentage Change in Budget, FY1995–FY1996 and FY1995–FY1997, CDC and Other Federal Health Agencies. *Sources:* Reprinted from Office of Budget, Office of the Assistant Secretary for Management and Budget, U.S. Department of Health and Human Services; Office of Budget, Environmental Protection Agency; Office of Budget, Occupational Safety and Health Administration, 1997.

1996. Somehow, CDC and NIH were immune to the budget slashing that Congress, led by House Speaker Newt Gingrich, was conducting as part of its perceived mandate to cut big government.

There was some correction of these budget trends during fiscal year 1997, but CDC and NIH were still the only agencies shown that received a real (adjusted for inflation) increase in budget from fiscal year 1995 to fiscal year 1997.

Of note, although funding for CDC's infectious disease programs increased most dramatically between 1995 and 1997, the overall funding level for CDC increased (even excluding funding for the National Center for Infectious Disease). Similarly, the funding increases for NIH were across the board. For example, both the National Institute for Allergy and Infectious Diseases (NIAID) and the National Cancer Institute (NCI) saw a 13% increase in budget from 1995 to 1997.

Deserving emphasis are two points that may not be evident in the excerpts. First, the Ebola virus has not yet infected a single person in the United States. But using this killer virus as a framing strategy to demonstrate the need for public health in general and for CDC in particular was quite effective in helping to frame the legislative debate over CDC's budget in a way that made increasing CDC's funding a way to reinforce the most important core values of policy makers. Rather than focusing on big government, government interference, infringement of civil liberties, interference with free enterprise, and economic hardship, the debate focused on the threat posed to the health and security of the entire nation if CDC was not funded to continue and expand its work in protecting the public from Ebola and other killer viruses.

Thus, it was not truly the importance of improving health that motivated increased CDC funding. Had this been the case, the debate should have focused on the diseases that are really the major causes of suffering for Americans: those related to tobacco, alcohol, motor vehicle accidents, acquired immunodeficiency syndrome (AIDS), and firearms. Instead, the debate focused on diseases affecting relatively few Americans, including one disease (Ebola virus infection) that has never been reported in a human being in the United States!

In reality, Ebola virus posed little threat to the health of anyone in America. As Dr. Margaretha Isaacson stated, "Ebola is of absolutely no danger to the world at large. It is a dangerous virus, but it's relatively rare and quite easily contained" (Regis, 1996, p. 235). And as Ed Regis (1996) noted in *Virus Ground Zero,* "the fact of the matter was that Ebola hemorrhagic fever, along with Marburg and Lassa, were diseases of poverty and bad hospitals. Although they thrived momentarily when they erupted in such environments, those same viruses were stopped cold every time they turned up in well-equipped medical institutions, whether in developed countries or elsewhere" (p. 235).

By reminding policy makers of our human frailty, our vulnerability, and our lack of control over our environment, the Ebola virus outbreak in Zaire did help public health practitioners to more effectively frame the important role that the institution of public health plays in our society. With a consistent theme, horrifying metaphors, recognizable and popular catch phrases, graphic visual images, and a strong appeal to the basic human desire for control over one's environment, the killer virus frame played a key role in CDC's success in securing funding for its role in preserving and protecting the public's health.

Second, although the framing of the debate over CDC's budget was influenced by many factors, including the many popular books and movies about Ebola virus and other emerging infectious diseases (the epilogue of the book *Ebola* was actually printed in the *Congressional Record*), the CDC itself made a calculated attempt to influence this framing. For example, an article on smoking initiation among youth in the United States (CDC, 1995b) was pulled from the *Morbidity and Mortality Weekly Report* two days before its scheduled publication to make room for a report on the Ebola virus outbreak in Zaire (CDC, 1995a). This article, which appeared on May 19, 1995, was strategically placed so that it would appear several days before Congressional budget hearings on CDC funding. The media coverage resulting from the Ebola virus article directly influenced the way that public health and CDC were framed in the Congressional hearings.

For example, a May 19, 1995, article from *The Los Angeles Times* was entitled "CDC Lab Sees Budget Cuts as Deadly Threat; Health Officials Warn That the Agency's Ability To Do Its Job as the World's Premier Facility for Tracking and Controlling Disease Is at Stake" (Cimons, 1995, p. A4). The article framed CDC funding as an issue of need to protect the security of the nation from devastating threats like that posed by the Ebola virus. Although only a small fraction of CDC's effort is dedicated to controlling Ebola virus, the article suggested that the Ebola virus outbreak in Zaire had exposed the need to bolster funding for the entire CDC. Not only CDC's role in preventing the spread of viral disease was in jeopardy, so was "the agency's ability to do its job as the world's premier facility for tracking and controlling [all] disease" (Cimons, 1995).

The release of CDC's article on the Ebola virus resulted in articles in several major newspapers that framed the outbreak as an indication of the need for greatly increased funding for CDC's laboratories, and as a sign of the important role that CDC plays not only in protecting health, but in protecting the nation's security. On May 20, 1995, articles that framed the issue in this way appeared in the *Austin American-Statesman* (Altman, 1995), *The Commercial Appeal (Memphis)* ("Cuts Threaten CDC's Health, Agency Warns," 1995), and *The Dallas Morning News* ("Key Disease-Fighting Lab Fears Fund Loss," 1995).

Perhaps more importantly, CDC's funding crisis was the topic of a May 20 feature news story on the Cable News Network (CNN; CNN, 1995). On this show, Dr. David Satcher, CDC director, stated that "people here will pack their bags at a moment's notice to go anywhere in the world to fight diseases. I mean, it's just the attitude of CDC people. It's a shame, you know, that people like that are not supported in terms of facilities and other things that they need" (CNN, 1995). The chair of the House Appropriations Committee, Representative John Porter, also was interviewed. He stated that "recently, and very recently, it seems as if people in Congress are becoming much more aware of the critical nature of emerging infections and the importance of the CDC strategy" (CNN, 1995).

The media's framing of the Ebola virus outbreak in Zaire as a potential threat to the widespread health of the nation resulted in CDC's Ebola hotline being flooded with hundreds of calls a day (Rochell, 1995). And the widespread concern, and in some cases paranoia, about the threat of emerging infectious diseases among the public translated into political pressure to increase CDC's funding, in spite of the budget slashing that affected nearly every other major federal agency during the 104th Congress.

Officials at CDC readily acknowledge that they "take advantage" of disease outbreaks to secure increased funding (Regis, 1996). In *Virus Ground Zero*, Ed Regis (1996) quoted former CDC director Justin Andrews: "We took advantage of every crisis. When Asian flu came along, we were at the door asking for more money. When the staphylococcus scare appeared, we asked for more money and got it" (p. 27). Regis (1996) stated that "any new disease outbreak, furthermore, could be turned into proof that the CDC was not yet big enough, and into an opportunity for making additional funding requests" (p. 27).

This strategy is actually an example of using marketing principles to sell public health more than it is one of political opportunism. In fact, by tying funding requests to new disease outbreaks, public health practitioners are able to effectively define, package, position, and frame their product and to remind policy makers just what it really is that public health offers them. They are able to use these disease outbreaks to remind policy makers that they are not just selling health; they are selling freedom from the unknown, control over a universal threat to survival, security against a national or global catastrophe that could occur at any time.

As Regis (1996) explained, Dr. Joseph Mountin, director of the office of Malaria Control in War Areas (MCWA, the predecessor of CDC), used this approach to convince Congress to fund a new Communicable Disease Center, the CDC, in 1946 when the end of World War II meant the closure of the MCWA office. "The new entity would be called the Communicable Disease Center and would concentrate on helping the states deal with a variety of local health problems. Congress would have to fund this new project, but who in the House or Senate could resist, especially after Mountin and his men went into action handing out photographs of MCWA sprayer-equipped jeeps rolling through peaceful suburban streets and parks, protecting Southern belles and fine American males from the *Anopheles* mosquito. It would be like voting against God or nature" (p. 28).

Note that although the image of Mountin's staff fighting malaria was the critical part of the frame that was successful in eliciting funding for the establishment of

CDC, the functions of the new agency would go far beyond the control of malaria. Similarly, the use of the Ebola virus scare to help frame the need for CDC resulted in increased funding not only for the level 4 laboratory that studies the virus, but for CDC divisions across the board.

Fred Kroger, director of CDC's Office of Health Communication, noted the intuitive use of marketing principles by public health leaders at CDC in their translation of the threat of emerging infections, including Ebola virus infection, into increased funding for all areas of CDC activity. In a chapter entitled "Marketing Public Health: The CDC Experience," Kroger and colleagues suggested that "a good topic for a future conference might be a case study of CDC's strategic efforts to translate the very real threat of emerging infections, as underscored by the recent outbreak of Ebola fever in equatorial Africa, into financial support for the hemorrhaging infrastructure of the U.S. public health system, from a Congress that has been openly hostile to funding increases for 'social' programs" (Kroger, McKenna, Shepherd, Howze, & Knight, 1997, p. 268).

In some ways, the marketing of CDC as an essential societal institution for protection of the public's health and the nation's security parallels the marketing of public health during its initiation as a societal institution in the nineteenth century. In both cases, it was not the threat of disease itself that led to public action. Rather, it was the threat of uncontrolled disease that could affect all citizens, rich and poor, and therefore constituted a universal threat to the ability of citizens to live in freedom from plague, independent of the yoke of epidemic disease, and in control of their lives. It is this sense of universal vulnerability and this sense of a threat to autonomy and control that resonated so deeply with the core values of policy makers.

As Frank Ryan (1997) explained in *Virus X*, it is not merely the concept of disease, but the fear induced by a threat of loss of control that makes infectious disease so alarming.

> It is an altogether normal reaction when the ordinary man or woman retracts in horror at the thought of microbes invading and destroying their body. Such microbes threaten us. Every parent knows the terror when a child develops a high temperature and the fear of loss strikes deeply into the heart. . . . For the moment, mercifully, most germs are still sensitive to antibiotics, and that means most bacterial infections remain eminently curable. . . . A new epidemic, caused by an emerging virus, is potentially more threatening because it does not lie within human control. (p. 139)

While substance abuse, violence, injury, and poverty can be viewed as affecting "other people," the newly emerging infectious diseases were seen as representing a threat from which no one could escape. As summarized by the Institute of Medicine panel on emerging infectious diseases, "as the human immunodeficiency virus (HIV) pandemic surely should have taught us, in the context of infectious diseases, there is nowhere in the world from which we are remote and no one from whom we are disconnected" (Lederberg, Shope, & Oaks, 1992). What a sensational marketing pitch for public health. And the Ebola virus presented a perfect opportunity to make that pitch. Because any two points on earth are within 24 hours of each other by airplane, "what that meant was that the Ebola virus was now no more than twenty-four hours away from you. Your own home—your very own neighborhood—was only a day away from the Ebola virus!" (Regis, 1996, p. 57).

To use this marketing strategy effectively, public health practitioners must first understand how policy makers and the public view public health as an institution and identify their needs and desires in terms of their views of public health protection. Formative research is needed specifically to identify ways that might be effective to market public health as an institution. This research process was initiated recently in three ways. First, the CDC initiated a long-term effort to better market public health. The first step was to conduct polling and focus groups to identify the public's perceptions of the role and function of public health. Fred Kroger and colleagues explains that the "CDC, in collaboration with a number of public health partners, has initiated a long-term effort to better tell the public health story. One of the initial steps was to task Macro International Inc. and Westat Inc., contractors for health communications evaluation, to gauge the public's understanding of public health's role, to identify misconceptions, and to identify potential strategies for strengthening the marketing abilities of these public health partners" (Kroger et al., 1997, pp. 273, 274). Second, a Harris poll was conducted to assess national public opinion concerning the role, function, and benefits of public health as an institution (CDC, 1998; Taylor, 1997). Third, the Field Institute conducted a similar survey of public opinion concerning public health in California (CDC, 1998).

The results of CDC's focus groups were encouraging. Although they "confirmed the belief that public health is largely invisible," they also revealed "a readily stimulated reservoir of appreciation for the services of public health, within the public in general and among elected officials in particular" (Kroger et al., 1997, p. 274). The research revealed that "personal health benefits can be seen, even by persons who do not use public health services directly" (Kroger et al., 1997, p. 274).

Similarly, the Harris and Field polls found that an overwhelming majority of Americans attach a great deal of importance to the core functions of public health. For example, 93% of adults believe that the "prevention of the spread of infectious diseases like tuberculosis, measles, flu and AIDS" is very important; 90% believe immunization is very important; 83% believe that improving the quality of education and employment is very important; 82% believe that ensuring that people are not exposed to unsafe water, air pollution, or toxic waste is very important; and 82% believe that conducting research into the causes and methods to prevent disease is very important (Taylor, 1997). Although the public recognizes these functions as being important, they do not appreciate the fact that these are the core functions of public health. Only 1% of adults listed health education and promotion of healthy lifestyles as a core public health function (Taylor, 1997). Similarly, only 1% of adults listed the prevention of infectious disease or immunization as core functions of public health. Instead, most people interpreted public health as referring to the provision and reimbursement of medical care or welfare (47%) or to the overall health of the public in general (36%).

In a recent article in the *Morbidity and Mortality Weekly Report* (CDC, 1998), the CDC Public Health Practice Program Office summarized the results of these polls and concluded the following:

> Interest in marketing public health has been stimulated by perceived low public support for public health activities, limited financial resources, and the impact of extensive restructuring in the health-care sector. The findings in this report indicate substantial public support for public health services and suggest the need to determine the extent to which this support is consistent across jurisdictions and whether it can be translated into policy. Finally, these findings suggest the need for strengthened methods to improve the polling of opinion about public health, including clarifications of the distinction between clinical care and community- or population-oriented disease and injury prevention, and the practical meanings of "public health," "community health," and other key terms. (pp. 72, 73)

These initial efforts to begin the formative research process for marketing public health as an institution are promising. They reveal the potential to use the principles of marketing to compete successfully for public attention and resources.

CONCLUSION

The way in which public health in general, and CDC in particular, were defined and framed during the 104th Congress demonstrates many of the principles in the preceding chapters of this book. It shows how public health practitioners must not rely on their own intuition to define public health and the role of their agencies, but must instead base their definition of the public health product on formative research that explores the needs and desires of policy makers. It illustrates how public health practitioners must frame their programs and institutions in a way that satisfies an existing need among policy makers. The public health practitioner must offer a benefit and communicate an image of the public health institution that reinforces the most influential core values of policy makers: freedom, independence, autonomy, control, and security.

The basic principles the public health practitioner must apply to successfully market changes in individual behavior, adoption of public health programs and policies, and support for public health as a societal institution are now outlined and illustrated. It is in the public health campaign that the public health practitioner has the challenge and opportunity to put the strategic marketing theory and principles into action. The second part of this book presents a detailed, step-by-step guide to the planning, implementation, evaluation, and refinement of public health campaigns. It shows how the principles discussed in this first part of the book can be applied to each of these components of a public health campaign.

REFERENCES

Altman, L.K. (1995, May 20). Cutbacks at U.S. agency strain aid for Ebola crisis. *Austin American-Statesman*, p. A5.

Cable News Network. (1995, May 20). *Centers for Disease Control building shows age*. Atlanta, GA: Author.

Centers for Disease Control and Prevention. (1995a). Outbreak of Ebola viral hemorrhagic fever—Zaire, 1995. *Morbidity and Mortality Weekly Report, 44*, 381–382.

Centers for Disease Control and Prevention. (1995b). Trends in smoking initiation among adolescents and young adults—United States, 1980–1989. *Morbidity and Mortality Weekly Report, 44*, 521–525.

Centers for Disease Control and Prevention. (1998). Public opinion about public health—California and the United States, 1996. *Morbidity and Mortality Weekly Report, 47*, 69–73.

Cimons, M. (1995, May 19). CDC lab sees budget cuts as deadly threat; Health officials warn that the Agency's ability to do its job as the world's premier facility for tracking and controlling disease is at stake. *The Los Angeles Times*, p. A4.

Cuts threaten CDC's health, agency warns. (1995, May 20). *The Commercial Appeal (Memphis)*, p. 5A.

Henig, R.M. (1997). *The people's health: A memoir of public health and its evolution at Harvard*. Washington, DC: Joseph Henry Press.

Key disease-fighting lab fears fund loss; CDC says cuts would hurt epidemic battle. (1995, May 20). *The Dallas Morning News*, p. 7A.

Kroger, F., McKenna, J.W., Shepherd, M., Howze, E.H., & Knight, D.S. (1997). Marketing public health: The CDC experience. In M.E. Goldberg, M. Fishbein, & S.E. Middlestadt (Eds.), *Social marketing: Theoretical and practical perspectives* (pp. 267–290). Mahwah, NJ: Lawrence Erlbaum Associates.

Lederberg, J., Shope, R.E., & Oaks, S.C., Jr. (Eds.). (1992). *Emerging infections: Microbial threats to health in the United States*. Washington, DC: National Academy Press.

McGee, D.E. (1996). Emerging meanings: Science, the media, and infectious diseases. *Journal of the American Medical Association, 276*, 1095–1097.

Peters, C.J., & Olshaker, M. (1997). *Virus hunter. Thirty years of battling hot viruses around the world*. New York: Doubleday.

Regis, E. (1996). *Virus ground zero: Stalking the killer viruses with the Centers for Disease Control.* New York: Pocket Books.

Rochell, A. (1995, May 19). "Hot Zone" author cool to Zaire trip: No desire to see Ebola firsthand. *The Atlanta Journal and Constitution,* p. A3.

Ryan, F. (1997). *Virus X. Tracking the new killer plagues out of the present and into the future.* Boston: Little, Brown.

Taylor, H. (1997). *Public health: Two words few people understand even though almost everyone thinks public health functions are very important.* New York: Louis Harris and Associates.

APPENDIX 8–A

Excerpts from the Congressional Record, 104th Congress

Why Africa Matters: Emerging Diseases (Page S9009)
United States Senate
July 29, 1996
Senator Nancy Kassebaum (R-KS)

Today, I will begin with an issue of particular concern to me—emerging infectious diseases. Last year, I chaired a hearing of the Senate Labor Committee on Emerging Infections: A Threat to the Health of a Nation. The focus of the hearing was on domestic vulnerability to disease, but international issues—especially those involving Africa–surfaced again and again.

It is impossible to isolate the domestic epidemiological situation from a larger global context. Microbes simply do not observe political boundaries.

Mr. President, the sheer volume of human contact at the approaching turn of the century creates a situation in which no country or class is immune from the threat of disease. In 1993, over 27 million people traveled from the United States and Canada to developing countries. The incubation period of most epidemic diseases far exceeds the duration of most international flights. No state can test all entering persons for every known disease. Even secure borders cannot stop contaminated water, food, or animal vectors from transmitting microbes across boundaries.

For example, international trade was the mechanism by which a strain of the Ebola virus, previously confined to central Africa, surfaced in Reston, VA, in 1989, and in Texas in 1996. The devastating effects of Ebola's hemorrhagic fever, and the mysteries surrounding its transmission, have created a sense of fear and insecurity around the world since the 1995 outbreak in Zaire. Yet Ebola represents

---

Source: Reprinted from The Congressional Record, 104th United States Congress.

only one of a number of new diseases which present a threat to all of mankind—at least 30 new infectious diseases have emerged in the last 20 years. . . .

In the 1990s, a review of CDC surveillance systems determined them to be woefully inadequate within the United States, and so haphazard as to be nonexistent abroad. . . .

Mr. President, at the Labor Committee hearing last year, Dr. David Satcher, Director of the Centers for Disease Control and Prevention, indicated that CDC received the first report of the 1994 Ebola outbreak in Zaire in May of that year, but the first case probably occurred in January.

Early warning systems simply did not exist. . . .

This is just one reason, Mr. President, why Africa does matter to us. I suggest it is a security threat, as well as a personal threat, and one that we should care about with interest and compassion, as we look to our own budgets, and as we look to our own strategists.

50th Anniversary of the CDC (Page E1197)
United States House of Representatives
June 27, 1996
Representative Henry Waxman (D-CA)

As CDC celebrates a half century of public health excellence, we are mindful of the skill and courage of these early public health pioneers, who risked their lives in order to address environmental hazards and control diseases such as smallpox, polio, malaria, and diphtheria. We are honored to continue on in their work and committed to the difficult challenges that lie ahead.

CDC has contributed to the control of infectious diseases such as the Ebola outbreak in Africa and tuberculosis in the United States. We also have protected workers from environmental hazards, improved early detection and control systems for breast cancer and cervical cancer, recommended fortification of foods with folic acid to prevent birth defects, and conducted research to identify potential dangers of airbags to infants. . . .

The anniversary is a milestone for our Nation. It is a sobering reminder of the challenges we face as we enter the 21st century, when, clearly, public health will be a global concern. Increased disruption to the tropical environment will result in diseases that are no longer contained in a localized habitat but, rather, migrate with their human hosts to cities and neighboring continents. The mobility of people, through air travel, natural disaster, or civil war, is reshaping the routes of infections and the course of epidemics.

The 50th Anniversary of the Centers for Disease Control and Prevention
   (Page S7298)
United States Senate
June 28, 1996
Senator Bill Frist (R-TN)

Mr. President, in the United States and around the world, the words "Centers for Disease Control and Prevention" are synonymous with public health. What started in 1946 as a small and comparatively insignificant branch of the Public Health Service, established to prevent the spread of malaria, is today one of the most highly regarded agencies in the Federal Government—an agency whose interests include every communicable disease known to man, and whose mission is to protect the public health by providing practical help whenever and wherever it is called upon to do so.

Over the years, the CDC has become more than just a center for disease control. As early as the 1950's, it became a center of epidemiology, providing surveillance of known diseases and ferreting out the cause of new ones wherever they occurred. From influenza, polio, tuberculosis, and smallpox in the United States to, more recently, Ebola fever in Zaire, the CDC has answered SOS calls from all over the world, and become not only a global leader in public health, but the Nation's and the world's response team for a wide range of health emergencies.

The 50th Anniversary of the CDC (Page S7298)
United States Senate
June 28, 1996
Senator Edward Kennedy (D-MA)

I commend the agency for its extraordinary contributions to the Nation and the world. We need its leadership now, more than ever. New public health challenges await us in the future. Diseases and disasters are no longer easily confined to their place of origin, and wars and natural disasters create new opportunities for the spread of infectious diseases. The lessons of the past 50 years have taught us that we must expect the unexpected. Whether the issue is fighting Ebola outbreaks in Africa, the reemergence of drug-resistant tuberculosis in the United States, or many other public health threats, we know the Centers for Disease Control and Prevention will be at the forefront of the worldwide effort to combat them.

Happy Birthday, Centers for Disease Control (CDC) (Page E1198)
United States House of Representatives
June 27, 1996
Representative John Dingell (D-MI)

Unlike many other excellent health institutions, such as the National Cancer Institute or the Food and Drug Administration, CDC is only infrequently in the limelight. But it is that very fact which provides confidence, for the lack of CDC headlines means that we are not facing a crisis requiring urgent expert action. When we do not hear about the epidemiologists, worker safety specialists, immunization gurus, laboratory scientists, and infectious disease experts of CDC, it is because they are doing quietly and efficiently what they have done every day for the last 50 years—protecting the public health.

But when we do hear about CDC, we know we are facing an urgent crisis—but that crisis is being handled expertly—whether it is the occurrence of a mysterious infectious disease, later called Legionnaire's disease in Philadelphia, or the first case of AIDS in San Francisco; illness and death from food contaminated with *E. coli* in the States of Washington, California, Idaho, and Nevada; measles epidemics in major metropolitan areas across the United States; *Cryptosporidium* in Milwaukee drinking water; serious illness from oysters in Florida; an outbreak of hanta virus in New Mexico, Utah, Arizona, and Colorado; the reemergence of tuberculosis as a serious health risk, especially in New York, Miami, and Los Angeles; or lead poisoning in children in Chicago and Rhode Island.

While CDC has been catapulted only recently onto suburban movie screens because it inspired "The Hot Zone," the agency has over its 50-year history, cooled off many hot zones with its unique expertise and capability. CDC assists governments and health officials all over the world in preventing and controlling disease and responding to crises that literally threaten the health and safety of entire populations of people—Ebola virus in Zaire; deadly chemical release in a Tokyo subway; disease-causing radioactive fallout in the Marshall Islands; outbreaks in Spain of illness from contaminated cooking oil; worldwide immunization efforts to prevent deadly childhood and adult illnesses such as smallpox—now completely eradicated because of these efforts; typhoid fever, and polio. . . .

I am proud to have supported the work of CDC over many of its 50 years. Congress and the American people have entrusted one of our most precious possessions to this remarkable agency—the public health.

Budget Impasse and Centers for Disease Control (Page S63)
United States Senate
January 4, 1996
Senator Sam Nunn (D-GA)

Mr. President, there are many examples of the harm being done by the shutdown. One example which has not drawn much attention is the fact that the U.S. Centers for Disease Control and Prevention, the CDC in Atlanta, GA, is virtually shut down. Today is the 50th year of operation of the Communicable Disease

Center, and it is effectively closed. Except for a skeleton staff, no personnel are available to fulfill the functions of the CDC.

This is bound to have an impact on the health and safety of the American people and, indeed, citizens around the world. The workers at the CDC are the same Federal workers who pinpointed the cause of Legionnaire's disease and toxic shock syndrome. These are the same men and women who risked their lives to investigate the recent outbreak of Ebola and track the course of influenza, AIDS, and TB across the nation and indeed the world. Their job is to investigate, to define, to monitor and to prevent disease—to get out in front of emerging infectious diseases, food and waterborne diseases, respiratory infections, birth defects, lead poisoning, air pollution, radiation, and other environmental health emergencies.

The problem in this area is you do not know it is an emergency if you are not out in front of it before it is too late. We will be lucky if we get by with this shutdown and closedown of the CDC without having some serious problem and erosion in the health of the American people.

In some cases, the CDC implements control measures during a critical time when minutes and even seconds count. Rarely a week passes by without the CDC directing the Nation's attention to important new research findings on public health issues. At this point, we do not know what public health crisis will emerge in 1996. With a CDC shutdown, we do not know what might be happening right now. What we do know is that the CDC plays a critical role in watching for signs and sustaining sophisticated surveillance and monitoring communications with medical health officers in our Nation and throughout the world. We do not know the impact of the Government shutdown on the health of the U.S. citizens. We may not know until it is too late.

Like other Federal employees, the people in CDC are deeply dedicated, hardworking persons, scientists, physicians, and public health professionals. Some even risk their lives to investigate outbreaks of unknown, sometimes even deadly diseases. These people are protecting the Nation's health and they are anxious to return to their jobs. . . .

We cannot afford to wait to open the doors at the CDC. The health of the Nation and the world could be at stake.

The 50th Anniversary of the Centers for Disease Control and Prevention
   (Page E1193)
United States House of Representatives
June 27, 1996
Representative Edward Markey (D-MA)

CDC has been faced with a host of challenges over the last half century, and the many scientists and public health professionals who make this relatively small agency a force to be reckoned with have never failed to rise to those challenges. Utilizing a technique for investigating disease outbreaks, "Hot Zone" author Richard Preston has called the marriage of great labs with shoe-leather disease detective work, CDC has taken on epidemics around the globe. The threat of emerging infectious diseases that our Nation and the world now faces becomes somewhat less alarming when we remind ourselves of the unflagging courage and unfailing efforts of the devoted professionals at CDC who stand ready to fight back.

Departments of Labor, Health and Human Services, and Education, and
   Related Agencies Appropriations Act (Page H8316)
United States House of Representatives
August 3, 1995
Representative Dan Miller (R-FL)

Mr. Chairman, this bill is an integral part of our effort to balance the budget, the moral and economic challenge of our time. This bill meets its share of the burden and therefore deserves every Member's support. These are the tough choices we are having to make to balance this budget. . . .

By setting priorities, we eliminated programs that do not work and strengthened ones that do. Spending taxpayer dollars on useless programs is not compassion. Balancing the budget and setting priorities is real and true compassion. There are many programs which we found to be essential.

Some of these include the five prevention programs within the Centers for Disease Control which all received increases above their 1995 funding levels. The first is the breast and cervical cancer screening program. The subcommittee's recommended increase of $25 million, which goes from $100 to $125 million, will provide enough funding to permit the expansion of this program into all States, thereby allowing greater access for low-income, high-risk women to receive screening and referral services for the detection of breast and cervical cancer at earlier and more treatable stages.

The prevention program of infectious disease received over a 20-percent increase. This additional funding is intended to provide sorely needed resources to the CDC for addressing such monumental problems as the Ebola virus and *E. coli* which we have all heard so much about lately.

Additionally, the bill increases funds for chronic and environmental disease prevention and sexually transmitted disease prevention by $15 million. This will permit enhancement of programs such as diabetes control and education, cancer registries, birth defects, disabilities, and other diseases.

Finally, the subcommittee provides additional protection for our most important resource: Children. The Childhood Immunization Program has gone from $465 million to $475 million, a $10 million increase, which will permit the CDC to purchase more vaccines, expand clinic hours, and provide increased outreach opportunities ensuring vaccination for previously unreachable children.

Mr. Chairman, this bill does fund those items in which the Federal Government has a legitimate and necessary role. AIDS prevention has gone from $569 million to $595 million. The Ryan White Program, the AIDS Treatment Program, goes from $633 million to $656 million. Overall, the bill increases funding for prevention programs by $63 million. This is $63 million which will go toward assisting low-income women and children to achieve better health care and $63 million which will go toward securing the safety of our Nation by protecting us from infectious diseases.

Statements on Funding for the NIH
United States Senate
May 25, 1995
Submitted by National Institutes of Health

The National Institutes of Health (NIH) is establishing a "New and Re-emerging Infectious Disease Initiative." This initiative addresses the threat of new microbes (such as Ebola virus and HIV), re-emerging infectious diseases (such as cholera and hantavirus), and drug-resistant strains of previously treatable infections (such as tuberculosis and streptococcus). The focal point of this initiative will be the development of vaccines, the most cost-effective and dependable method to combat new and re-emerging infectious diseases, particularly in light of increasing resistance to virtually all of the currently available antibiotics.

The NIH is uniquely positioned to launch this initiative because of its many infectious disease research collaborations with the World Health Organization, the Centers for Disease Control, the Agency for International Development and many individual nations. All of these collaborations assist in the attempt to identify and to control outbreaks of emerging and re-emerging microbes. . . .

Effects of a Budget Cut: A budget cut would curtail or significantly slow all of these efforts, both the launching of the "New and Re-emerging Infectious Diseases Initiative" and the continuation of NIH's network of national and international tropical, parasitic, and primate research centers. International collaborations are especially vulnerable to budget cuts, but the ongoing crisis concerning the Ebola virus demonstrates the obvious need for sustained, stable funding.

The seriousness of this challenge cannot be overstated. Events of the past year have demonstrated our increasing vulnerability to infectious diseases that may rapidly assume epidemic proportions. Many new and re-emerging microbes threaten our Nation's health. Vaccine development, continued international collaboration, and rapid identification of new strains are our best hope for the future.

Unanimous Consent Agreement
United States Senate
May 22, 1995
Senator Barbara Mikulski (D-MD)

Let us go to the Centers for Disease Control. We now know Ebola virus threatens Zaire and could even possibly threaten the world.

We had a near outbreak in something called The Hot Zone in northern Virginia. If you read the book, you know what the story was. It was Federal employees at Fort Dietrick who were willing to risk their lives—who were willing to go into the hot zone to kill the monkeys that carried this disease.

When you read the newspaper accounts—this is not Mikulski memos, this is newspaper accounts—that talk about how skimpy the resources are at CDC and in infectious diseases, they are stretched so thin that they are now afraid an accident could happen at the CDC exactly at the same time when we are asking for their help. The world is asking for their help to come and take care of the Ebola virus.

Let us talk about other threats to the safety and security of the United States.

Concurrent Resolution on the Budget
May 24, 1995
United States Senate
Senator Mark Hatfield (R-OR)

If my friends are not interested in the humanitarian aspect of reducing suffering and putting the value on human life—and quality life, not just quantitative life—I hope we would support this because I am convinced it is the answer. If you are not impressed with that factor, then look at the cost. We have saved billions of dollars per year in what we have been able to accomplish in medical research with TB. Now we are having a revival of TB. We have Zaire and the Ebola problem over there, that is a threat to this country. Every time we used to want to get an increase in military spending we could say, "The Russians are coming," and, boy, everybody would jack up another $1 million. I want to tell you, "The viruses are coming." They are here. And we better get ready for that warfare because we need this kind of weaponry to fight it.

Senator Barbara Boxer (D-CA)

Now, it hurts my heart to vote to cut other domestic programs. It breaks my heart. I think it is outrageous that we do not have the votes here to include defense in a small cut, but like the Senator from Oregon I am a realist. I am a realist, and I wish to see this funding be restored to the NIH. We are one plane ride away from a major epidemic. We read with horror about this Ebola virus. Anyone who has read the book "The Hot Zone" understands the tenuous position we are in in this very world in which we now live. As we lose the rain forests of the world, what scientists are discovering is that viruses that live in the rain forests are looking for other hosts, and they are finding us. So to cut back on the National Institutes of Health, which is our first line of defense against these diseases, would be worse than outrageous.

Concurrent Resolution on the Budget
United States Senate
May 18, 1995
Senator Barbara Boxer (D-CA)

Under current funding, for every four grants that are approved—in other words, if scientists come forward with a good possibility of finding a cure for a disease, one in four of those applications is approved. I wish we could approve and fund all four. We can fund one in four. Under this Republican budget, we will be lucky to fund 1 in 100 new applications—1 in 100. Now, you do not have to be too smart to know that this is shortsighted. We are one plane ride away from disaster. You have read about this Ebola virus. We are one plane ride away from disaster, and we are unilaterally disarming our scientists in this country.

PART II

Using Marketing Principles To Design, Implement, and Evaluate Public Health Interventions

Planning

Adequate planning is at the heart of marketing social change. It is during this stage that the types of changes needed to address a specific problem are identified and prioritized. These changes might include modifications in individual behaviors and lifestyles, improvements in social and economic conditions, and reforms to social or organizational policies. Once changes have been identified and prioritized, a strategic plan for addressing them is developed.

The first two chapters in this section will review the major marketing concepts and present a strategic planning process. The last two chapters will cover activities that are used to support the strategic planning process: conducting formative research and developing strategies to frame messages that appropriately position a social change.

CHAPTER 9

Applying Marketing Principles to Public Health

The principles of marketing provide a disciplined, consumer-focused, research-based process to plan, develop, implement, and assess many different types of social change initiatives designed to improve the public's health. Although marketing social change is much more difficult than marketing commercial products, the basic premise is the same: Develop a solid, strategic approach by positioning and packaging the product (whether it is an individual behavior change, program, policy, or public health itself) and framing messages about it to address the needs, wants, and values of target audience members. Then use this strategy to guide the selection and development of all components of the initiative. However, the traditional marketing concepts of product, price, place, and promotion must be adjusted to address the environment in which social change takes place—and an additional factor must be considered: partners.

——— ઢ ———

THE ROOTS OF MARKETING SOCIAL CHANGE

The idea of using marketing principles to "sell" social changes as diverse as health practices, recycling, volunteerism, and voting has been around for a long time. In an oft-cited article, Weibe noted in the early 1950s that nonbusiness managers see private-sector marketing communications and ask, "Why can't you sell brotherhood like soap?" We see the answer as twofold: First, unfortunately, it isn't that easy; selling social change is much more difficult than selling soap, for reasons presented in Chapter 2 and later in this chapter. Second, 25 years of adapting basic marketing principles to public health interventions has taught us that the marketing approach, augmented with tools from other disciplines, provides a sound framework for developing, implementing, and refining social change efforts.

In 1971, Kotler and Zaltman published their landmark article, "Social Marketing: An Approach to Planned Social Change," in which they defined social marketing as "the design, implementation, and control of programs calculated to influence the acceptability of social ideas and involving considerations of product planning, pricing, communication, distribution, and marketing research" (p. 5). The first practical public health applications took an advertising approach (providing informational, or "what to do" messages, such as "stop smoking—it might kill you" but not "here's how to do it" information directed at overcoming barriers or building skills based on research with the audience), as Fox and Kotler observed in a 1980 retrospective. They noted that the social advertising approach then evolved to social communication (making greater use of personal selling and editorial support in addition to mass advertising), and finally, a true marketing approach characterized by (1) marketing research—what we refer to in this book as formative research—to understand the potential size of the market, the major groups or segments within it, and their corresponding behavioral characteristics; (2) product development, in terms of searching for the best product to meet the need, rather than using a sales approach of trying to sell an existing product; (3) using incentives; and (4) facilitating behavior change by considering ways to make adoption of the behavior easier.

In the intervening years, many investigators have analyzed how applying marketing principles to social change differs from commercial product marketing. Most contemporary definitions of social change marketing emphasize behavior change as the product being marketed and social good as the motivation of the marketer. The definition that may be used most often today was put forth by Alan Andreasen in 1995:

> Social marketing is the application of commercial marketing technologies to the analysis, planning, execution, and evaluation of programs designed to influence the voluntary behavior of target audiences in order to improve their personal welfare and that of their society. (p. 7)

This definition embodies five principles for applying marketing to social change and distinguishes the marketing approach from other approaches often used:

1. conducting formative research to understand the consumer
2. influencing behavior change (rather than simply trying to increase knowledge or change attitudes)
3. developing programs specifically for carefully selected audiences
4. constantly monitoring and refining implementation

5. influencing social behaviors "not to benefit the marketer but *to benefit the target audience and the general society*," as Kotler and Andreasen wrote in 1996 (p. 389)

As we have discussed in earlier chapters, marketing public health can involve (1) marketing individual health behavior changes; (2) marketing specific public health programs; (3) marketing policy changes, including laws and regulatory changes; and (4) marketing public health as an institution. The first type of marketing targets primarily members of the public. The last three types target policy makers as well.

At the most basic level, all of these scenarios involve an individual changing a behavior: a member of the public choosing low-fat foods or getting an immunization; a policy maker supporting a public health program, a proposed law that will protect public health, or the role of public health in the health care system. The same process can be used to develop interventions for each scenario. However, the tools used to bring about change often differ for each scenario, and public health interventions usually include many components in addition to traditional marketing activities. For example, efforts to induce individual behavior change may involve health education, training and technical assistance, and continuing medical education in addition to the marketing tools most visible to nonmarketers (such as packaging and promotion through mass communication). Efforts directed at policy makers often involve media and/or grass-roots advocacy and lobbying.

Our premise in this book is that the marketing approach provides a basic framework from which to develop strategic interventions to bring about social change:

The principles of marketing provide a disciplined, audience-focused, research-based process to plan, develop, implement, and assess interventions designed to influence the behavior change of target audiences in order to improve their personal welfare and/or that of their society.

This statement emphasizes some key aspects of the marketing approach that are often misunderstood or ignored by marketers of social change:

- Marketing (for commercial products or social change) is a *process*, not a theory. In fact, as described in subsequent chapters, marketing encourages the use of many appropriate theories and models of human behavior and behavior change. The marketing process is often depicted as a circle or wheel, to emphasize its cyclical nature, as shown in Figure 9–1.
- The marketing approach emphasizes extensive research in order to understand the point of view of the target audience (whether it is composed of policy makers or members of the public) and develop programs that address their needs and wants rather than only the desires of the sponsoring organization. It also emphasizes evaluation and refinement throughout the life of the program. Hence, research and evaluation are at the core of the process.

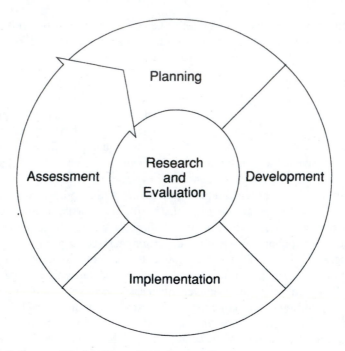

Figure 9–1 Stages of Social Change Initiatives

KEY CONCEPTS FROM COMMERCIAL MARKETING

To successfully apply marketing principles to public health programs, one must first understand some of the key concepts underlying commercial marketing. In particular, the cost benefit exchange; the emphasis on behavior change and the consumer; and the role of product, price, place, and promotion (the four Ps that form the marketing mix) must be grasped.

The Cost Benefit Exchange

As discussed in Chapter 2, marketers believe that the notion of exchange plays a central role in the choices people make: A person gives something in order to get something in exchange. For example, if you are walking down the street on a hot day and you pass a lemonade stand, you might pay $1 and get a glass of lemonade. But you are actually buying much more than the glass of lemonade. The glass of lemonade provides a specific benefit—a way of quenching thirst—and you determine that quenching thirst is worth $1. When marketers think of exchanges, they think of what is given as the cost, or price, of that which is received, which is the benefit. The actual product is often merely a means of obtaining the desired benefit.

To illustrate benefits further, let's change our example a bit. You're still walking down the street on that hot day, but instead of a lemonade stand, you encounter a convenience store with many types of drinks. When deciding which drink to purchase, you weigh the costs of each against the benefits of each. The costs may be more than financial; for example, calories are a cost if you are watching your weight; therefore, water or a diet soft drink would be a low-cost choice. And benefits beyond thirst-quenching ability are likely to come into play. Perhaps you like one type of drink better than another, or perhaps one is 100% fruit juice and therefore has the added benefit of being better for you than others. But perhaps the 100% fruit juice is also more expensive. Now you must compare the water, diet soft drink, and juice and decide whether the juice's added health benefit outweighs its additional calories and higher price.

As these examples illustrate, regardless of the type of exchange, people go through a process of weighing the benefits they attach to a product (tangible and intangible) against the costs (again, costs may be tangible, such as money, and intangible, such as time or status) before making an exchange. The benefits must outweigh the costs for a person to complete the transaction. These mental transactions can become quite complex, particularly when (as is often the case) people are being asked to replace an existing behavior. In such cases, they must calculate the costs and benefits associated with their existing behavior and the costs and benefits associated with the new behavior, then compare the two before making a decision. Chapters 3 and 6 discussed the important role that core values—such as freedom, independence, autonomy, and control—play in how people perceive and evaluate costs and benefits.

This notion of trading off benefits and costs is not unique to the marketing approach; many commonly used models and theories of health behavior change incorporate similar concepts. For example, one of the most widely used models of health behavior, the health belief model (Strecher & Rosenstock, 1997) posits that individuals

> will take action to ward off, to screen for, or to control an ill-health condition if they regard themselves as susceptible to the condition, if they believe it to have potentially serious consequences, if they believe that a course of action available to them would be beneficial in reducing either their susceptibility to or the severity of the condition, and *if they believe that the anticipated barriers to (or costs of) taking the action are outweighed by the benefits* [italics added]. (p. 44)

Similarly, the transtheoretical model of stages of change includes a decisional balance construct described as the pros and cons, or benefits and costs, of changing a behavior (Prochaska, Redding, & Evers, 1997). The model will be described in greater detail in Chapter 10. The basic premise is that individuals go through a series of stages in making a behavior change (precontemplation to contemplation to preparation to action to maintenance and, for some behaviors, finally to termination). After studying 12 problem behaviors, Prochaska concluded that progression through the stages—to the point of taking action—is related to quantifiable changes in the cost benefit equation. More specifically, progressing from precontemplation to action involves approximately a .5 standard deviation decrease in the cons, or costs, of changing; progressing from contemplation to action involves approximately one standard deviation increase in the pros of changing (Prochaska, 1994; Prochaska et al., 1997). Discussing these changes, Prochaska (1994) noted that

> the pros and cons of behavior change are likely to be crucial for progress across the first four stages of change, in part because they represent an interaction of individual psychology and public health policy. The pros and cons for the 12 behaviors [studied] are assumed to assess the individual's internal representations of the actual consequences of changing high-risk behaviors. Those representations are clearly related to the individual's stage of change. The internal representations are probably also related to the society's readiness to change public policies, to increase the pros of healthy behavior changes and the cons of not changing. (pp. 50–51)

Another theory that includes the concept of costs and benefits is the social cognitive theory, which is often used to shape public health interventions. Its basic premise is that behavior is determined by a series of reciprocal interactions among the behavior, personal factors, and environmental influences (Bandura, 1986). It will be discussed in more detail in Chapter 10, but one of the concepts incorporated in the theory is the notion of outcome expectancies (or what Bandura called *incentives*), which are defined as "the *values* that a person places on a particular behavior. . . . Expectancies influence behavior according to the hedonic principle; that is, if all other things are equal, a person will choose to perform an activity that maximizes a positive outcome or minimizes a negative outcome" (Baranowski, Perry, & Parcel, 1997, p. 163).

It is important to point out that from both a marketing standpoint and from the standpoint of the health behavior models described above, the only relevant costs and benefits are those that are important to the consumer—and, in some instances, one consumer's cost might be another's benefit. In our example above, calories were considered a cost by our hypothetical consumer. Another consumer might consider calories a benefit, and a third might not think of them at all when assessing the costs and benefits of different beverages. It is easy to make the mistake of assuming that benefits to the public's health will be perceived as benefits by individuals being asked to make a change. Often they are not—or are not important enough to affect the balance of a transaction.

The marketer's job is to

1. get to know the potential consumers, to find out what their current behaviors are and what benefits and costs they attach to a particular exchange.
2. make any needed adjustments to the product, its price, or where customers can obtain it.
3. promote the exchange to consumers such that perceived benefits are maximized and perceived costs are minimized.

As Kotler and Andreasen (1996) put it, "for the marketer to be successful, the customer must believe that the exchange that the marketer is promoting is better than any reasonable alternative—including doing nothing" (p. 111).

Emphasis on Behavior Change

Kotler and Andreasen (1996) noted that "in our view, the bottom line of all marketing strategy and tactics is to influence behavior. Sometimes this necessitates changing ideas and thoughts first, but in the end, it is behavior change we are after. This is an absolutely crucial point. Some nonprofit marketers may think they are in the 'business' of changing *ideas,* but it can legitimately be asked why they should bother if such changes do not lead to action" (p. 110).

Commercial marketers have an obvious reason for wanting to influence behavior—and a singular goal: to increase sales. Ultimately, the behavior they want to influence is what product or service the consumer buys. Social change goals and objectives often are not so clear-cut. There may be a variety of behavior changes that people could make that would lead to reduced morbidity and mortality. There often is not a direct relationship between the action of an individual and reductions in incidence or death. Sponsoring institutions may not see their role as influencing behavior change; rather, their mission may be to "disseminate information" or "educate." Or staff within the organization may have been trained in the knowledge-attitudes-behavior (KAB) paradigm, so they think that by increasing peoples' knowledge or changing their attitudes, behavior change will follow. Noting that interventions changing knowledge or attitudes do not usually result in behavior change, some researchers argue that the KAB paradigm is too simplistic and does not reflect our best understanding of how to influence behavior (Baranowski, 1997).

Bringing about social change means focusing on behavior change. Sometimes it is policy makers who need to change a behavior (such as how they vote or whether they craft a new regulation), and at other times individuals need to change personal behaviors. If a variety of behaviors could be changed, they usually can be prioritized according to most significant public health benefits or consumer willingness to make the changes. If an organization's mission is to "disseminate information" or "educate," why? What do the organization's mission-writers think will change if people have the information or become more educated? A little thinking usually will reveal a link to a behavior.

This is not to say that social change programs should never make an effort to increase knowledge or change attitudes. Rather, behavior change should be the end goal. Sometimes more knowledge is necessary before behavior can change— for example, parents are unlikely to immunize their children unless they know that they need to. However, the information needs to be related to the behavioral goal and tailored to the target audience's needs based on how ready they are to change their behavior. For example, in a review of nutrition education interventions, Contento and colleagues (1995) found that many of the interventions emphasized "how-to" knowledge or skills information, when the audience members were not yet ready for such information. They needed motivational information about personally relevant positive or negative consequences of behavior or other motivators of change before they were ready for "how-to" information.

One of the challenges public health practitioners face is selecting a specific behavior to change; often a number of behaviors can lead to desired outcomes. Using appropriate models and theories of behavior change can help practitioners make such choices. This process will be discussed in greater detail in Chapter 10.

The Importance of the Consumer

Marketing has been defined as the planned process of exercising influence on customer behavior. In order to influence a customer, one must first understand the customer and the determinants of his or her behavior. Therefore, marketers make consumers the focal point of their efforts and analyze all aspects of the exchange transaction from the consumer's viewpoint. Commercial marketers place enormous emphasis on learning all they can about their customers and potential customers. Their mission in life is to know who their consumers are, what they want and need, and where and how to reach them.

Marketing is often described as being *consumer driven*. In commercial marketing, that usually means identifying a consumer need and then developing or positioning a product to fulfill that need, although there are instances when a product has been developed or discovered and then a "need" is identified. In public health, we usually have to "create" need, but we often have a harder job: We start with a product people don't want and must then ferret out benefits they can or do associate with it in order to find a way to position it as superior to competing products. This makes solid consumer research—especially in terms of core values and benefits that people can associate with a product or behavior change—even more important for public health practitioners than it is for commercial marketers.

Public health organizations using a marketing approach often have difficulty being truly customer driven. A number of factors contribute to this difficulty. First, the structure of most public health organizations is not conducive to the marketing mind-set. Public health institutions typically are not run by individuals with a marketing background, and priorities are not set from within a marketing or behavior change framework. Unlike commercial marketers, who develop products based on what customers are most likely to purchase, public health institutions often allocate resources based on legislative priorities as reflected in mandates or current funding streams (i.e., if tax money or grants are available for tobacco control, then the institution focuses on tobacco control), rather than on an analysis of what behavior changes might best impact a population's health—let alone what changes are most likely to be made by the population served. Rather than driving the effort, marketing is usually only one component of it.

The position of staff within the organization attempting to develop a marketing-based effort leads to the second factor that affects a public health institution's ability to be customer driven: Because staff are often part of communication or public information departments, they often have little or no ability to influence priorities or institute other changes needed to support a marketing approach. While Andreasen (1995), among others, has criticized many social change marketers for effectively defining marketing as communications, it is not surprising that social change efforts often center around communication activities, given the background and organizational position of the staff. For example, a governor announces a new campaign to improve mammography rates among women age 50 and older. The communication staff can use marketing principles to develop the campaign: They can conduct consumer research to identify appropriate audiences, learn the benefits and barriers the audiences associate with mammography, and learn the ideal places to deliver mammograms and messages about them. They can develop, pretest, and produce a thorough promotional effort to be delivered through mass media and health care facilities. But most likely they will be able to do almost nothing about the financial cost of a mammogram, and/or about whether insurers will cover the cost. Similarly, they will be unable to overcome accessibility barriers, such as those faced by women who live far from the nearest mammography facility or who cannot afford to take time off from work to visit such a facility during business hours. Addressing these barriers would require working in partnership with local providers, something that may not be encouraged under the staff's organizational structure.

The third factor that affects many public health institutions' ability to be customer driven is a hesitancy to focus on specific groups of customers because of a mandate to serve "the general public." Trying to appeal to everyone is problematic for a number of reasons. One, it wastes resources because not everyone needs a particular intervention. Often, particular subgroups of the population are reached by other entities, have a very low incidence of the problem the intervention addresses, or have already embraced the behavior being promoted. Two, key to being customer driven is identifying and understanding the customer in question. Even if "everyone" needs a particular intervention, some subgroups are likely to be closer to actually changing their behavior (perhaps they have even tried to change) while others are not nearly ready (maybe they have not even thought about it). And different groups will associate different costs and benefits with the behavior in question. An intervention designed for "everyone" will likely either

- persuade no one because it is too scattered and resources are wasted promoting costs and benefits to audiences who do not perceive them as the most important costs and benefits, or
- focus on specific costs and benefits and therefore be relevant to only particular segments of the population (in other words, targeted by default rather than by intention).

Finally, social change resources are often extremely limited. By trying to stretch them to include "everyone," no audience group will be reached with any intensity. Consider an advertising analogy: What would happen if an automobile manufacturer decided that the target audience for a new station wagon was everyone? Let's say the manufacturer wanted to produce an ad and buy 10 prime-time (8 to 11 PM) placements over the course of a week. Using a targeted approach, the advertising agency would determine who is most likely to buy the car, develop an ad that promises them the specific benefits they desire, and place the ad during television shows that reach the most members of the target audience possible, without going over budget. This approach would maximize both the number of target audience members reached and the frequency with which they are reached. Using the "everyone" approach, the advertising agency would try to buy time on the shows that have the largest audiences, although they probably won't be able to include the top-rated shows and stay within their budget. Given the total number of prime-time programs each night, most people might see the ad only once or twice, if at all. By contrast, targeted consumers are likely to see it every night they watch TV. The next time they shop for a car, they are much more likely to think of the new station wagon if they saw the ad multiple times and not just once.

The Four Ps: The Marketing Mix

In commercial marketing, *product, price, place,* and *promotion* are referred to as "the four Ps" and constitute what is termed the marketing mix—the group of variables that a marketer can alter to successfully sell a product. Together, these four form the core building blocks of marketing strategy. A brief description of each variable and some of the issues surrounding its conceptualization in social marketing is presented below. Chapter 10 will describe how a program's strategic planning process can address the marketing mix variables.

Product

The product is the idea, behavior, good, or service that is exchanged with the target audience for a price. The product can be tangible or intangible. When social changes are involved, the product is most often a behavior and is therefore intangible, although the behavior may be linked to use of a particular product or service. For example, in a family planning program the desired behavior may be to space pregnancies out, rather than having one birth immediately after another. Contraceptives are an obvious tangible product likely to be involved in this exchange—even though spacing is what is actually being sold. Similarly, the 5 A Day for Better Health program encourages increased consumption of particular products—fruits and vegetables. Other programs, such as those promoting increased physical activity, decreased fat consumption, or violence prevention, often cannot easily tie their behavior changes to a product or service.

Sometimes widespread social change will not or cannot occur until laws, regulations, or other government policies either change to facilitate new services or add a measure of enforceable behavior change. For example, seat belt use in the United States did not increase significantly until a large number of states passed laws mandating their use. In 1983, seat belt use prevalence was only 15%; by 1995, all but two states had seat belt laws in effect and use prevalence had increased to 67% in 1994 (Nelson, Bolen, & Kresnow, 1998). Similarly, nonsmokers had no real way of escaping cigarette smoke until regulatory changes were widespread, such as bans on smoking on domestic flights and mandates for smoke-free workplaces.

Policy changes can be marketed to policy makers using the same principles that are used to market behavior change to individuals. Formative research should be done to identify the benefits *to the policy maker* of embracing the policy or program—and the drawbacks he or she associates with being characterized as a supporter of it. The program or policy can then be repositioned and messages about it reframed accordingly. (Chapter 6 discussed this process in more detail.) What are often thought of as marketing techniques can play a role in building support for policy changes, for example, through promotional activities that encourage the desired behavior and support changing cultural norms. But other techniques, such as lobbying and grass-roots organizing, are often necessary to change policy.

Sometimes the lack of a tangible product or service causes program planners to get caught up in defining the social change product. Asking the following questions can help:

- What are the benefits of the behavior change to members of the target audience—what needs or wants do they have that our behavior change (product) can fulfill?
- What is the competition for the behavior?

As we discussed earlier, when people buy something they receive a benefit in exchange. The product is just the means of obtaining the benefit. It is vital to define the product in terms of the benefit it will provide to consumers; in effect, it will satisfy an existing need in a new way. The benefit must override the benefit of the current behavior to the person and must be something the person perceives to be a benefit, not just something that is beneficial to public health. Some public health programs try to sell the long-term public health benefit (e.g., reduced risk of cancer, lives saved from seat belt use, etc.), rather than short-term individual benefits. While some people will change a behavior to benefit society if it is at very low cost to them, most people will not be sufficiently motivated to change health-related behaviors because society might derive a benefit or because they may derive a benefit in the distant future. They are more likely to change their behavior because they will achieve a short-term benefit for doing so (Backer, Rogers, & Sopory, 1992; Baranowski et al., 1997). And they must perceive the change to be consistent with their core values and with the person they want to be.

Part of understanding a product is understanding its competition. *Every* proposed behavior change has competition: the existing behavior. Andreasen (1995) has noted that target audiences often have very good reasons for maintaining their behavior patterns. The benefits they receive from their current behavior—or the drawbacks associated with a new behavior—may outweigh the benefits associated with the new behavior. When a public health program or policy is the product, the competition may have to do with resources (other funding needs are more of a priority to the policy maker), philosophy (such as a belief that there are too many government programs already or that government should not intervene in personal decisions), or pressure from interests that are not related to health (i.e., businesses saying increased regulations to safeguard the public's health would be "bad for business"). Sometimes it is necessary to restructure the product in order to overcome problems related to competition.

Another aspect of understanding a product is identifying how often people have an opportunity to "buy" it—and their circumstances when such opportunities arise. In many instances, people don't change their behavior by making one decision. Some lifestyle changes may get made dozens of times a day. For example, deciding "I am going to start eating five servings of fruits and vegetables each day" is only a starting point. Actually changing the behavior involves a decision every time the person considers eating something: "Am I going to have the apple or the candy bar?" As marketers, in order to persuade our target audience to choose the apple, we have to understand what the competition is—and what the audience finds appealing and unappealing about each option.

Identifying how frequently target audience members will have to make the behavior change and the circumstances under which they will make it can help program planners assess its feasibility and ease of adoption. Sometimes asking people to try the behavior change "the next time" they are confronted with it is less threatening to them than telling them to do it every time, and therefore more likely to be embraced. For example, if target audience members think they can't possibly eat five servings of fruits and vegetables, telling them to try a fruit or vegetable the next time they're looking for a snack (rather than every time, or rather than trying to eat five servings) may be more successful. They may say to themselves, "I can do that."

Similarly, asking a target audience member to perform an action only under particular circumstances can be helpful. Chapter 3 included an example discussing how human immunodeficiency virus (HIV) prevention programs targeting gay men usually focus on risk elimination ("use a condom every time you have sex for the rest of your life"), rather than on risk reduction. However, condom use is associated with a lack of trust and with decreased pleasure, and as the example notes, some men engage in unprotected sex precisely because it is self-destructive. These competing benefits may combine to overshadow the benefit of potentially preventing HIV infection by using a condom. A more realistic behavior change may be to ask gay men to use a condom with all new or casual sexual partners, situations in which the behavior's competition is not nearly so great. While this strategy may be difficult from a public health standpoint (where consistent condom use with all partners is the goal), it may result in more progress toward the desired behavior than a message to "use a condom every time."

Finally, program planners must identify all changes that are needed to reach public health goals and determine the appropriate approach or combination of approaches for each change. As noted throughout this book, personal behavior does not take place in a vacuum. To effectively change behavior, it is necessary to consider the historical, cultural, political, and social environments in which change will take place. As Fox and Kotler noted in 1980, there are four broad approaches to producing social change: legal, technological, economic, and informational. Effectively bringing about social change often requires several of these approaches. Some practitioners argue that many social change efforts devote too many resources to informational approaches and not enough to legal and technological approaches (such as new regulations and new products or services; see, for example, Smith, 1997).

To illustrate, consider the problem of child safety seats in cars. In 1996, almost 80% of child safety seats were used improperly (National Highway Traffic Safety Administration [NHTSA], 1996). Many are not properly secured with seat belts, and many are put in the wrong position in the car (for example, in an airbag-equipped passenger seat). Solving the problem involves a combination of approaches. The informational approach is a short-term solution that involves providing parents with information on how to install the seats properly; directions are included with the seat itself and with the car, and many federal, state, and local agencies make information available. Many communities also demonstrate proper installation by publicizing days on which police officers will be available to check, and, if necessary, correct installation.

The technological approach involves

- persuading car manufacturers to provide a standard easy-to-use mechanism for restraining child safety seats. (Currently a cumbersome latch clip must be used with most shoulder/lap belts. The clip can easily be misplaced, and if parents don't have the original car seat directions, they may not know it exists.)
- persuading manufacturers of child safety seats to standardize their designs enough that the same installation steps can be used for all seats.

Implementing the technological approach will likely require a regulatory approach. To that end, in 1997 NHTSA issued a notice of proposed rule making, the first step in creating a new federal regulation. The proposed rule outlined a system for anchoring child safety seats that would require specific, standardized components in vehicles and on child safety seats (NHTSA, 1997).

Program planners should strive to ensure that they identify all approaches—legal, economic, technological, and informational—that could be used to bring about change and that adequate resources are put behind all necessary changes. To ensure that relevant issues are considered and that, if necessary, program components are developed to help bring about policy changes, these questions should be asked during the planning stage:

- What legal, technological, and/or economic policy changes can facilitate individual behavior change?
- How can marketing-based efforts support these changes?
- What accomplishments can reasonably be expected, independent of policy changes?

Price

Price is the cost to the target audience of making an exchange. In commercial marketing, price almost always has a financial component; if consumers are considering trying a new product or service, the associated risk of change creates a psychological component as well. With social changes, the price is more likely to be time, effort, lifestyle, or psychological cost. Fine (1992) has termed these *social prices*. For example, insisting that a sexual partner use a condom has a high potential psychological cost: The partner may reject the one insisting or make assumptions about promiscuous behavior or lack of trust. Being the first policy maker to change from opposing to supporting a policy can create a high psychological or social cost. Many consumers perceive various health behaviors, such as increasing physical activity, as costing a great deal of time. And some behaviors require effort, such as obtaining more nutritious foods if they are not readily accessible. Rothschild (1979) argued that these nonmonetary costs "may be perceived as greater than monetary costs which dominate the price of consumer products" (p. 13).

When the product is a public health program or policy, the perceived psychological price may include an infringement on basic values, such as that resulting from government interference or limitations on freedom. Laws mandating seat belt use and restrictions on smoking are two examples that fit both categories.

Asking the following questions may help program planners work through the price of their social marketing product:

- What will the behavior change "cost" each target audience member in money, time, effort, and psyche?
- Do target audience members perceive the costs to be a fair exchange for the benefit they associate with the behavior change?
- How can costs be minimized?

Usually, the only way to answer these questions is through careful formative research as will be outlined in Chapter 11. Costs are often referred to as barriers, because they stand between the consumer and the behavior change.

Place

In commercial marketing, place is the outlet or outlets through which products are available. Place is often the most difficult commercial marketing "P" to conceptualize in social change programs—and the one that can be most difficult to control. Behaviors that involve a tangible product usually have a clear place, but others do not. For example, if the goal is to increase usage of services provided by a health clinic, marketers can conduct consumer research to assess how physically accessible the clinic is. (What are the hours? How can people get there? Do they have access to those modes of transportation? How difficult is it to make an appointment?) Marketers can also examine other aspects of the place that might affect usage, such as staff behavior, waiting times, crowding, temperature, cleanliness, and provisions for child care or for activities for children while they wait.

For other behavioral interventions, place is much more difficult to define. For example, consider the many public health programs that encourage lifestyle changes, such as increased physical activity, reduced consumption of total or saturated fat, and increased consumption of whole grains and/or fruits and vegetables. In these instances, no one physical place is associated with the behavior.

In social change programs, "place" often winds up being conceptualized as message delivery channels. It is more useful to define "place" as where the individual will be when he or she has access to the product or service, if one exists, and/or engages in the desired behavior. For interventions targeting policy makers, "place" is often twofold:

1. the environment where policy decisions are made (i.e., for elected officials, the legislature or the office that they hold) and
2. the constituency the policy maker represents.

Each of these "places" is likely to present distinct costs and benefits to the policy maker vis-à-vis the policy under consideration.

This conceptualization facilitates thinking through the aspects of "place" that impact strategy, namely

- What are target audience members' perceptions of the place?
- What barriers (costs) does place create, and how can they be overcome?

As an intervention is developed and specific behavior changes are selected, formative research can help identify situations in which the desired activities will take place. Armed with this knowledge, public health marketers can work to change the characteristics of these places or, through promotional activities and materials, to provide consumers with ideas for making their own changes. Changing place characteristics often necessitates approaches beyond marketing, such as changes in policy or regulations. For example, widespread smoke free public places would not have been obtained without changes in local ordinances. Providing children with adequate time to eat a healthful lunch or including sufficient instructional time for health education also requires policy changes at the school level and often at the district or state level. In situations such as these, a marketing approach can help identify the characteristics of the ideal place, and promotional activities often can support the need for such characteristics. However, techniques other than promotion are necessary to bring about such changes.

An example of using promotional activities and materials to help consumers modify their "places" can be found in the 5 A Day for Better Health program. Formative research conducted for the program revealed that two reasons people don't eat more fruits and vegetables is that they are not accessible (because vending machines don't contain them, for example) and that they don't think of them (because the fruits and vegetables are at the bottom of the refrigerator in a dark bin). Although the program planners could not control every place that someone might obtain fruits and vegetables, they could—and did—incorporate simple ideas into promotional activities and materials to help consumers improve their fruit and vegetables "places." For example, they included suggestions such as making fruits and vegetables accessible during the day by putting them into briefcases and lunch bags, and putting them out in a bowl or on a higher shelf in the refrigerator so that people can see them more easily when hunting for something to eat (Lefebvre et al., 1995).

Promotion

Traditional promotion consists of communicating to the target audience about the behavior change through some combination of advertising, media relations, events, personal selling, and entertainment. When policy change is the goal, promotion often includes techniques such as grass-roots advocacy, media advocacy, and lobbying.

All promotional activities have a common goal: to maximize the likelihood that target audience members will engage in the transaction by reaching them with messages highlighting the exchange's benefits to the consumer and minimizing—or providing methods to overcome—the costs.

Advertisements are perhaps the most visible form of marketing promotion. Examples of other types of promotion activities include

- framing of content of media coverage through media relations efforts, such as preparing print, audio, and/or video news releases or press conferences and conducting briefings with reporters;
- community events, such as promoting free blood pressure screenings to people attending minor league baseball games, as the National High Blood Pressure Education Program's Strike Out Stroke initiative did;
- personal selling, such as having physicians or nurses "talk up" a particular behavior related to family planning or the availability of a new vaccine; and
- entertainment, such as integrating public health messages into television series' story lines or producing popular entertainment with a public health message, such as the top-10 Latin American music hits written and produced as part of a U.S. Agency for International Development project (Braus, 1995).

In order to develop the promotion component of a public health effort, it is necessary to fully understand product, price, and place and then use that information to develop a communication strategy for each primary and secondary audience. (Chapter 12 will present a process for developing a communication strategy.) The communication strategy helps managers frame promotional messages by describing

- the action the target audience should take as a result of the communication.
- the barriers to the action.
- the benefit to be promised in exchange for the action.
- the support for the benefit.
- the tone communications should use.

- the openings through which target audiences can be reached with the communication.

After designing a communication strategy, the promotion plan is developed. This plan spells out the materials and activities that will form the promotion, as well as the timeline for development and implementation. Key questions that guide development of the communication strategy and promotion plan include the following:

- What is the current demand among target audience members for the behavior change?
- What messages can best influence demand?
- What promotional materials and activities are appropriate for the message?
- How can those materials and activities best be delivered to target audience members?

Public health marketers face the following unique difficulties related to each of these questions:

Negative demand. Commercial products and services are developed to meet a consumer need; if market research determines that there is little or no demand for the product or service, it will not be produced. In contrast, most public health "products" have few people clamoring for them. Although there are exceptions, if people wanted to engage in the behavior, often there would be no need for the public health program. Consequently, public health practitioners not only have the challenge of promoting a behavior change, they have to find a way of creating demand for it. Chapter 2 discussed the challenge of negative demand in greater detail.

Lack of funds to purchase time and space. For the advertising component of their promotional mix, commercial marketers usually have substantial budgets available to purchase time and space for their messages. This allows them to control both the content of the message and when, how often, and where it appears. Because most public health programs do not have the resources required to purchase comparable amounts of advertising time and space, their promotional efforts are inherently more difficult to target effectively and efficiently. Rather than using paid advertising as the backbone of a media campaign, public health marketers often must use a combination of public service advertising and media relations.

Limited control over message delivery. Because most public health programs are not purchasing advertising time and space from broadcast and print media, placement of public service advertising is at the whim of the public service director at each station or publication. Public health marketers cannot select the program and time slots most likely to reach the target audience, nor control the frequency with which an ad is shown. They can make suggestions to the public service director for optimal placement, but must make do with what the media offer. Generating news coverage of public health efforts also presents a challenge. Often, the behavior a public health organization is promoting is considered "evergreen," or not time sensitive, so reporters and producers feel no pressure to run a story. Even if a story runs, the organization cannot control the editorial content of it; key messages may be minimized, deleted, or changed. And the public health staff in charge of media efforts often have little experience with proactive media relations. They work in an environment where reporters call for comments or information on various topics, not where they call reporters to ask them to cover a particular story.

Limited ability to assess impact. Commercial marketers can tie many of their promotional activities directly to product sales, making it relatively easy for them to assess the effect of various activities and fine-tune their promotional mix. As Chapters 17 and 18 will discuss, it is often difficult to measure the impact of communications activities. Consequently, it is more difficult to determine what aspects of the promotion mix need refinement. However, Chapter 17 will suggest how to build evaluation activities into promotion components to help with program refinement. Chapters 13 through 16 will provide a more detailed analysis of some issues to consider and steps to take when developing and implementing promotional activities.

Social change efforts use many of the same promotional tools as commercial marketing efforts, but the need to induce policy change as well as individual behavior change often requires a different approach to using these tools. For example, the media advocacy approach is fundamentally a promotional approach: It relies on media relations and, often, paid advertising. But, as Wallack and Dorfman's description of media advocacy makes clear, it uses these promotional tools in a fundamentally different way:

> The purpose of media advocacy is to promote public health goals by using the media to strategically apply pressure for policy change. It provides a framework for moving the public health discussion from a primary focus on the health behavior of individuals to the behavior of the policymakers whose decisions structure the environment in which people act. It addresses the power gap rather than just the information gap. (1996, p. 293)

An Additional P: Partners

Beyond the traditional marketing mix of product, price, place, and promotion, social change efforts often have to consider an additional P: partners.

Social change efforts typically commence when there is scientific consensus that a particular behavior change will benefit the individual and society. By the time such consensus is reached, many organizations (often both public and private) may have an interest in promoting the behavior change and, if necessary, in developing technological and policy changes to facilitate individual behavior change. Unfortunately, what often happens is that each organization develops its own program and does not coordinate efforts with the other organizations. Completely separate programs can jeopardize success in a number of ways. First, each organization may target the same or similar groups with different messages, leading to confusion among consumers and policy makers as to the actions they should take. Second, if mass media efforts are involved, the organizations are usually competing for limited media time and space (both in terms of public service advertising space and editorial coverage of the issue). The media usually do not run multiple stories based on each organization's perspective, so someone's efforts will be for naught. This duplication of effort can result in wasted resources.

Often, a better solution is for organizations to recognize that others are also interested in promoting the social change. By combining or coordinating efforts, consumers and policy makers are reached by sources they trust with a consistent, clear message—and resources are maximized. Each partner organization can perform the activity for which it is best suited. Unfortunately, these types of partnerships are all too rare. At the conceptual level, partnerships are difficult because each organization has its own wants and needs. At the operational level, a host of practical difficulties can prohibit progress, including different fiscal years and institutional timetables, restrictions on government agencies working with private sector organizations, and organizational cultures.

Even if perfect partnerships cannot be formed, it is important for public health practitioners to know the other organizations involved with a social change effort and to coordinate activities with them when possible. Often, partners can provide access to or added credibility with key target audience segments. For example, the national 5 A Day for Better Health program includes a partnership between the National Cancer Institute (NCI) and the Produce for Better Health Foundation (PBHF), a nonprofit organization established and funded by the produce industry. The partnership gives NCI ideal access to the 5 A Day target audience: signs in grocery stores and labels on products, exactly where purchase decisions are made. And NCI gives PBHF additional credibility through messages encouraging consumers to eat more fruits and vegetables.

During the planning process, addressing the following questions should provide a starting point for ensuring that social change efforts are planned with potential partners in mind:

- What other organizations are addressing the social change?
- What organizations are credible to the target audience?
- What are the opportunities to work together with either type of organization?

Chapter 14 will provide additional information on this important social marketing variable. Exhibit 9–1 summarizes all of the Ps, and Appendix 9–A describes a social change effort that illustrates many of the concepts discussed in this chapter.

Exhibit 9–1 The Social Marketing Mix

Product
The behavior, good, service, or program exchanged for a price
- What are the benefits of the behavior change to members of the target audience—what needs or wants do they have that the product (behavior change, program, or policy) can fulfill?
- What is the competition for the product?
- What legal, technological, and/or economic policy changes can facilitate individual behavior change?
- What accomplishments can reasonably be expected independent of policy changes?

Price
The cost to the target audience member, in money, time, effort, lifestyle, or psyche, of engaging in the behavior
- What will the behavior change "cost" each target audience member in money, time, effort, lifestyle, and psyche?
- Do target audience members perceive the cost to be a fair exchange for the benefit they associate with the behavior change?
- How can cost be minimized?

Place
The outlet(s) through which products are available—or situations in which behavior changes can be made
- What are target audience members' perceptions of the place?
- What barriers (costs) does the place create, and how can they be overcome?

Promotion
A combination of advertising, media relations, promotional events, personal selling, and entertainment to communicate with target audience members about the product
- What is the current demand among target audience members for the behavior change?
- What messages can best influence demand?
- What promotional materials and activities are appropriate for the message?
- How can those materials and activities best be delivered to target audience members?

Partners
Other organizations involved with a social change effort or serving as conduits to target audiences
- What other organizations are conducting activities addressing the social change?
- What organizations are credible to the target audience?
- What are the opportunities to work together with either type of organization?

CONCLUSION

Marketing principles can be used to guide the process of developing, implementing, and refining a social change initiative. They can help select specific behavior or policy changes on which to focus and emphasize the importance of identifying the wants, needs, and values of a target audience—whether that target audience is a member of the public or a policy maker—and then packaging and positioning the product to satisfy those wants, needs, and values. Marketing principles and practice also provide techniques to constantly monitor and refine initiatives to respond to changing conditions.

REFERENCES

Andreasen, A.R. (1995). *Marketing social change: Changing behavior to promote health, social development, and the environment.* San Francisco: Jossey-Bass.

Backer, T.E., Rogers, E.M., & Sopory, P. (1992). *Designing health communication campaigns: What works?* Thousand Oaks, CA: Sage.

Bandura, A. (1986). *Social foundations of thought and action.* Englewood Cliffs, NJ: Prentice-Hall.

Baranowski, T. (1997). The knowledge-attitudes-behavior model and defining "behavior changes." In L. Doner (Ed.), *Charting the course for evaluation: How do we measure the success of nutrition education and promotion in food assistance programs? Summary of proceedings* (pp. 26–27). Alexandria, VA: U.S. Department of Agriculture.

Baranowski, T., Perry, C.L., & Parcel, G.S. (1997). How individuals, environments, and health behavior interact: Social cognitive theory. In K. Glanz, F.M. Lewis, & B.K. Rimer (Eds.), *Health behavior and health education: Theory, research and practice* (2nd ed., pp. 153–178). San Francisco: Jossey-Bass.

Braus, P. (1995). Selling good behavior. *American Demographics,* 60–64.

Contento, I., Balch, G.I., Bronner, Y.L., Lytle, L.A., Maloney, S.K, White, S.L., Olson, C.M., & Swadener, S.S. (1995). The effectiveness of nutrition education and implications for nutrition education policy, programs, and research [Special issue]. *Journal of Nutrition Education, 27*(6).

Fine, S.H. (1992). *Marketing the public sector: Promoting the causes of public and nonprofit agencies.* New Brunswick, NJ: Transaction.

Fox, K.F.A., & Kotler, P. (1980). The marketing of social causes: The first 10 years. *Journal of Marketing, 44*(4), 24–33.

Kotler, P., & Andreasen, A.R. (1996). *Strategic marketing for non-profit organizations* (2nd ed.). Upper Saddle River, NJ: Prentice-Hall.

Kotler, P., & Zaltman, G. (1971). Social marketing: An approach to planned social change. *Journal of Marketing, 35,* 3–12.

Lefebvre, R.C., Doner, L.D., Johnston, C., Loughrey, K., Balch, G., & Sutton, S.M. (1995). Use of database marketing and consumer-based health communications in message design: An example from the Office of Cancer Communications' "5 A Day for Better Health" program. In E. Maibach & R. Parrott (Eds.), *Designing health messages: Approaches from communication theory and public health practice* (pp. 217–246). Thousand Oaks, CA: Sage.

National Highway Traffic Safety Administration. (1996). *Patterns of misuse of child safety seats: Final report* (Rep. No. DOT HS 808-440). Washington, DC: Author.

National Highway Traffic Safety Administration. (1997). *Tether anchorages for child restraint systems; Child restraint anchorage system,* 62 Fed. Reg. 7858.

Nelson, D.E., Bolen, J., & Kresnow, M. (1998). Trends in safety belt use by demographics and by type of state safety belt law, 1987–1993. *American Journal of Public Health, 88,* 245–249.

Prochaska, J.O. (1994). Strong and weak principles for progressing from precontemplation to action on the basis of twelve problem behaviors. *Health Psychology, 13*(1), 47–51.

Prochaska, J.O., Redding, C.A., & Evers, K.E. (1997). The transtheoretical model and stages of change. In K. Glanz, F.M. Lewis, & B.K. Rimer (Eds.), *Health behavior and health education: Theory, research and practice* (2nd ed., pp. 60–84). San Francisco: Jossey-Bass.

Rothschild, M.L. (1979, Spring). Marketing communications in nonbusiness situations or why it's so hard to sell brotherhood like soap. *Journal of Marketing, 43,* 11–20.

Smith, W. (1997). Confounding issues in evaluations of nutrition interventions. In L. Doner (Ed.), *Charting the course for evaluation: How do we measure the success of nutrition education and promotion in food assistance programs? Summary of proceedings* (pp. 11–13). Alexandria, VA: U.S. Department of Agriculture.

Strecher, V.J., & Rosenstock, I.M. (1997). The health belief model. In K. Glanz, F.M. Lewis, & B.K. Rimer (Eds.), *Health behavior and health education: Theory, research and practice* (2nd ed., pp. 41–59). San Francisco: Jossey-Bass.

Wallack, L., & Dorfman, L. (1996). Media advocacy: A strategy for advancing policy and promoting health. *Health Education Quarterly, 23,* 293–317.

Weibe, G.D. (1951/1952). Merchandising commodities and citizenship on television. *Public Opinion Quarterly, 15,* 679–691.

Using Marketing Principles To Combat Telemarketing Fraud Victimization

BACKGROUND

Telemarketing fraud in the United States is a pernicious problem, estimated by Congress to cost consumers $40 billion a year. The actual cost may be much higher, because not all losses are clearly documented. Some consumers are too embarrassed to report having been defrauded; others do not realize that fraud occurred. The stereotypical victim of telemarketing fraud is a lonely widow, living alone and eager for any contact with the outside world, even if the price of such contact is her financial security, her independence, and her dignity.

Formative research indicates that this view is seriously distorted. While a disproportionate number of all victims are older, most are relatively affluent, well educated, and well informed; are socially active; and express many of the same attitudes about telemarketers that are widely held by nonvictims. Quantitative and qualitative studies show that the principal difference between victims and nonvictims is that those who avoid being victimized will hang up the phone or listen to signals during the call that alert them to a scam. Victims, on the other hand, are more reluctant to hang up on telemarketers, and they listen for signals that they believe confirm the caller's legitimacy.

Some policy changes have been made to protect Americans against telemarketing fraud. Most notably, Congress passed the Telemarketing and Consumer Fraud and Abuse Act in 1994, which resulted in a Federal Trade Commission (FTC) telemarketing sales rule addressing the predatory and abusive prac-

Source: Reprinted with permission from *Using a Social Marketing Approach To Combat Telemarketing Victimization,* by John Killpack (unpublished paper). Copyright © 1997, American Association of Retired Persons.

tices committed by some telemarketers and providing a basis for enforcement action by the FTC and the states.

CHALLENGES AND OPPORTUNITIES

Educating consumers about telemarketing fraud is complex because the behaviors involved are complex. Consumers cannot simply be told to hang up on all telemarketers because many telemarketers are legitimate. However, there is no easy way for consumers to separate legal telemarketing calls from illegal fraud. Even if a simple criterion could be identified and communicated, many victims lack the skills to end calls from fraudulent telemarketers even when they feel pressured by the caller. Many feel that it is rude to hang up on anyone, including telemarketers. In addition, victims often assume responsibility for being victimized in fraudulent schemes, an attitude that has been confirmed in past public education efforts that relied on simple directions such as "just hang up," and platitudes such as "if it sounds too good to be true, it probably is." Formative research indicates that other challenges include the following:

- Most victims and nonvictims say that it is hard to spot fraud when it is happening.
- Most victims and nonvictims do not understand that fraudulent telemarketing activity is illegal and take a "buyer beware" attitude toward telemarketers.
- Most consumers do not know where to call to find out if a telephone offer is legitimate.
- Most victims do not report the matter to anyone.

The recently passed federal legislation indicates that telemarketing fraud is on public and policy agendas, providing an opportunity to educate consumers about protecting themselves from telemarketing fraud and to work toward additional policy changes to better protect them. In addition, the FTC rule provides a supportive environment for additional policy changes: The rule provides states with a basis for enforcement action and specifically allows states to enact provisions that provide greater consumer protections, as long as they do not conflict with the federal law.

GOAL

To help reduce telemarketing fraud victimization by giving consumers tools (including legal remedies) and helping them develop a skeptical attitude toward telemarketers so that they can recognize fraudulent callers and shorten and/or terminate questionable calls.

OBJECTIVES

To increase

- the proportion of older consumers who recognize that telemarketing fraud is a crime.
- the proportion of consumers who will shorten and terminate fraudulent telemarketing calls.
- the proportion of consumers who can cite strategies to avoid telemarketing fraud victimization.

TARGET AUDIENCES

For individual behavior changes:

- Americans age 50 and older who have been or are likely to be victims of telemarketing fraud

To support policy changes:

- federal and state policy makers
- general public
- mass media

STRATEGY

The program is a joint effort of national, state, and local consumer and law enforcement organizations. Behavior change will be brought about by (1) framing telemarketing fraud as a crime and (2) providing consumers with the skills they need to recognize potentially fraudulent calls and shorten or terminate them. Policy change will be brought about by (1) framing telemarketing fraud as the crime that it is on the media, public, and policy agendas; and (2) providing state and grass-roots support for legislative advocacy issues.

PARTNERSHIPS

With the American Association of Retired Persons (AARP) assuming the lead, the program includes ongoing cooperative work with Royal Canadian Mounted Police and the following U.S. organizations:

- Federal Bureau of Investigation (FBI)
- U.S. Department of Justice
- Postal Inspector
- Administration on Aging
- National Consumer League's National Fraud Information Center
- National Association of Attorneys General

The partners played a significant role in developing the program, and they support implementation and help secure media coverage. In addition, corporate sponsors support specific program interventions and help disseminate antifraud messages to their customers and stakeholders. Consumer groups at the state and national levels are recruited to assist in lobbying for telemarketing legislation.

EDUCATION AND PROMOTION

The program positions telemarketing fraud as a criminal activity, but one that consumers can take steps to protect themselves against. This positioning was based on the research findings described above, as well as on qualitative research with telemarketing fraud victims that revealed that (1) taking action against telemarketing fraud can be linked compellingly to the core value of control (i.e., "learn how to protect yourself"); and (2) it is unrealistic to try to persuade all segments of the population to hang up on telemarketers; some do not want to or are not capable of doing so. The positioning is illustrated by the program theme line: "Fraudulent telemarketers are criminals. Don't fall for a telephone line."

Mass communication activities include public service announcements for television, radio, print, and outdoor, consumer fact sheets, community forums, and special events. These activities serve to position telemarketing fraud as a crime and provide basic education to target audience members who need to change their behavior while reinforcing positive actions taken by those who have developed adequate self-protection mechanisms. Interpersonal efforts that build on this foundation include cooperative work with local consumer protection groups, AARP chapter events, and one-on-one peer counseling.

Additional mass media tactics are used to help position the issue on public, policy, and media agendas. These tactics include using video and audio news releases, news conferences, and special events such as forums for the media that bring reporters and editors together with fraud victims and law enforcement officials. Media placements have included significant, ongoing coverage of both the issue and the campaign messages in national, major market, and local newspapers; on cable, network, and local television; and on network and local radio.

Community-based activities are designed to help target audience members follow through on behavior changes. Community activities include consumer education, consumer advocate training, and peer support. Community forums and "reverse boiler rooms" are two types of activities that have been particularly effective in reaching members and simultaneously garnering media attention. These activities will continue to be replicated in additional communities nationwide.

Reverse boiler rooms use the tools of fraudulent telemarketers to reach victims and those known to be at risk of victimization. Using prospect lists confiscated in law enforcement crackdowns, trained volunteers call victims and potential victims to alert them that they have been targeted by fraudulent telemarketers. Through

December 1997, 12 reverse boiler rooms were conducted in concert with federal and state law enforcement organizations. Court watches are used to support the aggressive prosecution and conviction of fraudulent telemarketers. During court watches, community volunteers amass outside courthouses and in courtrooms to demonstrate community support for prosecution and to dramatize community interest in the issue.

LEGISLATIVE ADVOCACY

AARP is working to enact state legislation to expand the consumer protections in the FTC rule and provides support to state legislative committees and grassroots advocacy efforts, tailoring that support to meet each state's needs. Legislation providing enhanced consumer protections was passed in Ohio and Pennsylvania in 1996 and introduced in nine state legislatures in 1997. Of these nine, two states (South Dakota and Vermont) have already approved the legislation; one (Oklahoma) passed a modified bill. Five others are still considering it.

EVALUATION

In addition to ongoing monitoring of all tactics, outcomes will be evaluated by comparing yearly tracking surveys with the results of a February 1996 baseline telephone survey of adults age 50 and older.

CHAPTER 10

The Planning Process

Adequate planning is essential to the marketing approach—and essential to successfully achieving social change. Planning begins with conducting a thorough analysis of the situation at hand: identifying and prioritizing the problems based on public health burden, assessing the environment in which the change will take place, and determining interventions most likely to be effective given the type of problem and the environment for change. The next step is to set goals and objectives by specifying behaviors, conditions, or policies to be changed. Then planners must determine target populations for each desired social change and develop a thorough understanding of each audience. In particular, planners must identify and prioritize the audience's basic needs, desires, and values and then identify how the current behavior satisfies each and explore how the desired behavior can be framed to reinforce core values. Based on this information, a strategic plan addressing all aspects of the marketing mix—product, price, place, promotion, and partners—is developed.

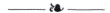

Developing a strong, effective social change effort is an iterative process. To facilitate understanding, this book presents the process as a series of discrete, sequential activities (Exhibit 10–1), but in reality, the steps often overlap or repeat based on new information or changing conditions. This iteration is a defining characteristic of the marketing approach, providing the flexibility to adapt to different issues, environments, resource levels, and conditions.

As is evident from the number of activities shown in Exhibit 10–1 for each stage (and the number of chapters in this book devoted to aspects of planning), adequate

Exhibit 10–1 Planning Social Change Efforts

Stage 1: Planning
- Analyze the situation:
  - –Identify and prioritize problems based on public health burden.
  - –Assess the social change environment, including competition.
  - –Identify interventions most likely to be effective.
- Set goals and objectives: Specify behaviors, conditions, or policies to be changed.
- Segment and select target audiences: Determine the target populations for each desired social change.
- Understand target audiences:
  - –Identify and prioritize basic needs, desires, and values.
  - –Identify current behavior and attributes of the behavior that satisfy those needs, desires, and values.
  - –Explore ways of framing the desired behavior to reinforce core values.
- Develop strategic plan addressing product, price, place, promotion, and partners:
  - –Redefine the product as offering a desired benefit.
  - –Package and position the product as offering the benefit.
- Develop communication strategy:
  - –Frame the communication to reinforce (not to conflict with) audience's core values.
  - –Focus on the promise (the benefit) and support for it.
- Conduct message concept testing.

Stage 2: Development
- Develop product and/or promotion plans.
- Develop prototype products and/or communication materials.
- Pretest with target audience members.
- Refine products and materials.
- Build in process evaluation measures.

Stage 3: Implementation
- Produce products and materials.
- Coordinate with partners.
- Implement intervention.
- Conduct process evaluation.
- Refine products, materials, and delivery channels as needed.

Stage 4: Assessment
- Conduct outcome evaluation.
- Refine program.

---

planning is vital to market social change successfully. Consumer and market research are integral parts of the planning process. Allocating sufficient resources to ensure adequate planning and development can prevent costly mistakes and will result in a stronger, more effective initiative.

In the United States, public health interventions that use marketing techniques often center on health communications (promotion). As a result, planning activities are often conducted in the context of developing a communications campaign. However, because all aspects of the marketing mix interrelate, it is important to think through all of them generally before filtering them through the prism of communications. Doing so also helps to ensure that program managers develop clear and reasonable expectations of what marketing approaches can accomplish in the larger realm of social change. Therefore, this book is structured so that an overall strategic plan is developed first, followed by development of a communication strategy, messages, and plans. This chapter discusses developing the strategic plan; Chapter 11 will discuss some of the qualitative and quantitative research techniques that can be used during planning; and Chapter 12 will discuss developing a communication strategy to properly frame the initiative.

THE IMPORTANCE OF SOUND STRATEGY

The planning process is designed to give project staff the background they need to develop a comprehensive framework for the intervention. The emphasis is on learning everything needed to develop a sound strategic approach. Understanding the difference between strategy and tactics—and knowing when to develop each—is a key aspect of successfully using marketing principles.

A strategy is "the broad approach that an organization takes to achieving its objectives" (Andreasen, 1995, p. 69). An initiative may have one or more strategies, depending on its objectives. Strategies are usually long term, meaning that they are developed with the intention of using them for 3 to 5 years. Once strategies have been developed, the tactics—short-term, detailed steps that will be used to implement each strategy—can be developed for each program component.

- Strategies are more abstract: for example, communicate how to easily add two daily servings of fruits and vegetables to people who already eat three and are trying to eat more; offer parenting classes for pregnant women; motivate parents to express their support of school health to administrators and policy makers.
- Tactics are concrete: a product launch, a community event, the content of a specific parenting class, or speaking to community groups.

Investing time up front in solid planning, and then using the plan to assess individual tactics, ensures that all aspects of the implementation are cost efficient and appropriate to the objectives and the target audience(s). It is often very difficult for everyone involved with an initiative, particularly the tactical experts, to be disciplined about assessing tactics against the strategy. However, this assessment is very important. No matter how exciting a tactic is, if it does not fit with the strategy, it will waste precious resources.

In order to construct a strategy, program planners need to

- understand the environment in which the intervention will operate;
- understand the science behind the potential change(s); and
- identify appropriate target audiences, and understand their wants, needs, values, and capabilities related to the target behavior.

The challenge is to balance each of these factors and come up with a strategy that will result in the social change that will have the most positive impact on the public's health. All of these factors interrelate, so choices are rarely clear-cut. The public health practitioner's natural inclination is to begin with a consumer behavior change. This choice may not be appropriate in some situations. For example, target audience members may be unable to make the change solely as a result of marketing or communication efforts. Consider the example of child safety seats discussed in Chapter 9. There is substantial evidence that 80% of child restraints are not installed correctly (National Highway Traffic Safety Administration [NHTSA], 1996). The reason is not lack of knowledge or lack of desire. It is physically very difficult to anchor a car seat in a way that would provide maximum protection in a crash. The long-term solution is to work with car seat and automobile manufacturers to improve and standardize installation mechanisms—a regulatory approach.

In other situations, the consumer target audience may be unwilling to make the behavior change. For example, the surest way to prevent sexual transmission of human immunodeficiency virus (HIV) is abstinence. Few members of at-risk populations are willing to make such a behavior change, so interventions often emphasize safe practices instead. But even these behaviors cannot be promoted in some environments. An HIV-prevention program strategy that focuses on telling adolescents "if you're sexually active, use a latex condom" and increasing the accessibility of condoms (i.e., by providing them in school-based clinics) simply will not be acceptable in many American communities. The planning process must provide enough information to assess each potential behavior change in terms of likelihood of adoption and appropriateness for the environment in which it will be implemented.

PLANNING PRINCIPLES

The following key principles can help guide the planning and development of a social change effort.

Craft an intervention that will impact behavior. Particularly among programs focusing on mass communications, the focus is too often on building awareness about an issue, rather than on providing target audience members with the tools and motivation to make efficacious behavior changes.

Be theory driven. Using theory wisely is a hallmark of effective marketing practice. Theories and models of behavior change and learning can play important roles in shaping public health interventions. They can help program managers select target audiences, set reasonable objectives, and tailor intervention components to each target audience's unique needs. Many different theories and models can help practitioners structure their interventions. Some that have broad applicability include diffusion of innovations (Rogers, 1983), the transtheoretical model of stages of change (Prochaska, Redding, & Evers, 1997), and social cognitive theory (Bandura, 1986; Baranowski, Perry, & Parcel, 1997). Core concepts of these will be discussed in the next section of this chapter.

Understand the target audience. Its members are people, not a bunch of statistics. What are they doing now? How will they react to the action you want them to take? What is motivating? What stands in the way? What products or services can be developed to aid the behavior change? How can communications be crafted so that they speak to each target audience member and deliver a relevant attention-getting message?

Set realistic expectations. Creating and sustaining a social change often takes a long time. Commercial marketers are usually pleased if they can increase market share by 2% or 3% in a year. Yet public health practitioners routinely set themselves up for failure by expecting to see 20% to 30% of the population change lifelong behaviors within a couple of years.

Create a unified strategic program. A program will maximize impact and achieve significant results only if all media relations, materials development, liaison activities with partners or the community, and other program components follow a common strategy and reinforce each other.

Leverage resources and relationships. It is crucial to work aggressively to leverage resources for maximum impact. Both dollars and reach can be stretched through collaborations among government, voluntary, and private sector organizations that share a common goal.

Build in evaluation from the start. A well-thought-out evaluation framework, developed in tandem with the project itself, results in activities that are well targeted, resource efficient, and more likely to result in the desired outcomes. Chapters 11 and 16 will discuss formative evaluation techniques; Chapters 17 and 18 will provide discussions of potential process and outcome evaluation activities.

THE ROLE OF THEORY AND MODELS OF BEHAVIOR

Theories or models of how change occurs should guide development of the strategic plan and, ultimately, the components of the intervention. The role of theory is to help determine how change will occur and the role that the intervention can play in facilitating that change. It can also help planners set reasonable objectives; if one expects change to occur very quickly and easily, objectives are likely to be quite different than if one expects change to be gradual and difficult. There is no one theory or model that will work for every situation. It is not unusual for interventions to be guided by the constructs of a number of different models; examples of this occur throughout this book. The following sections discuss some of the most prominent theories and models used today.

Diffusion of Innovations

An *innovation* is an idea, practice, or object that is perceived as new by an individual or other unit of adoption, such as an organization or community (Rogers, 1983). *Diffusion* is the process by which an innovation is communicated through certain channels over time among the members of a social system (Rogers, 1983). Diffusion of innovations has been widely studied in a variety of settings and disciplines. Combined, these studies give a clear picture of what happens when an innovation—or a public health "solution"—is introduced to a population. While the basic sequence of events is the same across settings, the amount of time diffusion takes and the ultimate success of a diffusion effort vary widely and depend on factors unique to the type of innovation.

Backer, Rogers, and Sopory (1992) discussed two types of innovations relevant to public health: *incremental* and *preventive.* With incremental innovations, an individual takes an action now in order to receive a short-term benefit. With a preventive innovation, an individual takes an action to lower the probability that an undesired event (such as developing heart disease or cancer) will occur over the long term. They note that preventive innovations are more difficult to diffuse successfully. Various authors have identified other characteristics of the innovation that affect its likelihood of being successfully diffused and implemented (Green, Gottlieb, & Parcel, 1991; Kolbe & Iverson, 1981; Orlandi, Landers, Weston, & Haley, 1990; Leonard-Barton, 1988; Parcel et al., 1989; Rogers, 1983; Smith,

Howell, & McCann, 1990; Zaltman & Duncan, 1977). Characteristics common to many innovations are included in Table 10–1.

Classic diffusion theory divides members of a population into six categories based on their rate of adoption: innovators, early adopters, early majority, late majority, late adopters, and laggards (Rogers, 1983). These six categories are defined mathematically, by plotting time of adoption on a normal curve and dividing it into standard deviations from the mean time of adoption (Green et al.,

Table 10–1 Characteristics Affecting Successful Diffusion of an Innovation

Characteristic	Description
Relative advantage	The extent to which the innovation is better—faster, cheaper, or more beneficial—than existing practice
Compatibility	The degree to which the innovation is congruent with the potential adopters' existing practices, values, and realities
Complexity	The degree to which an innovation is simple or complicated—those that are less complicated usually require fewer changes and are more likely to be implemented
Communicability	The ease with which the innovation can be clearly communicated
Observability	The degree to which target adopters can watch someone model the innovation before adopting it themselves
Trialability	Also termed *divisibility* or *flexibility*—the extent to which an innovation can be divided to allow trial or piecemeal adoption and implementation
Cost efficiency	The degree to which tangible and intangible benefits outweigh cost
Time	The amount of time that must be invested to make the change
Commitment	The quantity of resources that must be invested to make the change
Risk and uncertainty	The amount of vulnerability and doubt associated with adopting the innovation
Reversibility	The ease with which an adopter can discontinue the innovation and revert to previous practice
Modifiability	The innovation's capacity to be changed as updates to it become available
Emergence	The extent to which an innovation is still being developed—those that are still changing may diffuse more slowly due to confusion, concerns about scientific merit, and the need for continual changes or adjustments

1991). Green and McAlister (1984) pointed out that some innovations, such as health practices requiring voluntary individual action, typically will not be adopted by the last 50% of the population unless adoption is required by law or by an employer.

The Transtheoretical Model of Stages of Change

Researchers from a number of disciplines have developed various models of behavior based on the idea that individuals move through stages of readiness as they change behavior. The transtheoretical model developed by James Prochaska and his colleagues is used extensively by practitioners seeking to change health behaviors. A thorough introduction to the transtheoretical model is provided in the second edition of Glanz, Lewis, and Rimer's *Health Behavior and Health Education* (Prochaska et al., 1997). The model is based on four core constructs: stages of change, decisional balance, self-efficacy, and processes of change. Descriptions of each of these constructs are provided in Table 10–2.

The transtheoretical model has been used to develop interventions targeting smoking cessation and a range of chronic conditions. The model is often used to segment audiences by their stage of change and then to develop interventions tailored to each stage (also called stage-matched interventions). An alternative is to segment audiences by stage, but then select one or two of the stages to target, as was done for the 5 A Day for Better Health program's media campaign.

As program components are developed, the transtheoretical model can provide guidance on the emphasis and content of these components, both in terms of decisional balance (what marketers would call the cost benefit equation) and in terms of processes that will promote change at each stage—the actions that people take to progress through the stages. Prochaska and colleagues (1997) argued that for a person to progress from precontemplation to contemplation, the pros—or benefits—of changing must increase, so interventions should focus on the pros. In contrast, to progress from contemplation to action, the cons—or costs—of changing must decrease, so program components targeting people at this stage should focus on reducing costs.

Prochaska and colleagues (1997) have also used the transtheoretical model to determine what type of change process to emphasize based on the stage people are in. They argue that practitioners need to use processes such as consciousness raising, dramatic relief, and environmental reevaluation to help people move from precontemplation to contemplation. In contrast, self-reevaluation processes are most helpful as people move from contemplation to preparation, when self-liberation processes take over. Once people take action, contingency management, helping relationships, counterconditioning, and stimulus control help them make the transition to maintenance.

Table 10–2 Transtheoretical Model Constructs

Constructs	Description
Stages of change	
Precontemplation	Has no intention to take action within the next 6 months
Contemplation	Intends to take action within the next 6 months
Preparation	Intends to take action within the next 30 days and has taken some behavioral steps in this direction
Action	Has changed overt behavior for less than 6 months
Maintenance	Has changed overt behavior for more than 6 months
Decisional balance	
Pros	The benefits of changing
Cons	The costs of changing
Self-efficacy	
Confidence	Confidence that one can engage in healthy behaviors across different challenging situations
Temptation	Temptation to engage in the unhealthy behavior across different challenging situations
Process of change	
Consciousness raising	Finding and learning new facts, ideas, and tips that support the healthy behavioral change
Dramatic relief	Experiencing the negative emotions (fear, anxiety, worry) that go along with unhealthy behavioral risks
Self-reevaluation	Realizing that the behavioral change is an important part of one's identity as a person
Environmental reevaluation	Realizing the negative impact of the unhealthy behavior or the positive impact of the healthy behavior on one's proximal social and physical environment
Self-liberation	Making a firm commitment to change
Helping relationships	Seeking and using social support for the healthy behavioral change
Counterconditioning	Substituting healthier alternative behaviors and cognition for the unhealthy behaviors
Contingency management	Increasing the rewards for the positive behavioral change and decreasing the rewards of the unhealthy behavior
Stimulus control	Removing reminders or cues to engage in the unhealthy behavior and adding cues or reminders to engage in the healthy behavior
Social liberation	Realizing that the social norms are changing in the direction of supporting the healthy behavioral change

Source: Reprinted with permission from K. Glanz, F.M. Lewis, and B.K. Rimer, *Health Behavior and Health Education: Theory, Research and Practice, 2nd edition,* p. 62, © 1997, Jossey-Bass Inc., Publishers.

Social Cognitive Theory

Social cognitive theory (SCT) is the modern incarnation of social learning theory. SCT views behavior as "dynamic, depending on aspects of the environment [anything external to the person] and the person, all of which influence each other simultaneously" (Baranowski et al., 1997, p. 158). The interaction among self, environment, and behavior is termed *reciprocal determinism*. The idea is that changes in any one of these three areas influence the other two.

SCT encompasses a number of concepts; the essence of it involves the aforementioned reciprocal determinism, as well as (1) increasing self-efficacy, or a person's confidence in his or her ability to perform a particular behavior; and (2) modeling positive outcomes of healthful behavior using credible role models and incentives.

Basically, using SCT to plan an intervention involves identifying appropriate *environmental changes* (similar to what marketers do when they adjust place or product) to support the desired behavior change, providing opportunities for *observational learning* by modeling appropriate behaviors for the target audience, and increasing *self-efficacy* by providing audience members with an opportunity to practice small changes and therefore increase their confidence in their ability to engage in the desired behavior. A more thorough discussion of the theory as it applies to health behaviors is provided in a chapter by Baranowski and colleagues (1997) in *Health Behavior and Health Education*.

THE OUTCOME: A STRATEGIC PLAN

Although many activities occur along the way, the results of the planning process are boiled down into a strategic plan that provides overall guidance for the program. This plan is sometimes referred to as a marketing plan or strategy statement. Using the end plan as a road map throughout the planning process helps ensure that planning efforts stay focused on "need to know" issues, rather than on going off on "nice to know" tangents. Exhibit 10–2 provides a sample outline of a strategic plan. There are probably as many ways of constructing a strategic plan as there are people who write them; the approach presented in this chapter closely follows the planning process outlined here.

The strategic plan should outline how the intervention is expected to work: who it should reach, what action people are expected to take as a result of the intervention, and how the strategies are expected to bring this action about. Once the strategic plan has been completed, it is used as a guide to develop separate plans for

Exhibit 10–2 Outline of the Strategic Plan

Executive Summary
Background and Mission
Challenges and Opportunities
Goals
Objectives (Measurable Outcomes)
Target Audiences
Core Strategy
Components for Implementing and Monitoring Strategy:
    Product Development
    Managing Perceived Price
    Improving Access (Place)
    Promotion
    Partnerships
    Evaluation

---

each strategy and to develop evaluation plans. The plan serves not only as a blueprint for the program, but as an organization's memory, reminding managers (or informing new staff or partners) of the history and rationale underlying the approaches selected. However, strategic plans are never finished. They should be dynamic living documents, revised to reflect changing audiences and environments. The next few sections of this chapter will outline the activities that culminate in the strategic plan. The activities to be outlined in Chapters 11 and 12 support strategic planning efforts.

ANALYZING THE SITUATION

The first step of planning is to collect and analyze information that will provide an understanding of the environment in which the program will operate. This process is referred to by various names, including "background review," "market survey," "market audit," "environmental scan," and "situation analysis," the term used here.

A situation analysis can vary in its level of detail, depending on the resources available and time allotted. Constructing it is a two-step process: first, information must be collected, and then it must be analyzed and turned into conclusions and recommendations to help make decisions for the next steps of the planning process.

Collecting Information

Collecting information for the situation analysis usually involves some or all of the following activities:

- reviewing the current science;
- reviewing the social environment;
- reviewing past activities and the results of those activities;
- identifying complementary and competing activities;
- analyzing how public policy issues are framed; and
- identifying sources of information about potential target audiences.

The situation analysis is usually constructed by using secondary research, that is, information or data originally collected for some other purpose.

Reviewing the Current Science

Planning an intervention begins with an understanding of the science upon which the effort will be based. A summary of this information should include

- morbidity and mortality data: These include the quantities and types of people most likely to develop or die from the condition and recent trends.
- known risk factors and, if possible, information on the quantities and types of people most likely to be affected by these risk factors: For example, one risk factor for breast cancer is bearing a first child after age 30. What percentage of women bear their first child after age 30? What other characteristics describe these women? What percent are married compared with women overall? What percent are of high, medium, or low socioeconomic status? Are there differences in education levels? All of this information helps to define potential target audiences.
- current behaviors: What are women doing now? What behavior will the recommended behavior replace? Why do people engage in their current behavior—what benefits and values do they associate with it?
- recommended behaviors: What should people do, and what is the likely impact if they do it? Recommended behaviors may involve treatment regimens for existing conditions, such as asthma or hypertension; screening for early detection of disease; or lifestyle changes to prevent disease (such as increasing physical activity, decreasing fat or salt intake, using condoms, or stopping smoking).
- known or suspected barriers to solving the problem: For example, do people lack information about what they should be doing? Is competition for the behavior too great? Must a policy change occur before people can change their behavior? If the behavior change involves using a product or program, is the product or program accessible to everyone who could benefit from it?

Scientific data often come from the institution sponsoring the program. Supplementary sources include state and local health department data, epidemiological and surveillance data collected by the Centers for Disease Control and Prevention (CDC), and other large federal studies, some of which will be discussed in more detail in Chapter 11. Relevant academic articles can often be obtained by searching MEDLINE, the National Library of Medicine's database (http://www.nlm.gov). In addition, CDC, the National Institutes of Health, and the major health professional organizations (e.g., the American Medical Association, the American Academy of Family Practitioners) and health voluntary agencies often provide information on risk factors, treatment guidelines, and the like.

Reviewing the Social Environment

Social conditions, social norms, and current policy play a large role in health behaviors. How do various aspects of the environment facilitate or hinder behavior? For example, what are the social norms of acceptable behavior? What laws or policies come into play? In their current form, do they help or hinder the program? Are there any new policies or changes in the pipeline? What is their likely impact? How important is the health issue to the community?

Taking a broader view, it can be useful to look at what the community believes to be the biggest social problems. Sometimes a particular health issue is actually at the root of many social problems. For example, Green and Kreuter (1991) noted that in 1989 a number of public opinion polls showed that the three leading concerns of Americans were crime, drugs, and acquired immunodeficiency syndrome (AIDS). They noted that "this list could be interpreted as drugs, drugs, and drugs" (Green & Kreuter, 1991, p. 91).

Information on the social environment can be obtained from academic studies. (The social science databases at most libraries can help in a search for them.) Existing surveys of public opinion and some of the studies conducted by governments will contain key economic indicators and other measures of social problems. Analyzing media coverage can also provide insight into the social environment and the current public agenda; this type of analysis will be discussed in more detail later in this chapter and in Chapter 17.

Reviewing Past Activities and Results

For ongoing programs, information should be collected on what has been done before—and what the results have been. It is important to identify not only what has been done, but also what has been working well and what has not, so that future plans can capitalize on past successes and avoid past mistakes. Ideally, the program will have included sufficient process and outcome evaluation measures to provide such information. If not, insight can be gleaned by talking to people involved with implementing the program. Try to identify the target audience(s);

goals and objectives; specific products, messages, materials, and distribution channels; and results. Materials used in the past, such as pamphlets and public service announcements, often have a longer life than program planners realize. If the materials are effective and consistent with the new strategy, planners can capitalize on their presence by using them in future efforts.

Identifying Complementary and Competing Activities

Often other organizations have programs that address the same issue. Identifying their activities can facilitate cooperation instead of competition by promoting synergy and preventing duplication of effort. Sometimes another group will already have a particular target audience adequately covered. At other times, working with another group to address the same audience may maximize both groups' resources. Perhaps materials can be shared or responsibility for needed materials can be divided up among the partners.

"Competition" for a public health initiative is anything that limits its resources, diverts attention from the subject of the initiative, or calls for contrary behaviors. There are three main sources of competition: other organizations conducting programs on the same subject, other social changes, and commercial sources. Why view the first two as competition? Because social issues compete for very limited resources, space, time, and audience attention. And in some instances, a group may be promoting a product, message, or practice in conflict with your organization's goals. Identifying "competition" allows planners to position and focus a program appropriately. Later, when tactics are being developed, knowing the competition's tactics allows program managers to maximize the attention their issue can command.

While many commercial entities promote healthy behaviors, some public health activities, such as preventing or stopping tobacco use, have a direct commercial opponent encouraging the very behavior that public health practitioners are trying to stop. More often, there are commercial institutions that emphasize behaviors or choices that are detrimental if not moderated or balanced by other behaviors. For example, a glance at Saturday morning television or the cereal aisle from a child's height will reveal far more products containing the "added fats and sugars" at the top of the Food Guide Pyramid than the whole grains, fruits, and vegetables that form the base of healthful eating. Similarly, the popular media tend to focus on violence and positively portray characters engaging in high-risk behaviors, such as smoking and nonmonogamous sexual activity. With the possible exception of physical activity, the media rarely picture everyday healthful behaviors such as using condoms or wearing seat belts.

Identifying "competing" activities helps program planners make informed decisions about how to proceed. They may decide

- to cede particular ground and focus on reaching target audiences through other channels.
- to try and counter the competition by increasing the presence of public health messages in the same places the "competitive" messages appear.
- in some instances to work with the authors of the "competitive" messages so that they present a more balanced message or at least decrease the frequency of messages or images that are detrimental to health.

Program planners often know of complementary or competing activities being conducted by other groups. Some activities also can be identified by phoning or writing to likely organizations and asking for copies of their materials addressing these audiences, through clearinghouses (such as those sponsored by federal agencies; http://www.healthfinder.gov is a good starting point for such a search), and through reviews of media coverage. Retrospective media coverage of particular topics can be obtained through electronic databases such as Nexis, Dialog, and UMI's ProQuest. Many libraries subscribe to these services (or see Chapter 11, Appendix 11–D for contact information). These databases usually include full text of articles from major national magazines and newspapers, as well as many local newspapers. Nexis also includes transcripts from major national television news shows and Cable News Network (CNN). In addition, Nexis, Dialog, and ProQuest include a large number of industry trade publications and scientific journals.

Ongoing media coverage can be monitored through these electronic databases or through traditional clipping services, such as Burelle's, Luce's, and Bacon's. These services employ staff who read through every page of every newspaper, looking for editorial content and advertisements containing the topics a client specifies. A more thorough discussion of electronic databases and clipping services will be provided in Chapter 17.

Analyzing How Public Policy Issues Are Framed

To help public health practitioners identify and evaluate potential ways of framing an issue, Ryan and others have developed the framing memo (Certain Trumpet Program, 1996; Ryan, 1991; Winett, 1995). In essence, a framing memo lists all potential ways an issue could be framed (by opponents and proponents of a policy) and the attributes of each and then provides a strategic analysis based on evaluation of each frame. The framing memo outlines the "arguments, images, and appeals to widely-shared principles that many people use to define and discuss an issue" (Winett, 1995, p. 1). It provides a "map and assessment of the range of arguments on an issue, so advocates may better make their case, and better anticipate what their opponents may say" (Certain Trumpet Program, 1996, p. ii).

To prepare a framing memo, public health practitioners must conduct a systematic search and review of newspaper articles on the public health policy topic of interest. Databases such as Nexis can be used to search and retrieve the text of relevant news articles. Practitioners can then review them to identify how both sides frame, or position, the policy issue. In identifying framing strategies, a matrix is prepared that summarizes, for each strategy,

1. the core position (main argument, summarized in one sentence);
2. the metaphor (the analogy used in the frame, with which the audience is familiar from another policy issue);
3. catch phrases (phrases used repeatedly to describe the argument);
4. symbols;
5. images (visual images evoked by the argument);
6. source of problem (who the frame implies is the source of the problem); and
7. appeal to principle (the individual core values to which the frame's arguments appeal).

Once all the framing strategies used in arguing for and against a proposal are outlined, they can be analyzed. Practitioners can compare the strength of frames used by the health advocate and the opposition. In particular, practitioners should evaluate how compelling the metaphors, symbols, catch phrases, and images evoked by the frames are for proponents versus opponents of the policy. What are the core values to which proponent and opponent frames appeal, and how do these core values compare in terms of how salient and influential they are to the target audience?

The analysis in the framing memo can provide guidance on which frames to emphasize or de-emphasize, which opposition frames need to be specifically countered, and whether it is necessary to develop new proponent frames. The framing memo can guide the development of new issue frames, and it can also help the practitioner to reframe opposition frames so that they support, rather than oppose, the proposed public health policy. Chapter 6 discussed these issues in greater detail. Chapter 12 will discuss using the framing memo to help craft a strategy for communications. Exhibit 10–3 illustrates how framing memos have been used to evaluate media coverage of the tobacco policy debate.

Identifying Potential Target Audiences and Sources of Additional Information

Selecting target audiences begins with determining the type of social change that will have the greatest impact on the public health problem. Do members of the public need to change their behavior? Does a new program, product, or service need to be developed to help individuals change their behavior? Do social conditions or policies need to change, either to support individual behavior change or to

Exhibit 10–3 The Tobacco Policy Debate

BACKGROUND

Menashe and Siegel (1997) prepared a framing memo on tobacco policy issues, attempting to identify and analyze the frames used to support and oppose tobacco policy interventions during the past decade. They identified these frames by analyzing all front page articles relating to tobacco that appeared in *The Washington Post, The New York Times, The Los Angeles Times,* and *The Wall Street Journal* from 1985 to 1996. A summary table from their framing memo outlines the five dominant tobacco industry frames (Table 10–3) and the five dominant tobacco control frames (Table 10–4) Menashe and Siegel identified.

In their analysis of how pro-tobacco control and anti-tobacco control groups framed the issue, Siegel and Menashe found that the tobacco industry has been much more successful in developing frames that appeal to the most compelling core values of the American public: freedom, independence, civil liberties, individual rights, control, autonomy, equality, fairness, economic opportunity, capitalism, and democracy (Table 10–3). In contrast, most of the public health community's frames have been based on the core value of health (Table 10–4).

TOBACCO INDUSTRY APPROACHES

The tobacco industry has been steadfast in framing tobacco policy in terms of core human values. Their dominant framing strategies—big government/civil liberties, moralizing/hostility, accommodation, choice, and health vs. wealth—elicit more of a passionate gut response than those put forth by tobacco control frames. The core frames of the tobacco industry conjure up images of a free America, anti-Big Brother sentiment, freedom of the American citizen, the freedom of choice, strengthening the economic prosperity of America and its citizens, supporting the economic livelihood of the tobacco farmer and the farmer's family, and also concern about America's youth. With the power of these images, it is no wonder that the tobacco industry has been able to remain so supported and successful.

TOBACCO CONTROL APPROACHES

Over the past decade, tobacco control advocates have increasingly used frames that appeal much more to the most compelling core values. For example, the deceit and manipulation frame (Table 10–4) appeals to the core values of fairness, equality, and justice. Its core position is that the tobacco industry intentionally manipulates people to smoke by control of nicotine levels, deceptive advertising, denial of tobacco's harmful health effects, and targeting of specific population subgroups. The core position of the nonsmokers' rights frame is that exposure to secondhand smoke violates people's right to a safe working environment and clean air in public places, and this frame appeals to the values of individual freedom, individual rights, and equality.

continues

Exhibit 10–3 continued

In addition, tobacco control frames that have been used most recently tend to attribute responsibility for the problem to society—that is, to the tobacco companies for
producing, marketing, and selling an addictive product and to the government for failing to control the sale and marketing of this drug to youth. For example, the smokers at
risk frame and illicit drug for minors frame attribute responsibility for the tobacco problem to individual smokers, individual youth, and individual merchants. In contrast,
frames such as deceit and manipulation, nonsmokers' rights, and drug delivery device
attribute responsibility to the tobacco companies and to the government.

CONCLUSIONS

The increased use of frames that are based on the most deeply ingrained core
values and that shift the attribution of responsibility from the individual to society
may, in part, explain the increased success of the tobacco control movement in obtaining unprecedented policy gains at the federal, state, and local levels. As Wallack,
Dorfman, Jernigan, and Themba (1993) suggest, "one of the great successes of the
antitobacco movement has been to win the framing battle with the tobacco companies and erode the credibility and legitimacy of the tobacco interests. As a result of
the movement's efforts', the general public increasingly views the tobacco industry
as 'merchants of death'" (p. 71).

Now that the dominant tobacco industry and tobacco control frames have been
identified and analyzed, tobacco control practitioners can use formative research to
test the effectiveness of alternative frames in garnering support for specific tobacco
policies. They can also test the effectiveness of new tobacco control frames and
attempts to reframe tobacco industry arguments so that they support, rather than
oppose, tobacco control policies.

---

support a new program, product, or service? If policies need to change, then the
true target audience is policy makers, although sometimes it is most effective to
convince a secondary audience, such as policy makers' constituents, to persuade
the policy makers.

Ideally, the situation analysis should include as much of a target audience portrait
as planners can paint with secondary information. In addition to a demographic description of potential audiences, planners will need detailed information on target
audiences' knowledge, attitudes, practices, and behaviors (KAPB) related to the public health problem. They will also need information on target audience members'
media habits, lifestyles, leisure activities, and general outlook, in order to identify
how best to construct and deliver products and/or messages they find appealing and
relevant. Chapter 11 will discuss this information in more detail.

However, this level of specificity usually is not possible at this stage in the planning process. The role of the situation analysis is to present some potential target

Table 10-3 Dominant Tobacco Industry Frames, 1985–1996

Frame	Big Government/ Civil Liberties	Moralizing/Hostility	Accommodation	Choice	Health vs. Wealth
Core position	Big government is interfering with personal lifestyle decisions, taking away smokers' rights.	Antismoking zealots are moralizing to us, discriminating against us, telling us what to do.	We can and should accommodate both smokers and nonsmokers.	Smoking is a matter of choice like any other choice in life.	Business will suffer if tobacco is regulated.
Metaphor	Big Brother Prohibition	Puritanism Holocaust	Accommodation of customers Negotiation Etiquette	Drinking alcohol Sex	Government regulation of small businesses
Images	Prohibition era 1984	Puritan era Holocaust Prohibition era	Negotiation Hospitality Environments	Prison cell	The Depression Small "mom and pop" stores
Catch phrases	Prohibition, big government, Big Brother, government off our backs, goes too far, red meat, candy, fat	Second-class citizens, cultural war; hostility; accommodation, tolerance, bombarded, antismoking zealots, fascists, health Nazis, attacking smokers, under siege	Accommodation, fair, balanced, reasonable, compromise, customers, clientele, hospitality	Choice, mature adults, judgments, clientele, already know the risks	Economic impact, jobs, out of business, tourists, making a living, difficult times, recession, suffering, hardship
Attribution of responsibility for problem	Big government Bureaucracy	Antismoking zealots	Hard-nose, uncompromising antismoking advocates	Individual smokers who make bad choices	Antismoking advocates who don't care about business
Implied solution	Keep government out of tobacco regulation.	Demand tolerance for smokers.	Demand accommodation of smokers and nonsmokers.	Let people decide whether to smoke, where to eat and work.	Let the market operate without intervention.
Core values	Freedom Civil liberties Autonomy Control	Freedom Civil liberties Autonomy Control Democracy	Fairness Equality	Freedom Autonomy Control	Free enterprise Capitalism Economic opportunity

Table 10–4 Dominant Tobacco Control Frames, 1985–1996

Frame	Smokers At Risk	Illicit Drug for Minors	Drug Delivery Device	Deceit and Manipulation	Nonsmokers' Rights
Core position	Smokers are putting themselves at great risk by smoking.	Cigarettes are not legal until age 18; thus we must punish merchants who sell them and youth who smoke.	Companies manipulate nicotine levels; therefore FDA must regulate the product for consumer safety.	The tobacco industry now manipulates people to smoke through deceptive advertising and lies.	Nonsmokers have a right to be protected from secondhand smoke in workplaces and public places.
Metaphor	Unhealthy habits, like drinking alcohol, eating high-fat foods	Illegal drugs: marijuana, alcohol	Regulation of medical devices and drugs, deceptive packaging, food labeling	Untruthful advertising	Environmental toxins; workplace hazards
Images	Making love with death; disgusting, dirty habit	Undercover investigations, law enforcement, speeding tickets, fines	Corporate fraud and deceit; painstaking investigation; vultures out to addict people	Secret plans; lying under oath; hiding	Smoke, hazardous workplaces, chemicals, pollution
Catch phrases	Unhealthy habit, discourage smoking	Crack down, sting operations, possession, use, supply, caught, punishment	Manipulation, fraud, deceit, jurisdiction, addictive, consumer watchdog	Lies, deceit, manipulation, targeting, denial, conceal, hide, secret	Nonsmokers' rights, health hazard, protection, danger, secondhand, involuntary, passive, smoke-free
Attribution of responsibility for problem	Individual smokers	Merchants Teenagers	Greedy, sneaky corporations that lie, mislead, and deceive	Tobacco industry	Workplace owners; government
Implied solution	Smokers should quit.	Merchants should not be allowed to sell cigarettes to youth; kids should not smoke.	Public must be protected by federal government.	Advertising and other aspects of tobacco business must be regulated.	Voluntary or legislative policies should restrict smoking in public places.
Core values	Health	Health	Health	Equality Fairness Justice	Freedom Civil liberties Equality Justice

audiences and identify additional sources of information that can be used to flesh out the audiences selected for the program. Program planners then need to weigh factors associated with each audience, such as the audience size (in terms of a percentage of the total population) and the impact on the public health problem of various actions the audience could take. As planners consider these factors, they will set behavioral objectives and select specific target audiences for each objective.

The best starting point for identifying target audiences is to segment the population of interest based on the behavior the program will seek to change. Dividing the population into those who already practice the behavior ("doers") and those who do not ("nondoers") provides some of the information needed to set goals and objectives and to define specific program target audiences. For consumer audiences, the health statistics reviewed earlier may include this information. For example, planners of an intervention to address youth smoking might divide children and teens into "never smoked," "tried it," and "current smoker." If the audience is policy makers, dividing them into those who have supported similar initiatives and those who have not is a logical starting point.

When consumers are the target audience, public health data sources usually lack much of the other information marketers need. With any luck, data may provide some information on knowledge and attitudes, but they almost never include information that helps determine how to reach an audience, such as their television, radio, and print media habits and leisure activities. Public health data also usually do not include information on the benefits and barriers people associate with the proposed behavior. When professionals or policy makers are the target audience, the public health practitioner encounters other problems locating needed information. Obtaining material produced by the policy makers can help assess how they are likely to think about an issue, as can reviewing media coverage for policy makers' comments.

The next step is to identify sources of information that could help further segment the target audience or answer some of these questions once the target audience is refined. Sources of additional information on consumer target audiences and some professional audiences can include

- past situation analyses or target audience profiles (prepared for an organization or for others addressing the same topic; federal agencies, voluntary health agencies, professional societies, and trade associations are also possible sources).
- government data sources, such as the National Health Interview Survey, the Behavioral Risk Factor Surveillance System, the National Health and Nutrition Examination Survey, and others.
- syndicated commercial market research studies, such as those conducted by Mediamark Research, Inc. (MRI) and Simmons Market Research Bureau, for

information on demographics, lifestyle, media habits, product purchase behavior, and leisure activities.
* public opinion polls, many of which are archived at The Roper Center for
Public Opinion Research at the University of Connecticut.

Chapter 11, Appendix 11–D will provide contact information for a variety of
secondary resources. While many of these sources are national, they can be useful
for local programs when no local data are available.

Assessing the Situation

Once program planners gather information, they must analyze and present it in
a way that helps them make decisions and shape the initiative. It is important to
identify and prioritize problems based on the public health burden they create,
assess the environment in which the social change will take place, and identify the
interventions most likely to bring about the particular type of social change.

The starting point of the analysis may be the public health burden or the social
environment; this depends on whether one is trying to prioritize the order in which
public health problems are addressed or developing an initiative to address a particular problem (e.g., cancer, nutrition, drug abuse). If the goal is to determine the problem an initiative (or initiatives) should address, it is best to begin with the social
environment and prioritize the problems in that context (e.g., what problems are
contributing to the worst, or most pernicious, social problems?). Green and
Kreuter (1991) called this the *reductionist* approach. If instead the goal is to understand the social environment in which a particular initiative will be put into place,
it is best to begin by looking at the public health burden associated with that problem and then work outward toward understanding the environment around the
problem. Green and Kreuter (1991) referred to this as the *expansionist* approach.

Identifying and Prioritizing Problems Based on Public Health Burden

The public health statistics and scientific recommendations gathered as the first
step of preparing the situation analysis provide a starting point for identifying and
prioritizing problems that an intervention could address. While identifying problems is relatively easy, the prioritization process is not clear-cut. Planners must
consider a number of factors when prioritizing, such as, What population groups
are affected most? What changes could be made that would have the most impact
on the problem? Can individuals make these changes now or will policy changes
be needed? What is the mission of the public health organization?

Reviewing information on competing and complementary activities, as well as
public opinion on the issue, can also help planners assess priorities. If other organizations are doing a sufficient job of addressing a problem, there may be no need

for another organization to make it a priority. On the other hand, multiple organizations focusing on a problem is often an indicator that the population as a whole considers it important or that the time is right to meet the challenge the problem presents.

Another important factor to consider when prioritizing public health problems is the current rate of adoption of each problem's solution. Diffusion of innovations, introduced earlier in this chapter, provides a framework to make such assessments.

Assessing the Social Change Environment

There are a number of ways to assess the social change environment. Kotler and Roberto (1989) outlined three methods: (1) scenarios construction; (2) analysis of strengths, weaknesses, opportunities, and threats (SWOT); and (3) issue identification and analysis. All involve examining trends and determining the potential opportunities and threats as well as the types of change that may need to occur (e.g., technological, political/legal, or economic).

The scenarios construction method involves building up multiple possible scenarios from the available data and then calculating the likelihood that each will occur. In the SWOT approach, the strengths and weaknesses of both the organization that will sponsor the intervention and of the social change itself are assessed. This information is then used to identify opportunities, or openings, for an intervention to make a difference. At the same time, potential threats to the success of the intervention are identified. This process helps point the intervention in promising directions, rather than wasting time on efforts that are not likely to succeed. Early identification of threats to success allows program managers to proactively address many of these threats or at least factor them in when setting expectations and objectives. With issue identification and analysis, technological, political/legal, economic, sociocultural, and demographic trends are analyzed to determine what the next major issue (i.e., potential change) is likely to be in each category and then who (what groups) are likely to support and oppose the issue.

Identifying Interventions Most Likely To Be Effective

In addition to understanding the environment in which the intervention will take place, it is important to assess, in a global sense, the type of change people will be asked to make (whether they are consumers, professionals, or policy makers) and to identify the types of interventions most likely to be effective in a particular situation. Although every intervention faces unique challenges, identifying the commonalities between the planned intervention and others allows an organization to conserve resources by focusing on approaches that have proven effective in the past. A number of social change classification approaches have been developed for this task.

Rangan, Karim, and Sandberg (1996) have developed an interesting framework for categorizing a social change and determining appropriate marketing strategies based on the costs and benefits the target audience associates with the change. They recommend categorizing the social change along two dimensions: (1) low cost to high cost and (2) tangible, personal benefits to intangible, societal benefits. As Figure 10–1 illustrates, this process results in the ability to assign the social change to one of four cells or types. Each type of change is characterized by corresponding marketing problems and solutions.

Low cost

Cell A	Cell B
Problem: Audience doesn't oppose behavior, but doesn't have needed information about it.	Problem: Audience doesn't oppose behavior, but it has no direct, compelling benefits for them.
– Benefits are clear and direct.	– Benefits are intangible and indirect.
– Change is easy.	– Change is easy.
– There is no need to address deep-rooted beliefs or attitudes.	– There is no need to address deep-rooted beliefs or attitudes.
Solution: Communication and information are key.	Solution: Communication should emphasize convenient, practical behaviors. Facilitator may be needed.
Trap: Using threat appeals in an attempt to change attitudes.	Trap: An overly moralistic tone or attempts to evangelize.

Tangible, personal benefits ———————————————————————— Intangible, societal benefits

Cell C	Cell D
Problem: Change is difficult; audience needs help doing it.	Problem: Change is difficult, and there is no individual benefit.
– Benefits are clear and direct.	– Benefits are intangible and indirect.
– Change is difficult.	– Change is difficult.
Solution: Balance communication to inform and affect social norms with strong community support system.	Solution: Try to reposition to Cell C by providing a direct benefit; if impossible, try (1) leveraging enthusiasm of early adopters or (2) supply-side persuasion.

High cost

Figure 10–1 The Cost Benefit Dimensions of Social Change. *Source:* Adapted and Reprinted by permission of *Harvard Business Review.* From "Do Better at Doing Good" by V. Kasturi Rangan, Sohel Karim, and Sheryl Sandberg, May–June 1996. Copyright © 1996 by the President and Fellows of Harvard College; all rights reserved.

Cell A: Easy Change, Direct Benefits. Cell A social changes have few costs to the target audience and provide tangible personal benefits. Providing motivational information may be enough to encourage change. Behavior changes that can be categorized as Cell A probably are more likely to be "onetime" or low-involvement behaviors, rather than ongoing or high-involvement behaviors. By onetime behaviors we mean those for which the target audience makes a decision to engage in the behavior, engages in it, and then does not have to think about it for some substantial period of time, as opposed to behavior changes that must be made frequently. For example, a low-involvement behavior like getting a flu shot or cancer detection test involves making a decision, making the appointment, and getting the shot or test—and then (assuming the test result was negative) not thinking about it again for a year or more. In contrast, ongoing or high-involvement behavior changes must be made on a regular basis. For consumers, changes in lifestyle, such as sexual practices, eating habits, or physical activity levels, fall into this category; target audience members often face myriad situations in which they must decide whether to engage in the behavior change. For policy makers, supporting public health as an institution is likely to fall into this category as well.

Cell A changes are usually the only type of social change in which a communication campaign alone can be expected to stimulate behavior change—and then only if there are no problems with accessibility. For example, consider childhood immunizations. For many parents or guardians in the United States, getting a child immunized is a low-cost direct-benefit behavior. Persuading them to get their children immunized is often as simple as informing them of the availability of the vaccine (assuming that health care providers have adequate supplies). But immunization may not be a Cell A problem for some parents and guardians. Perhaps they live far from the nearest physician or health center. Or perhaps they are too poor to afford the vaccine.

Cell B: Easy Change, Indirect Benefits. Many public health prevention initiatives can be categorized as Cell B efforts: The change is relatively easy, but a direct, compelling benefit to each individual cannot be guaranteed as a result of making the change. For example, taking steps to reduce the risk of developing cancer or heart disease does not guarantee that an individual will not develop such diseases. As Rangan and colleagues (1996) noted, the key to success for Cell B is to provide practical, convenient ways for the target audience to engage in the desired behavior. Cell B programs often require a communication campaign and some type of a facilitator that works more directly with target audience members.

The 5 A Day for Better Health program is an example of a Cell B program: Communication efforts focus on easy ways to add servings of fruits and vegetables, and a partnership between the produce industry and the National Cancer Institute (NCI) augments NCI's communication efforts and facilitates change by providing consumers with the information they need at the point of purchase. The produce industry also creates new products that increase convenience—such as prepackaged salads and carrot sticks. In many communities, the program provides nutrition education activities for children and/or adults.

Cell C: Hard Change, Direct Benefits. Other public health prevention and treatment efforts fall into Cell C: There are clear benefits to the individual, but the changes involved are exceedingly difficult. For example, smoking cessation, abstinence from drug use, and HIV prevention are most often Cell C problems. Among teens, abstinence from drug use and HIV prevention necessitate peer refusal skills that many teens do not have—skills that a communication campaign alone cannot build.

Cell C changes require a combination of intensive support provided at the community level and a communication campaign. Rangan and colleagues (1996) argued that many Cell C programs are hopelessly one sided, relying on a communication campaign or community efforts but not a combination of both. The skills needed for the behavior change must be built one on one or in small groups; the role of the communication campaign is to influence social and cultural norms surrounding the behavior.

Cell D: Hard Change, Indirect Benefits. Cell D changes are the most onerous; target audience members associate very high costs with making such changes and do not associate any personal benefit with doing so. Individuals in such situations often risk ostracism if they make the change; organizations risk putting themselves at a competitive disadvantage. Rangan and colleagues (1996) advocate repositioning Cell D problems into Cell C if at all possible. Their example was family planning efforts in Bangladesh. Targeting men resulted in a Cell D problem: Men could not see a personal benefit of fewer children, and the cultural costs of changing behavior were very high. By targeting women, program planners shifted it to a Cell C problem: Although women had many barriers to change (most notably access to contraception, since men usually do the shopping), they could see the personal benefit for themselves and their other children of making the change. The program used a two-pronged approach: (1) communication targeted to men to position support of family planning as acceptable and (2) provision of contraceptives to women through rural medical practitioners, who were trusted and who made house calls, thus saving women the embarrassment of buying contraceptives in public.

If repositioning a Cell D problem is impossible, Rangan and colleagues (1996) recommended trying to leverage the enthusiasm of early adopters (those most willing and likely to make the change), arguing that if they become committed to the cause, it is in their best interests to become active agents for change. However, those working in public health settings must carefully weigh the ethics of such a strategy; as we have already noted, one of the defining characteristics of Cell D problems is that the early adopters have much to lose by engaging in the behavior. "First, do no harm" should be a guiding principle when considering Cell D strategies that target early adopters. It is important to note that addressing Cell D problems will likely require broad interventions, repeated over a long time. Progress is likely to be slow, so expectations should be set accordingly.

An alternative strategy applicable to some public health problems is what marketers term "supply-side persuasion." In other words, rather than trying to get consumers to change, try to get manufacturers to change. While in some situations this strategy seems destined to fail (consider smoking and cigarette manufacturers), it works in others. Some regulations are in effect supply-side persuasion. For example, the Food and Drug Administration's recent decision to add folate to grain products can be thought of as supply-side persuasion: Rather than putting all the burden of consuming enough folate to avoid birth defects on pregnant women, the food processors will play a role. Supply-side persuasion might also consist of strategies such as persuading restaurant chefs or food processors to decrease the amount of fat or sodium in their foods.

It is important to remember that an intervention's classification into Cell A, B, C, or D may shift—or be repositioned by program managers—depending on the target audience. In fact, as discussed above, Rangan and colleagues (1996) recommend repositioning Cell D problems to Cell C if at all possible.

While not all social changes can be easily assigned to one of the cells described by Rangan and colleagues (1996) using such a framework helps program planners estimate the complexity of the social change and the corresponding structure of the intervention that will be required to bring about substantial change. Knowing whether an initiative is addressing a Cell A problem or a Cell D problem can help a manager be realistic about the potential impact of marketing efforts and the resources required to instigate change. It also provides an easy way to examine the social change along two important dimensions and assess the possibilities of repositioning it to increase success rates—through target audience selection, cost reduction, increased incentives, or more personalized benefits.

Social changes can also be classified along other dimensions, some of which were discussed in Chapter 2. For example, Kotler and Roberto (1989) analyzed social changes along three different dimensions that have to do with the type of product and its corresponding type of consumer demand.

Kotler and Roberto's first dimension is *difficulty of market penetration.* They divide social changes into the type of product or service that must be developed— new, superior, and substitute—depending on the state of consumer demand. New products fill a *latent* demand; in other words, target adopters have an unfilled need that the product or change addresses. An example would be behavior changes to prevent high blood pressure or heart disease. In contrast, superior products are appropriate when there is *underfilled* demand—the current behavior itself, or its accessibility, does not satisfy target adopters' needs. Their example is rural areas where physicians are too few and far away. Finally, substitute products or behaviors must be developed to address the *unwholesome* demand that occurs when target adopters are engaging in harmful behaviors, such as drug abuse. The challenge is to "de-market" the existing behavior and provide a substitute that the target adopters will accept.

Kotler and Roberto (1989) also divided behavior changes into those tied to a tangible product, such as family planning and contraceptives, versus those that involve the behavior change alone. They argued that if a behavior is tied to a tangible product, the marketer must market both the behavior and the product, a situation they characterize as *dual* demand. They noted that dual demand can take a number of forms, each requiring a different marketing strategy. For example:

- The product may already be embraced by the target adopters for reasons other than the behavior change (e.g., condoms may be used to prevent disease but not as a method of family planning).
- The behavior change has been adopted but the particular product has not been.
- Both product and behavior change are at the same stage of adoption.

Their final classification system is based on whether the target adopters must embrace an idea, make a single behavior change, or make a sustained behavior change. For single behavior changes, such as getting a flu shot or donating blood, they note that demand is *irregular*—the change only needs to happen at certain times or under certain conditions. Therefore, the marketing task is to convince people to do something once. Community tragedies sometimes create a different sort of irregular demand: The public and policy makers suddenly clamor for a public health program previously thought to be unimportant. With sustained behavior changes, marketers who have successfully convinced target adopters to try the behavior will eventually face a *faltering* demand situation when compliance with the behavior drops. Those marketing disease prevention frequently have this problem: When prevention programs are successful, nothing bad happens—indeed, nothing appears to happen at all—and policy makers are often tempted to reallocate resources to burgeoning crises.

Using approaches such as these to classify the social change and identify the problems, solutions, and marketing strategies needed will provide a foundation and focus for subsequent planning efforts.

SETTING GOALS AND OBJECTIVES

After completing a thorough situation analysis, planners should set measurable goals and objectives for specific target audiences. Of course, this is much easier said than done, since appropriate objectives may differ somewhat depending on how the target audience is defined. Since goals and objectives are two terms used almost interchangeably and differently by different people, both should be defined.

Goals translate a program's mission into specific behavioral outcomes (Andreasen, 1995). For example, the goal of the 5 A Day for Better Health program is to increase Americans' fruit and vegetable consumption. The U.S. Department of Health and Human Services' Year 2000 health objectives for the nation are often used as program goals (as is true for the 5 A Day program).

Objectives quantify the goals and describe the specific intermediate steps to take to make progress toward them. In the private sector, objectives are typically defined in terms of product or service trial, brand awareness, or sales. Public health efforts often include health objectives (such as reductions in morbidity or mortality) and corresponding behavioral objectives that address how the health objective will be achieved.

Objectives should be measurable, solidly linked to a behavioral outcome, associated with a specific target audience, and associated with a specific time period. As Green and Kreuter (1991) noted, "objectives are crucial; they form a fulcrum, converting diagnostic data into program direction" (p. 118). They note that objectives should answer these questions:

1. *Who* will receive the program (health objective) or make the change (behavioral objective)?
2. *What* health benefit should be received or action should be taken?
3. *How much* of that benefit or action should be achieved?
4. *By when* should it be achieved?

Exhibit 10–4 presents some possible behavioral objectives for a mammography program targeting women age 50 and older. The goal of this hypothetical program is to increase the rates of screening mammography among older women, since research has shown that rates decreases with age (Marchant & Sutton, 1990).

In this example, many of the other social changes necessary to support increased use of mammography had already been implemented: Medicare and other

---

Exhibit 10–4 Sample Objectives for Mammography Program

1. By 2002, increase by x% the number of women age 50 or older who received their first mammogram in the past year.
2. By 2002, increase by x% the number of women age 50 or older who received a mammogram in the past year.
3. By 2002, increase by x% the number of general practitioners, family practitioners, and internists who discuss mammography at all office visits by female patients over age 50 and provide them with a referral if necessary.

insurance reimbursements for mammograms had been established. The first objective in Exhibit 10–4 is actually a product trial objective: Get women who have never had a mammogram to do it once. The second objective is trying to increase population compliance with the recommended schedule of annual mammograms.

The third objective addresses the behavior of a secondary audience: physicians. This objective illustrates one aspect of the iterative nature of the marketing process: how research conducted during the planning phase of a program can result in objectives and audiences that may not have been considered at the outset. In this instance, secondary research had shown that three-fourths of women went for a mammogram because their physician recommended it (Marchant & Sutton, 1990) and that overall visits to physicians increased with age (National Center for Health Statistics, 1990). So, if women got mammograms because their physicians recommended them and if older women were more likely to see a physician, why were screening rates lower for older women? A survey of women revealed two factors that likely played a role: (1) Obstetricians/gynecologists are more likely to recommend mammograms than are other physicians, but visits to obstetricians/gynecologists are less frequent for older women; and (2) women who went for a checkup were more likely to get mammograms than those who went for a specific problem, which suggests that physicians were less likely to discuss screening tests with women who were there only for a problem (Sutton & Doner, 1992). Therefore, increasing the percentage of physicians who recommend mammograms to all female patients, regardless of whether the office visit is for a checkup or a specific problem, is likely to increase the percentage of women who get them.

To measure progress toward objectives, baseline and follow-up data must be available. In some instances, previously conducted studies can supply baseline data (and help program planners set reasonable objectives by examining current behavior and, with any luck, recent trends over time). In other instances, a custom study must be conducted. When objectives are set, evaluation plans should be developed that spell out how progress will be measured against the objectives.

Green and Kreuter (1991) also outlined a number of other factors that planners should consider when setting objectives, namely that

1. progress toward meeting objectives should be measurable.
2. individual objectives should be based on relevant, reasonably accurate data.
3. objectives should be in harmony across topics and levels.

This third factor is particularly important; occasionally programs will inadvertently establish two objectives that conflict with one another.

When setting behavioral objectives, one should consider the type of change most likely to result in progress toward a health objective. That is, if the health objective is to reduce by x% the number of people who die in car accidents each year, a behavioral objective might be to increase by x% the number of people who wear seat belts. That might be supplemented by a regulatory/legal objective of increasing by $x\%$ the number of states that have primary seat belt laws in effect. It is very important to assess what can be accomplished, given the program's resources, and to refrain from setting objectives that the program cannot possibly address or attain. A thorough situation analysis coupled with a sound theoretical framework for the intervention should help avoid such problems.

SELECTING PRIMARY AND SECONDARY TARGET AUDIENCES

Identifying target populations for each social change is nearly as much art as science. It also tends to be an iterative process. As additional secondary and primary research is conducted, more is learned and the audiences are refined—or new audiences may be introduced, as the example in the discussion of objectives illustrates.

A program's *primary target audience* is the group that needs to make the behavior change. There can be more than one primary target audience, although each should form a distinct group. If "everyone" who has certain broad characteristics (e.g., American adults, policy makers) needs to make the change, then program planners need to identify a subset of this group who is either most willing to make the change or will have the most impact on overall public health by making the change. Some of the theories discussed earlier in this chapter can provide guidance in making such choices.

Secondary target audiences are people who can help the primary target audience(s) make the change. For example, family members of persons with hypertension can help them adhere to treatment regimens. Health care providers can counsel patients about various behavioral risk factors or recommend tests for early detection of disease. Health teachers or school food service personnel can help students change their eating habits. Constituents can help policy makers understand the importance of a particular initiative.

Target audience selection usually begins by dividing the population into groups based on some criterion and then looking at the differences between the groups. This process is called audience segmentation. The assumption behind segmentation is that each group is unique. Each has different current behaviors and reasons for those behaviors, and each associates different benefits and barriers with the behavior the program is promoting. Additionally, each group may be reached more efficiently through different channels, may need different products for support, and may respond to different types of message appeals. Programs that attempt to target "the general public" or "policy makers" risk being weak because they are designed to appeal to everyone (and therefore cannot focus on the benefits and barriers relevant to a particular group) or appeal only to managers who are not members of the population the program is supposed to address.

The goal of audience segmentation is to identify subgroups whose members are similar to each other and distinct from other groups along dimensions that are meaningful in the context of the program. Audiences can be segmented on a variety of dimensions, such as demographic, geographic, behavioral, or lifestyle characteristics. For most public health programs, behavioral segmentation is key to successfully bringing about social change. Chapter 11 will discuss various audience segmentation approaches and provides guidance on how to select target audiences based on the results of the segmentation process.

UNDERSTANDING TARGET AUDIENCES

Once target audiences have been identified, planners must develop a thorough understanding of them to craft an intervention that results in social change. Planners must identify and prioritize the audience's basic needs, desires, and values. What is important to the audience? Mapping potential target audiences' behavior is a good way to help identify their needs, desires, and values, as well as potential catalysts for their behavior change. A useful starting point is to compare "doers" (those who engage in the appropriate behavior) with "nondoers" (some segment of which will become the target audience). On what characteristics do the two groups differ? Some of these characteristics are the factors that determine each group's behavior. Understanding *why* each group engages in their respective behaviors helps us understand the needs, desires, and values that underlie the behavior. Chapter 11 will discuss qualitative research techniques that can be used to develop this understanding; Chapter 12 will present a more thorough discussion of processes to use in the context of crafting communication strategies to reach target audiences.

Once these basic needs, desires, and values have been identified, it is time to explore ways of framing the desired behavior to reinforce the target audience's core values. At this point, mapping the *proposed* behavior is very important. What is an audience member going to need to do in order to engage in the desired public health behavior? It is helpful to walk through the steps an audience member would have to take. What stands in the way? What is the benefit *to the individual* of engaging in the behavior? Sometimes secondary research can be used to answer these questions, but at other times primary research is required. Chapters 11 and 12 will provide information on approaches to gathering this type of information.

After planners have a sense of the barriers to the behavior (and the benefits of it from the target audience's perspective), they can examine what an intervention can do to make the behavior easier. One way to do this is to make a list of each barrier and what would need to change in order to reduce or eliminate the barrier. Then these changes can be assessed in terms of the marketing mix and the intervention's capabilities and resources. What changes can program components be designed to address? How will these components be delivered? If all changes cannot be addressed, will the intervention be strong enough to affect target audience behavior? To help think through all of the issues, Exhibit 10–5 summarizes some challenges to accomplishing social change. Many of these were discussed in detail in earlier chapters of this book.

At the end of this process, it is time to make some realistic decisions about the shape of the intervention—and whether to conduct it at all. For example, if the real problem is that clinics aren't open late enough for working parents to take their children there for immunizations, can the clinic hours be changed? If not, promotional efforts are unlikely to result in increased immunization rates.

PUTTING IT ALL TOGETHER: THE STRATEGIC PLAN

The changes planners decide to address through an intervention become the program strategies. It is very important to assess all aspects of the marketing mix (product, price, place, promotion, and partners) in terms of how they affect the

---

Exhibit 10–5 Some Challenges to Social Change

Obstacles associated with using a marketing approach in a noncommercial setting:
- Consumer data are more difficult to obtain and often of poorer quality.
- Financial cost is difficult to manipulate, so managers must rely on changing other costs (i.e., psychological, time, effort, or lifestyle costs).
- Communication strategies are more difficult to implement because channels cannot be controlled and messages may be complex.
- Results of marketing efforts are often difficult to evaluate.
- Organizations may not be marketing-savvy and/or control all components of the marketing mix.

Obstacles associated with changing ingrained behaviors:
- Negative demand—the target audience may oppose the change being advocated.
- Legal and regulatory changes may be required to support behavior change.
- The change may involve highly sensitive issues or may conflict with culture.
- The costs of the behavior change often exceed tangible benefits.
- The benefits may accrue to third parties, rather than to the individual making the change.
- Early adopters risk ostracism (for individuals) or losing a competitive standing in the marketplace (for companies).
- Change may take a long time.

target audience(s) and target behavior—and what will need to be in place for social change to occur. This is particularly important if the intervention will focus on
communication and promotion about a specific product or service. One of the
worst mistakes one can make is to stimulate demand for a product or service that is
not available or does not work as promised. Once disappointed, the audience will
be unlikely to come back and try again.

The easiest way to ensure that all aspects of the marketing mix are considered is
to address them in the strategic plan. The plan should present initial approaches to
redefining the product (or behavior) in terms of the key benefit it offers the target
audience through appropriate positioning. The plan can be relatively short, but
should outline how change is expected to occur and should include the information presented in the outline in Exhibit 10–1. For many social change initiatives,
enlisting the aid of a range of partners will be critical to achieving success. An
important part of developing the strategic plan is thinking through what makes
sense for your organization to do versus what other organizations may be able to
do more effectively and efficiently. Chapter 14 will discuss identifying and working with partners.

Once a strategic plan for the intervention has been developed, planners' attention must turn to developing the components—or tactics—that will constitute the
intervention. Part II, Section II discusses many aspects of this process.

CONCLUSION

Thorough planning is essential to successful social change endeavors. Planning
begins with an extensive analysis of the situation, including identifying and prioritizing problems based on public health burden and assessing the environment for
social change. These factors must be considered together in order to identify the
types of interventions most likely to be effective for a particular public health
problem. The next step is to set goals and objectives based on the specific behaviors, conditions, or policies to be changed; this process should be guided by a
theoretical framework or model of how change is expected to occur.

Target populations must be identified for each social change; a logical starting
point for their identification is to compare those who do not engage in the appropriate public health behavior with those who do engage in it. In order to design an
effective intervention, target populations must be thoroughly understood. In particular, the needs, desires, and values underlying their current behavior must be
identified, and then alternative ways of framing the desired behavior so that it is
consistent with or reinforces audience members' core values must be explored.

Once the appropriate positioning for the social change has been determined, a
strategic plan is developed. The strategic plan should outline how change is ex-

pected to occur and how the intervention will support that change. The plan should address all aspects of the marketing mix—product (behavior), price, place, promotion, and partners.

REFERENCES

Andreasen, A.R. (1995). *Marketing social change: Changing behavior to promote health, social development, and the environment.* San Francisco: Jossey-Bass.

Backer, T.E., Rogers, E.M., & Sopory, P. (1992). *Designing health communication campaigns: What works?* Thousand Oaks, CA: Sage.

Bandura, A. (1986). *Social foundations of thought and action.* Englewood Cliffs, NJ: Prentice-Hall.

Baranowski, T., Perry, C.L., & Parcel, G.S. (1997). How individuals, environments, and health behavior interact: Social cognitive theory. In K. Glanz, F.M. Lewis, & B.K. Rimer (Eds.), *Health behavior and health education: Theory, research and practice* (2nd ed., pp. 153–178). San Francisco: Jossey-Bass.

Certain Trumpet Program. (1996, September). *Framing memo: The affirmative action debate.* Washington, DC: Author.

Green, L.W., Gottlieb, N.H., & Parcel, G.S. (1991). Diffusion theory extended and applied. In W.B. Ward & F.M. Lewis (Eds.), *Advances in health education and promotion* (3, pp. 91–117). Greenwich, CT: Jessica Kingsley.

Green, L.W., & Kreuter, M.W. (1991). *Health promotion planning: An educational and environmental approach* (2nd ed.). Mountain View, CA: Mayfield.

Green, L.W., & McAlister, A. (1984). Macro-interventions to support health behavior: Some theoretical perspectives and practical reflections. *Health Education Quarterly, 11,* 322–339.

Kolbe, L.J. & Iverson, D.C. (1981). Implementing comprehensive health education: Educational innovations and social change. *Health Education Quarterly, 8,* 57–80.

Kotler, P., & Roberto, E.L. (1989). *Social marketing: Strategies for changing public behavior.* New York: Free Press.

Leonard-Barton, D. (1988). Implementation characteristics of organizational innovations: Limits and opportunities for management strategies. *Communication Research, 15,* 603–631.

Marchant, D.J., & Sutton, S.M. (1990). Use of mammography: United States, 1990. *Morbidity and Mortality Weekly Report, 39,* 621–630.

Menashe, C.L., & Siegel, M. (1997). *The power of a frame: An analysis of newspaper coverage of tobacco issues—United States, 1985–1996.* Boston: Boston University School of Public Health.

National Center for Health Statistics. (1990). Medical care survey. Unpublished raw data.

National Highway Traffic Safety Administration. (1996). *National drunk and drugged driving prevention month program planner* (Rep. No. DOT HS 808-455). Washington, DC: Author.

Orlandi, M.A., Landers, C., Weston, R., & Haley, N. (1990). Diffusion of health promotion innovations. In K. Glanz, F.M. Lewis, & B.K. Rimer (Eds.) *Health behavior and health education: Theory, research and practice* (pp. 288–313). San Francisco: Jossey-Bass.

Parcel, G.S., Eriksen, M.P., Lovato, C.Y., Gottlieb, N.H., Brink, S.G., & Green, L.W. (1989). The diffusion of school-based tobacco-use prevention programs: Project description and baseline data. *Health Education Research, 4*(1), 111–124.

Prochaska, J.O., Redding, C.A., & Evers, K.E. (1997). The transtheoretical model and stages of change. In K. Glanz, F.M. Lewis, & B.K. Rimer (Eds.), *Health behavior and health education: Theory, research and practice* (2nd ed., pp. 60–84). San Francisco: Jossey-Bass.

Rangan, V.K., Karim, S., & Sandberg, S.K. (1996, May-June). Do better at doing good. *Harvard Business Review, 74*, 42–54.

Rogers, E.M. (1983). *Diffusion of innovations* (3rd ed.). New York: Free Press.

Ryan, C. (1991). *Prime time activism: Media strategies for grassroots organizing*. Boston: South End Press.

Smith, D.W., Howell, K.A., & McCann, K.M. (1990). Evaluation of the coalition index: A guide to school health education materials. *Journal of School Health, 60*(2), 49–52.

Sutton, S.M., & Doner, L.D. (1992). Insights into the physician's role in mammography utilization among older women. *Women's Health Issues, 2*, 175–179.

Wallack, L., Dorfman, L., Jernigan, D., & Themba, M. (1993). *Media advocacy and public health: Power for prevention*. Newbury Park, CA: Sage.

Winett, L. (1995). *Advocate's guide to developing framing memos*. Berkeley, CA: Berkeley Media Studies Group.

Zaltman, G., & Duncan, R. (1977). *Strategies for planned change*. New York: Wiley.

CHAPTER 11

Formative Research

Formative research is at the core of the marketing approach. At the outset, it is used to help determine the most appropriate audiences to target for change. As audiences are selected, formative research helps program managers find out what audience members want and need, so that they can create, package, or frame the public health product accordingly. Formative research helps identify what actions target audiences are willing and able to take and how to convince them to take these actions. It is used to explore the perceived barriers to and benefits of taking an action. And it helps identify how to best reach audiences with the product or messages about it.

Formative research is commonly used for public health initiatives to support problem identification, audience segmentation, and development of the strategies to be used in the initiative. Both quantitative and qualitative research techniques are used.

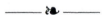

THE ROLE OF FORMATIVE RESEARCH

Formative research can be used in many ways. At times it is used as a situation analysis tool, to help identify the problems an initiative could address. It is essential to identifying and understanding the most appropriate audience(s) for a program to reach. It can also help identify the actions target audience members can take that will help them make the most progress toward addressing the public health problem. Once an intervention begins to take shape, formative research helps develop messages and materials that are original, relevant, and motivating to the target audience(s). It also helps shape products and services by providing feedback from target audience members on preliminary concepts or versions.

As an example of how formative research can be used, consider a situation in which immunization rates are lower than recommended. The first thing to do is identify the source of the problem: Why are immunization rates low? Formative research can help us understand (1) why people are not getting immunized and (2) under what circumstances physicians recommend the immunization to their patients. Armed with this knowledge, we can begin to investigate potential target audiences. For starters, should the target audience be unimmunized individuals, because for some reason they are not getting the immunization? Or should it be health care professionals—or both?

Once some of these issues are resolved, we will need to know when and where to intervene. Where are we losing people? What keeps them from engaging in the desired behavior? A useful analogy is that of an interstate highway. The desired behavior is at the end of the highway, but as a person embarks on his or her journey, there are many attractive exit ramps before the destination. If the person takes any of those ramps, he or she may never reach the destination. Another role for formative research is to find out who is being led astray and at what exit ramps. Then it can help us to understand why those ramps are more appealing than our destination, so that we can reposition the destination accordingly.

Formative research also provides information to help assess what actions we can reasonably ask the target audience to take. Returning to the highway analogy, can we ask target audience members to avoid the exit ramps on every trip, or only under certain conditions? We noted in Chapter 3 that human immunodeficiency virus (HIV) prevention efforts targeting men who have sex with men almost universally choose the former approach (always avoid the exit ramps), which in this context can be characterized as risk prevention: Use a condom every time you have sex. We also noted that many men found it impossible to comply with this guideline. Adequate formative research would have helped program managers realize that the latter approach is more likely to be successful: Use a condom in certain situations, such as with a new partner.

This chapter begins with a general discussion of the differences between quantitative and qualitative formative research techniques to provide a foundation for subsequent discussions of how formative research can be used to select audiences for and shape individual health behavior and policy change initiatives. Because many organizations conduct their own qualitative research, the final sections of the chapter discuss qualitative research techniques in greater detail. Chapter 16 will discuss using qualitative and quantitative methodologies to pretest messages and materials, and Chapters 17 and 18 will discuss some aspects of designing and implementing quantitative studies. Due to the complexity of the methodological issues involved, a detailed discussion of quantitative approaches is beyond the scope of this book.

Quantitative versus Qualitative Approaches

Quantitative research provides measures of how many members of a population have particular knowledge or attitudes, or engage in a particular behavior. In marketing, quantitative research is usually some form of survey, although at times elements of experimental design are incorporated. Quantitative surveys usually are conducted with large numbers of people scientifically sampled to be representative of the population. A structured questionnaire is used. Questions are always asked in the same order, and most questions have a fixed list of responses from which respondents must select their answer. Questionnaires can be self-administered (distributed to respondents by mail or in person) or interviewer-administered (in person or over the telephone). Quantitative research can be analyzed using a broad range of statistical techniques.

Quantitative data can also be collected using other methodologies. For example, observational methods involve literally observing people and counting how many engage in a particular behavior, such as smoking in a public place, fastening their seat belt, voting a particular way on a bill, or calling a telephone hot line. Other types of quantitative measures can include product sales and inventory tracking.

Depending on the type of data collected, quantitative studies can

- provide a baseline for tracking changes after a program is implemented.
- help segment a population for the purposes of identifying target audiences.
- provide information on how many people are in target audience segments or how many people think or behave a certain way.

In contrast, *qualitative research* provides insights into a target audience. The goal is to understand the reactions and motivations of the target audience. It addresses questions of "why?" rather than "how prevalent?" Most qualitative research takes the form of a discussion, with an interviewer asking questions that stimulate conversation in a group or one-on-one setting, rather than questions that require the respondent to choose from a fixed number of responses. Compared with quantitative studies, qualitative approaches are relatively unstructured; the interviewer works from a topic guide, rather than from a questionnaire, and the next question participants are asked often depends on their response to the previous one. Qualitative research usually takes place among a relatively small number of people, and the results should not be quantified, subjected to statistical analysis, or projected to the population from which participants were drawn.

Qualitative studies can provide:

- information on target audience perceptions and reactions.
- access to ideas or responses that researchers may not have considered.
- information on how target audience members view a process from beginning to end.
- insights into the core values underlying target audience beliefs, behaviors, and perceptions of behavior change.

Compared with quantitative research, qualitative projects are often less expensive and faster. However, choice of method should not be made based on cost or timing; each is appropriate—and inappropriate—for different types of research questions.

Table 11–1 presents distinctions between qualitative and quantitative approaches. Thinking about these distinctions when planning a study can help determine what type of approach is needed.

FORMATIVE RESEARCH TO SUPPORT HEALTH BEHAVIOR CHANGE

At times, formative research is used as a first step in planning, for example, to help identify which health problems to address, or to get a preliminary sense of what form a product or service might take. More often, initiatives seeking to change individual health behaviors use formative research in three ways. First, it is used to identify one or more target audiences for the initiative. Second, it is used

---

Table 11–1 Distinctions between Qualitative and Quantitative Research

Qualitative	Quantitative
Provides depth of understanding	Measures level of occurrence
Asks "Why?"	Asks "How many?" and "How often?"
Studies motivations	Studies actions
Is subjective	Is objective
Enables discovery	Provides proof
Is exploratory	Is definitive
Allows insights into behavior, trends, and so on	Measures levels of actions, trends, and so on
Interprets	Describes

Source: Reprinted with permission from M. Debus, *Handbook for Excellence in Focus Group Research,* © 1988, The Academy for Educational Development.

to develop an understanding of the needs, wants, and values of the target audience and how a behavior change can be positioned as fulfilling the audience's needs and wants and as something that is consistent with the group's values. Finally, formative research is used to develop and test products, services, messages, and materials designed to support the behavior change. This chapter discusses formative research to support development efforts; testing will be covered in Chapter 16.

Segmenting and Selecting Target Audiences

The process of dividing the population into groups based on one or more variables is termed *audience segmentation.* The goal of audience segmentation is to identify subgroups whose members are similar to each other and distinct from members of other groups along dimensions that are meaningful in the context of the behavior to be changed. Target audiences are then selected from these subgroups. Segmentation is a key aspect of effective programs. As Slater (1995) noted when discussing segmentation for health communication efforts, "success might not be assured by segmentation—there are too many other contingencies regarding resources, quality of implementation, and the inherent difficulty of the task. *Poor or nonexistent segmentation of audiences, on the other hand, is likely to doom public communication or education programs* [italics added]" (p. 186).

Types of Audience Segmentation

Audiences can be segmented on a variety of dimensions, such as demographic, geographic, lifestyle, or behavioral characteristics. The goal should be to segment them on variables that influence whether people will change the behavior of interest. Slater (1995) notes that these variables can "include attitudinal beliefs and perceptions of relevant social norms (Ajzen & Fishbein, 1980); self-efficacy and presence of behavioral models (Bandura, 1986; Strecher, DeVellis, Becker, & Rosenstock, 1986); salience of, and involvement with, the health behavior (Chaffee & Roser, 1986; Grunig & Hunt, 1984); perceived preventability and costs of alternatives (Maiman & Becker, 1974) and constraints regarding the behavior" (p. 189).

Unfortunately, many initiatives rely on what Slater (1995) calls "shortcuts" to segmentation. These shortcuts are taken for a number of reasons; one is that identifying the antecedents of behavior is a complex process. Even if the antecedents are identified, segmenting based on them often requires an expensive quantitative study and a great deal of time. A third reason may be a lack of behavioral science background among some practitioners.

A popular shortcut is *demographic segmentation,* or grouping people on characteristics such as gender, age, income, education, or race/ethnicity. As Slater (1995) notes, the potential flaw with demographic segmentation is that it often groups people together based on variables that are meaningless in the context of changing the behavior in question: two people can be demographically identical and yet lead totally different lives in terms of health behaviors and the factors that determine them. For example, consider two 23-year-old White males. Both have the same amount of education and income. Both are single. Both have the same type of job. One is gay and regularly practices unprotected sex with a variety of partners. The other has had the same girlfriend since 10th grade and practices abstinence. How would a demographic segmentation help a manager identify and understand the target audience member for a new HIV prevention program?

Sometimes *geographic* characteristics (i.e., whether a person lives in an urban, a suburban, or a rural environment; or the region, state, ZIP code, or neighborhood in which he or she resides) are combined with demographic and lifestyle information (i.e., product purchases, leisure activities, media habits, attitudes, interests, and opinions) to identify distinct neighborhood types. This process is referred to as *geodemographic segmentation* or *geoclustering* and is based on the old adage "birds of a feather flock together." That is, people who live near each other have similar attitudes, interests, and behaviors. This type of segmentation strategy can help in planning community outreach activities and services, as well as in delivering targeted messages through the mail. Research suppliers such as Claritas Corporation (Potential Rating Index by Zip Markets [PRIZM]) provide such analyses.

Although there are no hard and fast rules, for many public health programs the population should first be segmented based on current *behavior*. At a minimum, dividing the population into "doers" and "nondoers"—those who do and do not engage in the desired behavior—allows identification of determinants of behavior and other characteristics that distinguish the two groups. Individual groups can then be further segmented based on readiness to change or psychographic characteristics. Exhibit 11–1 presents a case study from the 5 A Day for Better Health program describing one application of this type of segmentation.

Sources of Segmentation Data

Ideally, audience segmentation and profiles would involve a custom quantitative study; however, time and resources often are not available for such endeavors. The usual starting point is to look at existing studies that include data on the health behaviors of interest. Federal data sources that may help include the National Health Interview Surveys (NHIS), the National Health and Nutrition Examination Surveys (NHANES), the Behavioral Risk Factor Surveillance System (BRFSS), and the Youth Risk Behavior Survey (YRBS).

In addition to measures of health behaviors, these studies include demographic information about respondents. With the exception of NHANES, all of the studies measure self-reported (not observed) behavior. Public-use data tapes are available from the National Center for Health Statistics for most of the studies, so custom analyses can be conducted.

Exhibit 11–1 Segmenting and Profiling the Audience for the 5 A Day for Better Health Media Campaign

BACKGROUND

The national 5 A Day for Better Health program, cosponsored by the National Cancer Institute (NCI) and the Produce for Better Health Foundation (PBHF), encourages Americans to increase their consumption of fruits and vegetables in order to decrease their risk of developing cancer. Rather than spend NCI's limited resources on all consumers and run the risk of diluting the impact of the media campaign, planners chose to follow marketing practice and segment the audience to maximize impact. The discussion below is based on the process outlined in NCI's media campaign strategy document (NCI, 1993) and in a chapter reviewing the campaign (Lefebvre et al., 1995).

METHOD

The first step was to segment based on behavior. A nationally representative baseline survey conducted in 1991 indicated that the average number of servings a day of fruits and vegetables consumed was about 3.5. Since this average intake is a point around which most people cluster, planners looked at this group in selecting a target audience. Next, they looked to theories of behavior change for guidance. The theoretical framework used was the transtheoretical model of stages of change (reviewed briefly in Chapter 10). Planners decided they wanted to first influence the largest number of people possible who would be open to the message (i.e., most ready to increase their fruit and vegetable intake) and who had not yet reached the objective of eating five or more servings daily. Therefore, they defined their target audience as people who were already trying to increase their consumption of fruits and vegetables (those in the contemplation or action stage) but who had not yet achieved the minimum of five servings a day.

Next, they used two different marketing databases to profile the psychographic and demographic characteristics of the target audience. The first database came from MRCA Information Services and linked information on demographics, food consumption (based on food diaries), dietary habits, attitudes, interests, media habits, and other lifestyle characteristics through an annual study of 2,000 households demographically balanced to represent the U.S. population. MRCA data were used to compare two groups. The target audience group was defined as those age 18 or older who reported increasing their consumption of both fruits and vegetables and who currently averaged two servings a day (range of 1.5 to 2.5). This group constituted about 14% of the total population. The comparison group was adults who were already eating 3.5 or more servings of fruits and vegetables per day.

The second database was DDB Needham's 1993 Life Style study, an annual survey of 4,000 consumers who are members of a mail panel study. Life Style includes nearly 1,000 questions related to attitudes, opinions, interests, activities, media habits, and demographics. Life Style results are demographically balanced to reflect the

continues

Exhibit 11–1 continued

U.S. population, but the sample tends to underrepresent the very poor, the very rich, minorities, and transient populations. Two groups were again compared, but they were defined somewhat differently, due to differences in the questions asked. The target group was adults who ate or drank two to three servings of fruits and vegetables on the previous day; desire to increase consumption could not be measured because the survey did not include such a question. Thus defined, the target group was about 50% of the population. The comparison group was adults eating five or more servings of fruits and vegetables on the previous day.

Findings from the two studies were consistent overall: The target audience is younger, married with children, employed full time, and generally concerned with good health. The comparison group is older, likely to be retired, and more concerned with a healthier diet. The Life Style profile provided additional insights into the target audience's psychographic profile: Target audience members tended to lead a faster-paced life and had less spare time; were more likely to suffer from stress-related conditions such as headaches, lack of sleep, and indigestion; and tended to be "impulse" buyers. In terms of media habits, target audience members tended to watch local news, news interview shows, and prime-time movies, and listened to soft rock, classic rock, easy listening, and country-western music. They were not as involved in volunteer and community activities as the comparison group.

The target audience profile built from the information in the two databases, coupled with previous qualitative research, was used to answer most of the strategic questions to be outlined in Chapter 12. However, planners did not know what the image, or personality, of the campaign should be. To find out, they sent a short questionnaire to members of the MRCA consumer panel who met the target audience definition. The questionnaire asked respondents to rate 29 adjectives in terms of how well the adjectives described themselves and then how well the adjectives described someone who eats five fruits and vegetables a day. Target audience members tended to describe themselves as dependable, sensible, concerned, and careful. In contrast, they viewed "5 A Day eaters" as smarter, more disciplined, healthier, and more fit.

RESULTS

Results were used to flesh out and shape the communication strategy for the program. The final strategy will be presented in Chapter 12.

Unfortunately, while these sources can provide useful behavioral and demographic data, they often provide very little information on respondents' lifestyles, leisure time activities, and media use habits—the information needed to design effective marketing efforts. In some instances, a commercial marketing study can fill the gap if it contains items that will allow appropriate behavior-based segmentation. Two well-known commercial marketing studies are the twice-yearly surveys conducted by Mediamark Research, Inc., and Simmons Market Research Bureau. These surveys include hundreds of items assessing what people do with their leisure time: what they read, watch, and listen to—and when they do it; and what products and services they buy—and how much they buy. These studies also contain full demographics for all participants. Appendix 11–D provides information on how to contact the vendors.

Other commercial marketing studies may address needs in specific areas. For example, MRCA's MenuCensus, mentioned in the 5 A Day case study in Exhibit 11–1, uses a food diary methodology to obtain detailed information on food consumption. The study also includes demographic details and information on participants' lifestyles and media habits.

The Audience Segmentation Process

In some instances, other completed studies may allow initial target audience profiling; at other times, it may be necessary to design and conduct one or more studies in order to collect the information needed. The following steps may be involved:

Step 1: Review the literature to identify (1) variables likely to be determinants of the behavior and (2) other studies that may have segmented the population based on these variables.

Step 2: If the determinants are unclear, consider conducting a qualitative study to help identify them. In fact, such a study may be a good idea because there may be determinants affecting behavior in a specific setting or group that theories would not include. An example that Slater (1995) relays is a focus group study that identified the perceived shortage of available Black men as a significant obstacle to HIV prevention among certain Black female university students.

Step 3: If custom analyses need to be conducted, determine the segmentation approach. According to what factors will the audience be segmented? Often a good starting point is "doers" versus "nondoers." Will a qualitative or quantitative approach be taken? This is often a function of whether adequate secondary data are available. Relying on qualitative techniques to identify the differences between audience segments is particularly problematic because of the lack of generalizability of the results—and because determinants can be identified, but not quantified, so it is difficult to isolate the critical ones. However, sometimes qualitative data can be collected more quickly and inexpensively than designing, fielding, and analyzing a major quantitative study.

Step 4: Collect—or analyze—the data and segment the audiences. Segmentation is often iterative; it must be revised as necessary until the segments make sense. The following sections provide guidance. This process also involves building profiles of each segment—their activities, lifestyles, and personalities. Segments need to be distinct from one another along these dimensions, or it will be impossible to target an intervention to reach them.

Step 5: Select the segment(s) to target with the program. The section below titled "Factors Influencing Target Audience Selection" provides some guidance on this process.

Choosing a Segmentation Strategy

This chapter discusses a number of segmentation strategies; in practice, every segmentation must be "custom fitted" to the problem at hand, and the resulting process is often a combination of approaches. As Slater (1995) noted, "the crucial point here is that it is more efficient, in terms of maximizing impact with given resources, to identify people who are similar in important respects and tailor one's communication content and delivery to them" (p. 187). To help assess potential segmentation strategies, Kotler and Andreasen (1996) identified six characteristics of an optimal segmentation strategy:*

1. *Mutual exclusivity.* That is, each person or organization fits the definition of only one segment.
2. *Exhaustiveness.* Every member of the population is included in a segment (even if not all segments are targeted by the program).
3. *Measurability.* Membership in a segment can be readily measured.
4. *Differential responsiveness,* which, as Kotler and Andreasen noted, is perhaps the most crucial criterion. Each segment should respond to different marketing strategies. If segments respond to the same approaches, then the segmentation strategy is not helping reach a particular audience.
5. *Reachability.* This is the degree to which the segments can be effectively reached and served.
6. *Substantiality,* or size. Segments should be large enough to be worth pursuing.

The last two characteristics apply to making decisions about which segments to target and are discussed in more detail in the next section.

Factors Influencing Target Audience Selection

Once the population has been segmented, it is time to select target audiences. One of two approaches can be used: Interventions can be tailored to each audience segment, or one or more audience segments can be chosen as the target audience(s). The approach used depends on the objectives of the program and on available resources; tailoring interventions for many audiences usually is an expensive proposition. This approach is most often used if most of the intervention will take place one on one; for example, hot line callers might receive different

---

Source: Kotler/Andreasen, STRATEGIC MARKETING FOR NONPROFIT ORGANIZATIONS, 5/e, © 1996. Adapted by permission of Prentice-Hall, Inc., Upper Saddle River, NJ.

materials depending on the audience segment they come from. Programs taking more of a mass approach, in which aspects of the intervention will be delivered to groups of people, usually select one or two audience segments and develop intervention components specifically for those segments.

When comparing different segments, a number of factors can be used to assess each group's suitability as a target audience, as shown in Exhibit 11–2.

Audience size. Sometimes program planners select a very small audience—often those most "in need" of a particular change. This decision can create two problems. First, if an overall goal is population-wide improvement, the program will have to work harder to show progress. Second, the channels available to deliver program messages, such as the mass media, may not reach the audience very effectively or efficiently. For individual health behaviors, those most "in need" are often defined as those farthest from the recommended behavior. Green and McAlister (1984) noted that mass media alone usually cannot effectively reach this group—interpersonal interaction is needed. And if mass media are used, there is likely to be a lot of "waste"—few people in the media audience will be members of the target audience.

Consider a private-sector analogy: If a commercial marketer wants to sell more of a product, it can target heavy, medium, or light users of the product. One school of thought is to target heavy users—since they already buy a lot of the product, they may be receptive to buying more. But if there are twice as many medium users as heavy users, to get the same impact on sales would require persuading the heavy users to buy twice as much more—they would need to buy two more packages a month to get the same impact as if the medium users bought one more package per month.

Extent to which the group needs or would benefit from the behavior change. For some populations, a particular behavior may be a hard sell because the group would derive little benefit from it. For example, it can be difficult to identify the benefits of early detection of breast or prostate cancer for very elderly people. In other instances, the group is already very close to the target behavior and may not see it as different enough from their current behavior to be worth changing.

Exhibit 11–2 Factors Influencing Selection of Target Audiences

- Audience size
- Extent to which the group needs or would benefit from the behavior change
- How well available resources can reach the group
- Extent to which the group is likely to respond to the program
- For secondary audiences, the extent to which they influence primary audiences

How well existing resources can reach the group. Many public health efforts rely in whole or in part on mass communication vehicles for promotional efforts. Does the target audience "tune in?" If materials will need to be produced in six or eight different languages, are sufficient resources available to do that? If the target audience is health professionals, does the program have access to channels that reach them effectively and efficiently?

Extent to which the group is likely to respond. If the group has no interest in the behavior change, the program will have to work much harder. Current behavior often can provide some insights into group members' likely interest. For example, if the 5 A Day for Better Health program had chosen to target people who currently eat no more than one serving of fruits and vegetables per day, it would have been targeting people who either did not like fruits and vegetables or could not eat them for some specific reason. Instead, the group selected already eats about three servings a day—an indication that they are not averse to the behavior in question.

For secondary audiences, the extent to which they influence primary audiences. Sometimes the best way to convince someone to change his or her behavior is to have someone else do the convincing. This is often true of behavior involving patient interactions with health care providers. When are people most likely to get an immunization or screening test or start treating a medical condition? When their physician tells them to do so. Secondary audiences can also form useful bridges to primary audiences for programs promoting the diagnosis of previously undiagnosed conditions or in circumstances when secondary audience members are more motivated to address a health problem than the person with the problem is.

Shaping Intervention Components

Once the audiences have been segmented and selected, managers should know whom they are addressing and how to reach them. As they begin to design the components that will constitute the intervention, additional formative research is used to shape each component, as discussed in the next two sections.

Developing Strategies and Tactics

One of the first tasks for formative research is to identify what *specific* action(s) audience members can take to move them toward the desired behavior. For example, the 5 A Day program learned that it was not enough to tell people to eat two more servings of fruits and vegetables; it was important to tell them exactly *how* to do so. Qualitative techniques can help at this point because they can identify obstacles specific to the behavior. In this instance, people said they didn't eat more servings because they didn't see fruits or vegetables when they were looking for a snack or opened the refrigerator, or that fruits and vegetables were not accessible at work. This information was turned into messages: Put fruits and vegetables in a bowl on the counter; move them up in the refrigerator; throw them in your bag on your way out the door to work. For programs with sufficient budgets, the issues identified in qualitative studies can be quantified with surveys.

Formative research can provide similar insights into product development or improving service delivery. For example, a focus group or even informal conversations with clinic users may reveal many reasons why they do not make more use of services: Perhaps they think staff are rude, perhaps hours are inconvenient, or perhaps they must travel too far. A training program can address the first problem; clinic hours might be adjusted to address the second problem. The third problem is a more difficult one, but in some instances it might be resolved by adding new locations, perhaps by using a mobile van if services could be delivered appropriately that way.

Framing Messages

The target audience profiles built as part of the segmentation process can be used in developing a communication strategy (see Chapter 12). However, they often do not include sufficient information about exactly what benefit to promise, how to support it, or what image to convey. Qualitative research is often used to explore these topics. Ideally, this research will then be quantified, but timelines and budgets do not always permit this final step. The case studies in Exhibit 11–1 (5 A Day) and Appendix 11–A (school health) describe different methods of obtaining some of this information. The moderator's guide (Appendix 11–C) was used for the school health project and provides an example of the type of questions that might be asked to help frame messages. Additional information is included in the section of this chapter on focus groups.

FORMATIVE RESEARCH TO SUPPORT PUBLIC HEALTH POLICY INITIATIVES

Formative research plays the same roles in initiatives to promote a public health program or policy as it does in campaigns to promote a change in health behavior. It helps to identify and understand the most appropriate audiences for the initiative to reach, and it helps to develop an initiative that is relevant and motivates the target audience.

Segmenting and Selecting Target Audiences

In most public health policy campaigns, there are three target audiences. First, there are the policy makers: those people who have the power to enact the public health program or policy. Policy makers are often elected government officials, such as town selectmen, city council or county board members, or state or federal legislators. At other times, they may be appointed government officials (such as the heads of government agencies and some school boards) or career administrators (such as city managers and school superintendents and principals). And sometimes policy makers are not affiliated with the government at all; employers in general and manufacturers in particular are two types of organizations that may play a role in policy.

Second, there are some members of the general public who can exert a strong influence on policy makers. Third, there are the mass media—newspapers, radio, and television—which can strongly influence the opinions of policy makers and the general public.

Wallack, Dorfman, Jernigan, and Themba (1993) explain that the policy agenda (those issues considered important by policy makers) is shaped by both the public agenda (issues important to the general public) and the media agenda (issues covered by the print and electronic news media). The media agenda can influence the policy agenda directly or by first placing an issue on the public agenda. An example of the media agenda directly influencing the policy agenda occurred in 1995 when *The Washington Post* reported that President Clinton had called for all states to enact legislation that lowered the legal blood alcohol limit for youth drivers to 0.02 mg/dL. The issue of more stringent youth drunk-driving laws was directly placed on the policy agenda in all 50 states (Harris, 1995). Policy makers could not ignore the issue once the President had embraced it and the national news media reported on it. In contrast, media coverage of the death of a teenage boy who was killed by a drunk driver in Gloucester, Massachusetts, put the issue of stronger drunk-driving legislation on the public agenda but not on the policy agenda (Langner & Laidler, 1993; Murphy, 1994). Only after a widespread public outcry did state legislators decide to do something about the problem (Wong, 1994a, 1994b).

So in contrast to health behavior change campaigns, in which the target audience usually consists of the people whose behavior is being targeted, the target audience for policy campaigns consists of three diverse groups: (1) policy makers, (2) the general public, and (3) members of the mass media.

Because of the diverse nature of these target audiences, the nature of public health policy campaigns is also diverse. Varying activities are needed to influence each of the audiences. For example, lobbying, making visits to elected officials, and testifying at hearings are all necessary to influence policy makers directly. Grass-roots educational activities and the effective use of the mass media are necessary to influence the general public. And efforts such as meeting with editorial boards, writing op-ed pieces and letters to the editor, issuing press releases, and holding news conferences and events are necessary to influence the media.

For each of these campaign activities, a clear understanding of the target audience is necessary to craft messages that will be most effective. But first, careful segmentation within each of these audiences is necessary.

Policy Makers

Policy makers may be segmented based on their likely position on the public health policy or program. For example, one way to segment policy makers is into three groups: those who will definitely support the policy, those who will definitely oppose the policy, and those who are in the middle. It often might be most efficient to focus a campaign on the third group. It may not make sense to use limited time and resources on legislators who are unlikely to change their voting positions. For example, in a campaign to promote a mandatory motorcycle helmet law, it may be a waste of time to focus lobbying efforts on a legislator who is a strong civil libertarian who has opposed all health behavior regulations in the past on ideological grounds. It may be equally wasteful to focus on a legislator who has repeatedly sponsored motorcycle helmet legislation in the past.

Formative research can provide several important pieces of background information on policy makers. First, what are the legislators' current positions on the bill in question? How have they voted on similar legislation in the past? What are their ideological views, especially as they relate to the proposed legislation? This includes not only party affiliation, but other aspects of political ideology as well.

Second, it is important to identify legislators who hold key positions of influence, such as chairpersons of committees to which a bill is likely to be referred. At the state and national levels, the Speaker of the House and Senate Majority Leader are almost always in a position to influence legislation. At the local level, the mayor or first selectman is almost always in a critical position of influence on ordinances. Leaders of the minority party and caucuses of legislators may be important to reach. For example, there is a tobacco caucus in Congress that would be expected to play a critical role in any federal tobacco legislation.

Third, it is important to identify potential sources of influence on critical policy makers. What district does the legislator represent? Who are the most influential individuals, institutions, and other organizations in that district? Could any celebrities in the district help influence the legislator? In Fremont, California, for example, the Smoke-Free Fremont coalition enlisted the help of Olympic ice skater Kristi Yamaguchi in convincing city council members to enact an ordinance eliminating smoking in restaurants. Business groups or key businesses in a district may be a particularly valuable source of influence in a public health policy campaign.

Fourth, it may be useful to identify the source of campaign contributions for legislators. For example, in promoting policies to regulate alcohol, tobacco, or firearms, knowledge of campaign contributions to legislators from the alcohol industry, tobacco industry, or the National Rifle Association may help to expose the degree of outside influence on the policy process.

Fifth, at the local level, it may be important to identify friends and family of council members, who may be the most effective liaisons to the policy maker on behalf of the health coalition.

There are many potential sources of this information. For state legislatures and Congress, library reference sections have guidebooks that list legislators, describe their districts, outline their committee positions, identify their political party, and provide addresses and telephone numbers. An increasing number of states have detailed information of this type on their World Wide Web sites, as does the U.S. Congress. (See Chapter 17 for more details.) Voting records and campaign contribution sources are usually available to the public.

Perhaps the best method to obtain information is to meet with each legislator, his or her staff, or both. This approach has the dual purpose of providing campaign representatives with an opportunity to tell the legislator their positions as well as learn about the legislator's. Too often, public health coalitions wait until late in a campaign to meet with legislators. It is usually too late, and important information that could have guided the development of the campaign has been missed.

Mothers Against Drunk Driving (MADD), in its *How To Compendium* (1991, p. 138), a policy manual for public health advocates, describes the importance of what it calls community analysis. MADD's description is a useful summary of many important formative research questions for promoting a public health policy:

> Know your community inside out, so that as you set goals and build an action plan, you can gauge the probable reactions of various constituencies, estimate your chances for success and build the power base you need to win. Community analysis means much more than being in command of facts about geography and governmental structures, ethnic and socioeconomic data. It means finding out what the power structure really is, not just what the table of organization says it is. It includes hard information on political make-up and party strength. It looks at the community for residential, business and industry concentrations and asks, "Who really runs which parts of town?" It searches out the ethnic, religious and organizational alignments, the loyalty groups, formal and informal. It finds out who's influential about what and with whom—maybe the local bank president at the state capital, the public works commissioner in the city council, it could even be the rock station disc jockey with his or her devoted listeners.... It is imperative to identify the hidden power structure affecting any specific issue you're working on, to line up allies within that power structure but also to spot opposition early in the game.... A careful community analysis can help eliminate the surprise and prepare the legislative committee to take the offensive.

General Public

It is particularly important to segment the general public, because a small number of individuals or groups may have a disproportionate amount of influence on public opinion, and on legislators. Geographic and sociodemographic segmentation, in addition to segmentation on the basis of political influence, may be important.

For example, if public health practitioners identify certain key legislators whose votes are likely to be pivotal, then it might be wise to focus educational, grass-roots, and media advocacy activities in that legislator's district. If a certain group is likely to be influential, like senior citizens in a campaign to regulate Medicare managed care plans, then practitioners may want to focus their public education and advocacy efforts at this segment of the population. Identifying and targeting citizens who are the direct beneficiaries of a public health program can also be critical. For example, in promoting a program that provides cigarette tax revenues for community tobacco prevention activities, it may be important to know what communities benefit from the tax revenue and to target these communities in grass-roots advocacy efforts.

The general public may also be segmented based on the way they are likely to vote on an issue. For example, in opposing a referendum to end affirmative action, it may be important to separately study the opinions of females, persons of color, and liberal and conservative White males. It may be, for example, that liberal White males are the key swing group whose votes will determine the ultimate fate of the referendum. Public education and advocacy efforts could then be conducted most efficiently by focusing on reaching this demographic group. With limited resources, it may not make sense to spend large amounts of money trying to influence the opinions of minority communities, which are likely to support affirmative action anyway.

Mass Media

The mass media should be segmented based on the results of the above formative research, which identifies key policy makers and segments of the general public. The geographic and sociodemographic reach of media outlets can then be studied, and those outlets whose reach matches the target audiences most closely can be selected for media advocacy efforts. In most states, and at the local level, the majority of the public is reached by one or two major media markets. It would be inefficient, for example, to run ads on every television station in Massachusetts, when television stations in Boston and Springfield reach the majority of state residents. If a particular legislator is important, then the media market that covers his or her district is essential.

Within a media market, it is important to decide which specific channel(s) are most useful (e.g., newspaper, radio, or television). Within each channel, it is important to identify the specific outlet(s) with the greatest reach and influence. It may be more efficient to meet with editorial boards of the three or four most important outlets than to try to visit every outlet in the media market. Information on the reach and audience composition of various media outlets is available through standard public relations and advertising resources such as Bacon's media directories, Standard Rate and Data Service (for profiles of all media outlets, including advertising rates for print media), Arbitron (for radio station ratings as well as audience size and composition), and Nielsen Media Research (for similar information on television stations and programs). Contact information for many of these resources will be provided in Table 17–1 in Chapter 17.

To be most effective, public health practitioners should segment their target audience down to the level of the individual reporter. It is important to identify which reporter's beat includes the topic of the public health policy in question and which reporters have taken an interest in this issue in the past. When planning a media event to promote the policy, the press release should be sent specifically to these reporters, and follow-up calls should be made directly to them, rather than to a general news desk. One formative research technique that is very easy, especially since most newspapers now have news archives that can be searched online, is to identify the authors of past news stories on the health topic of interest. Chapter 15 will provide more information on working with the media.

Shaping the Policy Initiative

As with health behavior change campaigns, once audiences have been segmented additional formative research is often needed to adequately craft the initiative. Sometimes this information can be gathered at the same time as the information used to segment the audiences; at other times it is gathered separately.

Developing Strategies and Tactics

The key to policy initiatives is to frame the message properly. This also is often true with health behavior changes. However, it is even more true with policy initiatives, since many are predicated on the assumption that in order to bring about policy change the issue must be on the public agenda, and it gets on the public agenda through the mass media.

However, some policy change initiatives have more components than others. In these situations, formative research can be used to shape many other tangible products and services that will be delivered as part of an initiative. For example, if a county health department is seeking to market public health as an institution, it might conduct formative research to determine what services residents are most interested in, and then focus on improving delivery of those services or, if necessary, creating new services to fill unmet needs. In other words, many traditional uses of market research—improving customer satisfaction, identifying unmet needs, and creating products to fulfill them—can also be used to support policy change.

Framing Messages

The formative research process plays three major roles in developing messages for a public health policy campaign: (1) assessing the existing level of support for the policy, (2) assessing the effectiveness of alternative ways of framing the policy issue to garner support for the policy, and (3) assessing the effectiveness of the ways opponents frame the issue to garner opposition to the policy. Public health practitioners can also use formative research to assess variation in support for a policy and the effectiveness of alternative issue-framing strategies by demographic characteristics.

As discussed in Chapter 7, the successful campaigns to promote cigarette tax increase ballot initiatives all used formative research early and often throughout the campaign. Support for proposed cigarette tax increases was assessed long before campaigns were initiated, and in some cases, before the language of the initiative was even drafted. But the level of public support for these policy initiatives was also assessed periodically throughout the campaign, allowing practitioners to refine their campaign strategies. Moreover, the health coalitions used public polling not only to assess the level of support for the initiatives, but to test various strategies for framing the initiative. These polls helped to identify what campaign themes, messages, and arguments would be most salient and influential on the voters.

Detailed examination of the framing of issues may be more valuable in strategic planning than simple data on public opinion about policies. Thus, public opinion polls should assess not only the general level of public support for specific policies and programs, but the degree to which various arguments for and against the policy or program resonate with voters. Chapter 10 discussed how to assess the way the issue is currently being framed by public health advocates and opponents. Once this assessment is available, existing and alternative approaches to framing the issue can be explored through public opinion polls. Practitioners must keep in mind that arguments that appeal to the core principle of health may not be as effective as those that appeal to more compelling core values, such as freedom, independence, and autonomy (see Chapter 6). Thus, practitioners should be receptive to many alternative frames.

There is no one formative research technique that is best for use in developing a public health policy campaign. For example, focus groups can serve as a valuable tool to explore a wide variety of potential frames, which can then be narrowed down and tested on the population as a whole in a survey. Ideally, formative research methods will be used in concert to achieve the three primary goals of assessing the level of support for a policy and the effectiveness of various ways of framing arguments for and against the policy.

Exhibit 11–3 describes how formative research was used to shape a campaign against a ballot initiative in California. Appendix 11–A provides a description of a very different type of policy initiative: how formative research was used to develop products designed to build community support for coordinated school health programs.

GAINING INSIGHTS: THE QUALITATIVE APPROACHES

Qualitative research is exploratory in nature. Rather than trying to measure how many people engage in a behavior or hold a particular opinion, qualitative research helps us find out *why*. Qualitative research can be used a number of ways:

- To provide insights for planning and product or service development. For example, the National Cancer Institute conducted focus groups with women likely to be at increased risk of developing breast and/or ovarian cancer as a way of informing their planning for breast and ovarian cancer prevention studies (Doner, Eisner, Giusti, & Nayfield, 1998).
- To help flesh out profiles of the target audience and identify perceived benefits, barriers, and misconceptions that target audience members associate with a behavior.
- To explore how to frame messages by testing message concepts with target audience members that link a specific benefit to various actions they could take that would bring them closer to the target behavior.
- To explore changes to the product, price, or distribution channels that will facilitate behavior change.
- To provide insights into the results of quantitative studies.

The two major qualitative research methodologies are focus groups and in-depth interviews. Each method is described in more detail below.

Focus Groups

Traditional focus group sessions are 1- to 2-hour structured discussions among 6 to 10 participants. They are led by a trained moderator working from a list of topic areas and questions (referred to as a moderator's guide or topic guide). People chosen to participate in the group meet certain criteria designed to ensure that they have the requisite target audience characteristics. The following section highlights some key aspects of the methodology; Morgan and Krueger (1998) and Krueger (1994) provide in-depth discussions of planning, developing, implementing, and analyzing focus group studies.

Focus group sessions are usually most productive when they are composed of homogenous groups. Participants are often divided into different groups based on

Exhibit 11–3 Using Formative Research To Frame Messages against a Ballot Initiative

---

BACKGROUND

The use of formative research in developing a policy campaign was illustrated by the California coalition that successfully defeated Proposition 188 in 1994. Proposition 188 was a ballot initiative sponsored by Philip Morris that would have repealed all 270 local antismoking ordinances in California, as well as the state's new law eliminating smoking in workplaces (including all restaurants), and replaced them with weak statewide smoking restrictions (Macdonald, Aguinaga, & Glantz, 1997). Most damaging, the initiative would have preempted the ability of cities and towns to enact more stringent regulation of smoking in the workplace in the future. Although the initiative was sponsored and promoted by the tobacco industry, the industry hid its involvement in the campaign from the public. Philip Morris used a public relations firm—the Dolphin Group—to run the campaign and formed a front group, Californians for Statewide Smoking Restrictions, to disguise its involvement and to mislead the public into thinking that this was an antismoking referendum. Using deceptive billboards that read "Yes on 188—Tough Statewide Smoking Restrictions—The Right Choice," the industry gathered enough signatures to qualify Proposition 188 for the California ballot in November 1994.

The public health community was in a difficult position. The anti-Proposition 188 coalition had only about $1.2 million to spend, as opposed to the $18 million spent by the tobacco industry to promote the referendum (Macdonald et al., 1997). The health coalition needed to be extraordinarily efficient in its campaign: It had to find the single most effective argument that would sway the most crucial voters. The coalition turned to basic marketing principles—and to formative research.

METHOD

The coalition conducted a public opinion poll to determine the baseline level of support for Proposition 188 and to test the effectiveness of various framing strategies for and against the initiative. The choice of a framing strategy to defeat the initiative was not intuitive. Many arguments could be made in opposition to the proposal: (1) It would set back public health by repealing local antismoking ordinances. (2) It would create weak statewide standards that were not adequate to protect nonsmokers from secondhand smoke. (3) It would prevent cities and counties from enacting more stringent secondhand smoke regulations in the future. (4) It would help the tobacco industry protect its profits.

The anti-188 coalition could have simply chosen one or more of these arguments to use as the basis of a campaign. But would such a theme have resonated widely with voters? The tobacco-industry-funded front groups promoting the initiative were making three arguments that could have swayed voters, even in light of the above arguments against the initiative: (1) Proposition 188 completely prohibits smoking in workplaces and restaurants unless strict ventilation requirements are met;

continues

Exhibit 11–3 continued

(2) Proposition 188 replaces the crazy patchwork quilt of local ordinances throughout the state and replaces them with one tough uniform state law; and (3) The uniform restrictions are stronger than 90% of the local ordinances currently in place—90% of communities in California would see an immediate increase in secondhand smoke protection as a result of passage of Proposition 188 (Macdonald et al., 1997).

Instead of relying on intuition to choose its campaign theme, the anti-188 coalition conducted extensive formative research. Public opinion polls were conducted to assess the reaction of voters to many alternative ways of framing the debate over Proposition 188 (Hypotenuse Inc., 1994; Marttila & Kiley, Inc., 1994). The results were striking. The initial support for the initiative was strong: about 60% of California voters supported Proposition 188. Although specific arguments about the negative impact of the initiative on protections against secondhand smoke did sway some voters, they did not change enough votes to predict defeat of the initiative. However, the poll revealed that simply mentioning that the initiative was sponsored by Philip Morris was enough to turn the vote around completely. In fact, when told that Philip Morris was behind the initiative, 70% of California voters stated that they would vote against it.

RESULTS

The coalition chose "Stop Philip Morris" as its campaign theme. It then conducted a coordinated campaign that included grass-roots advocacy, media advocacy, and paid advertising focused on this single theme. The goal was simply to educate voters about who was really behind Proposition 188, not to worry about making detailed arguments about why the initiative was bad for public health.

The coalition conducted not only an initial poll, but periodic public opinion polls throughout the 3-month campaign period to assess how well its approach was working. By mid-July, the initiative was ahead 52% to 38% (Macdonald et al., 1997). By mid-September, voters were about equally divided on Proposition 188. Seeing the dangerous level of support for Proposition 188, the health coalition stepped up its efforts to educate the public about the initiative's sponsor. The coalition hired Jack Nicholl to produce television advertisements using former Surgeon General C. Everett Koop as a spokesperson and paid to air these ads in the major California media markets during the last week of the campaign. The ads highlighted the deceptive nature of the pro-188 campaign, exposing that Philip Morris was behind the initiative and how Californians for Statewide Smoking Restrictions was trying to cover up this important fact. It was, in fact, the discouraging September poll results that convinced the national American Cancer Society and American Heart Association to make substantial contributions to the anti-188 campaign that allowed the Koop spots to be aired (Macdonald et al., 1997).

On November 8, Proposition 188 was defeated by an overwhelming margin of 71% to 29%. The coalition's strategy had succeeded. And it was careful formative research and subsequent tracking that allowed the coalition to develop an effective campaign, to monitor its progress, and to make necessary refinements along the way to increase the campaign's effectiveness.

demographic characteristics such as gender, age, and socioeconomic status. The reasons for such divisions are twofold: (1) People are more likely to speak openly in front of other people whom they perceive to be like themselves, and (2) any real or perceived hierarchy among group members will impact group dynamics. For example, if nurses and physicians are combined in one group, it is unlikely that much useful information will be obtained from the nurses. Many will defer to the physicians because physicians are viewed as more expert. If the nurses do participate, they will likely provide socially acceptable responses, describing what they are supposed to do as nurses. If they do something differently, they are unlikely to talk about it in front of physicians, and so many valuable insights may be lost.

Most researchers think carefully about topic matter before combining men and women in a group consisting of patients or members of the public, in part because there are many health topics that each gender will discuss more openly if members of the other gender are not present. Similarly, consumers with divergent socioeconomic status typically are not combined in one group. People with higher education often are more articulate than their counterparts with lower education, causing those with lower education to shut down. Additionally, people tend to use language differently when they are among members of their own "group," whatever group that happens to be, in part as a way of signaling group identity. This phenomenon is perhaps most pronounced with teenagers, but occurs with other groups as well. If one goal of conducting the groups is to learn how to talk to them or how to reference particular behaviors or products, mixing group members may thwart that goal because people may not use their normal word choices or speech patterns.

In addition to natural differences in conversational style, some demographic characteristics, particularly age and socioeconomic status, often lead to lifestyle differences. Depending on the subject matter, these differences may not only make it difficult for participants to relate to each other, but may in turn lead to differences in behavioral determinants and perceived benefits of and barriers to particular behaviors. For example, consider behaviors such as changing food preparation methods or increasing physical activity. In general, retirees can fit such changes into their schedules much more easily than middle-aged people with full-time jobs and children. But retirees may have many health-related barriers to such changes that most younger people do not have. Differences in socioeconomic status can have a similar effect: Among low-income people, product price (for example, for particular foods) is often the number one barrier; among high-income people, price is much less of an issue.

In general, discussion is more honest if participants do not know each other. However, in some instances it is nearly impossible to convene a group in which no one knows anyone else. This problem often occurs when groups of professionals are assembled, particularly in smaller geographic areas. For example, health care professionals are likely to know each other—or to have worked at the same places. Principals and teachers often know each other, as do business or community leaders.

Designing the Study

Step 1: Determine what you need to know and set research objectives. Some of the principles of "backward research" advocated by Andreasen (1988, 1995) can help at this stage. For example, determine what decisions will be made as a result of the study, and outline the research report as a way of coming to agreement on what information the study will provide. This process also helps identify any areas of miscommunication between researchers and program managers and keeps research costs down by separating "nice to know" areas of inquiry from "need to know" questions. More information on the backward research approach will be provided in Chapter 17.

There are two other important things to keep in mind during this process. First, there is a 2-hour window, at most, in which to discuss all of the topics. That may sound like a long time, but consider this: If the group has 10 participants, that gives each of them 10 to 11 minutes to talk (the moderator will spend a certain amount of time asking questions). Granted, every person won't respond to every question, but if you were doing an in-depth interview, instead of a focus group, how many topics would you expect to cover in 10 to15 minutes?

Second, remember that these are called *focus* groups for a reason. Make sure that the discussion is, in fact, focused, not a 2-hour omnibus study. If there are many topics to cover, prioritize them or break them into separate studies.

Step 2: Prepare proposed study design. The study design should spell out the research objectives, the total number of groups that will be conducted, the cities in which they will be conducted (and why they were selected), and the composition of each group or set of groups (recruiting specifications). It should also present a rough timeline and budget.

It is best to conduct groups in multiples of two. For example, if the audience of interest is Black men aged 25 to 34 who have a family history of high blood pressure, the study should include at least two groups with this audience in each location. Conducting two of each type of group helps to ensure that (1) comments from one anomalous group are not given more credence than they should be given and (2) if something disastrous happens (such as an uncontrollable participant or only three people show up for the group), there will be another group's input to use.

Consider conducting groups with "doers" (those who already engage in the desired behavior) and "nondoers" (the target audience). This approach can help you identify the determinants of doers' behavior and then find out to what extent these determinants and values can be tapped in the target audience.

Also consider the ideal size of the focus groups. In some situations, mini-groups or triads are preferable to full focus groups. For example, if the topic is such that much in-depth discussion will be required, sometimes mini-groups (four to five participants) are more productive. Mini-groups can also be useful for projects at the other end of the spectrum, when there is a lot of ground to cover and all participants would not have a chance to talk in a larger group. Triads can be a useful technique with children, many of whom are uncomfortable talking in a larger group of children they don't know.

Step 3: Prepare data collection instruments. The first task is to draft a recruitment screener based on the group composition criteria. The recruitment screener is a short questionnaire designed to determine whether people are eligible for the group and, if so, whether they are willing to participate. In addition to questions to ensure that participants meet the criteria for inclusion, recruitment screeners usually contain two questions used to exclude participants who might be more expert than others in the group. One question asks about occupation and disqualifies anyone who works in advertising, marketing, or market research (because they know too much about focus groups) or any occupation that would make them "expert" compared with the other group members. For example, nutritionists are usually excluded from groups discussing dietary behaviors, and health care professionals are excluded from consumer groups discussing health behaviors, particularly treatment issues. The other question is whether they have participated in a focus group before, and if so, how long ago it was held, to avoid getting "professional" focus group attendees. The increasing popularity of the methodology has made it much more difficult to identify people who have never participated in a focus group. Appendix 11–B contains a sample recruitment screener.

The next task is to draft a topic guide. Some topic guides include questions developed for other studies, but often much of a new guide must be developed from scratch. Exhibit 11–4 provides suggestions for developing the topic guide, and Appendix 11–C provides a sample guide. Remember that the guide is just that: a guide. People may agonize over every word in a topic guide, when the words that come out of the moderator's mouth may be quite different from those on the page.

Conducting the Groups

Step 4: Arrange logistical details, including a moderator and a facility in which to convene the group. Traditionally, focus group guidebooks recommended contracting with a professional moderator (unless, of course, staff members have such skills). However, recent trends have been toward greater community participation in the focus group process. There are a number of reasons for this trend; two pragmatic ones are quality of data and cost. As Krueger and King (1998) note, there are many situations in which an outside researcher may be unlikely or unable to collect the in-depth inside information that a community member volunteer can collect. Additionally, volunteers can help conduct a study when resources are scarce. (Professional moderators in major metropolitan areas often charge $1,000 or more

Exhibit 11–4 Suggestions for Developing the Topic Guide

- Open by thanking participants and explaining the process (i.e., there are no right or wrong answers; the goal is to get their opinions; the conversation is being taped). Provide a general description of the topic they will discuss and, if they may be anxious or suspicious, the reason why you convened this particular group.
- Begin by asking participants to introduce themselves; then ask one or two "warm-up" questions that get them talking and ease them into the subject matter.
- Most questions should be open ended. The goal is to stimulate conversation, not tally responses. The transition from writing structured quantitative questionnaires to relatively free-flowing qualitative topic guides is a very difficult one for most researchers to make.
- Build in exercises. They keep the group from getting bored and are a useful way of obtaining and capturing different kinds of information.
  1. Laddering exercises can be used to get at core values. Participants are first asked to name the positive attributes they associate with a behavior. The moderator records each attribute on a flip chart and, as each one is named, asks why that is important. The moderator continues asking why each subsequent attribute is important until the participant can no longer answer. For example:
     - What are the advantages of going for a 20-minute walk each day? It makes me feel good.
     - And why does it make you feel good? Because I have more energy the rest of the day, and I know I'm doing something good for my health.
     - And why is it important to have more energy? Because I can get more work done and feel more in control.
     - And what's good about doing something good for your health? Well . . . I want to be around for my kids . . . and I feel like I should . . . and I never have any time. There's so many things I don't do, so it makes me feel good when I accomplish taking the walk.

     Now we have learned that the walk makes the person feel more in control, is motivated in part by a need to meet family obligations, and increases self-esteem by making the person feel good.
  2. Free association is another technique to identify the attributes people attach to particular products or behaviors: "I'm going to say a word (or phrase) and I want you to tell me what comes to mind. The word is . . ."
  3. Participants can sort message concepts (provided on separate sheets of paper) from most compelling to least compelling (and then explain their rankings to you).
  4. Pictures can be used as stimuli in many different ways. For example, you can show participants a picture of someone engaging in the desired action and ask them to describe that person (another way of getting at values). You can also ask them to describe how they are different from, and similar to, the person pictured.

continues

Exhibit 11–4 continued

> Pictures of food can be extremely useful for exploring dietary knowledge. For example, show participants a variety of foods and ask them to "group" them into food groups, or ask them which ones are higher in fat or fiber, or lower.
>
> - Ask participants to recount a recent experience involving the behavior. Have them walk you through what happened and their perceptions of various aspects of the experience. For example, if you are trying to improve a health clinic, you might ask: Think about your last visit to the clinic. How did you make your appointment? (Probe for staff promptness and timeliness.) Was the appointment time that you wanted available? What happened when you arrived for your appointment? How were you treated by the front desk staff? What was the waiting room like? (Probes: What was good and bad about it?) How long did you have to wait to be seen? Was the wait longer or shorter than you expected? How was your experience with the nurse? Now tell me about the exam room. What was good and bad about it?
> - Close the group by asking whether people have any additional comments about any of the topics discussed, and then thank them for their participation.

per group; specialized moderators, such as those who are an ethnic minority or who work with children, can command much higher rates.)

Krueger and King (1998) outline the following additional situations in which a volunteer moderator is appropriate: when the required research is not complex or does not demand highly technical skills; when the process of research is more important than its product (i.e., the study can encourage people to think in new ways about a situation); and when the program or situation to be studied is not highly political. When none of these conditions is true, Krueger and King recommend using professionals.

When deciding whether to use a professional or a volunteer, be aware that moderating a focus group is not as simple as running a meeting. The moderator must perform a delicate balancing act of being detached in the sense that he or she asks questions but does not offer opinions, yet being able to persuade group members to open up. Moderating focus groups also requires substantial background in group dynamics and skill at handling a range of personality types. Additionally, an outside moderator's distance from the program is often a plus. Someone on the program staff is vested in how the groups turn out, particularly when ideas are being tested, and may have difficulty remaining unbiased and may unintentionally lead the group in the "right" direction.

If a professional moderator is used , the best way to identify a good one is to ask colleagues for recommendations. When you have identified two or three candidates, ask them for tapes (all will have audiotapes; many have videotapes as well) to get a feel for how they run groups. Generally speaking, it is a good idea to match the gender and ethnicity of the moderator to the gender and ethnicity of the group. Most moderators will not have as much health knowledge as program staff, but it is best if they have moderated groups on health topics with similar audiences in the past. In particular, if you are conducting focus groups with children, it is important that you use a moderator who specializes in working with children.

Moderators can have varying amounts of responsibility; most can draft the recruitment screener and topic guide, conduct the groups, and prepare a report. However, many moderators' reports are analytically weak; ask for examples of their reports before contracting out this critical aspect of the project. Moderators usually charge per group and may charge separately for writing a guide and report.

The easiest (but usually most expensive) way to conduct focus groups is to contract with a commercial focus group facility. These facilities feature rooms of an appropriate size, built-in audiotaping capabilities (with microphones located unobtrusively on the ceiling), and viewing rooms separated from the focus group room by a one-way mirror. Using your recruitment screener, commercial facilities can recruit most groups of consumers and professionals, unless the participants are very difficult to find in the general population (for example, if you need people recently diagnosed with asthma or women who use the services of a breast cancer clinic). However, it is important to monitor the quality of a facility's recruiting. In addition to checking references, one way to do so is to readminister the screener to participants when they show up, to ensure that they are qualified for the group.

When contracting with a vendor, the vendor will need the dates and times of the groups, the number of people to recruit for each, and whether videotaping is desired (audiotaping is automatically included). A general rule of thumb is to recruit two more participants per group than needed; that way, if a few people don't show up, the group will still be large enough. In addition to recruiting the participants, the facility staff will send confirmation letters with directions and make reminder calls a day or two before the group. Commercial facilities typically want to be paid for the incentives (payment to participants) before the groups take place; the balance is due after the groups (usually within 30 days). Incentive costs vary widely, depending on the locality and the type of participants; the facility can recommend an appropriate amount.

Groups can be convened at commercial facilities even if the recruiting is handled separately. Alternatively, if there are no facilities available (often true in smaller cities) or the program cannot afford commercial facilities, a focus group can be held in a hotel meeting room, a school classroom, or an office conference room. If you choose to conduct the groups yourself, you will need to handle the recruiting, confirmation letters, and follow-up calls; obtain a room and make sure it is set up properly (round or oblong tables are best); make sure participants have access to the room (if the group takes place after-hours in an office building, for example); make tent cards for all participants; handle audiotaping; and disburse the incentives.

Step 5: Conduct the focus groups. With a commercial facility and an outside moderator, all you need to do is show up and watch. You don't have to attend every group, but it is a good idea to attend at least one or two. Be forewarned that good moderators cover the topics on the guide, but they will not use the exact words and they may jump from section to section if participants make comments that make natural segues (and if the topic order is not critical). The first group is usually a pilot test; expect to make revisions to the guide afterward. Some sections may run long, some may need more probing, instructions to exercises may need revising, and some questions may just not work.

A note on videotaping: If the goal of videotaping is to be able to edit the groups into a brief highlights video, the audio quality will be mediocre at best and will not withstand being projected into a large room, unless participants were individually miked. Also, videotaping for wider use raises a number of ethical issues; participants are usually told that their comments are confidential. If there are plans to replay the videotapes to larger groups, participants should be informed of how the tapes will be used and asked to sign written release forms.

If the focus groups are conducted someplace other than at a commercial facility, no more than one person should observe the groups (unless a camera is set up and linked to a monitor in another room). The observer should sit at the table and take notes. He or she should be introduced to the participants, and his or her role should be explained. It is not acceptable to have multiple people sitting in the room watching; the effect on group dynamics is too adverse. If you are taping the groups, use the best tape recorders you can find, test them before each group, make sure the moderators know how to use them, and always carry extra batteries and tapes. It is safest to use two tape recorders per group, particularly if participants are seated at an oblong or oval table. Positioning the recorders near each end ensures that all voices, even those of soft-spoken participants, are captured.

Analyzing the Results

Steps 6 and 7: Analyze data and prepare report. Often it is best to prepare a "top line" (highlights) summary within a few days of the final group. The final report usually takes 4 to 6 weeks, in part because it cannot be completed until transcripts are ready. There are a number of approaches to analyzing focus group data. Some people present the results of each group separately; that is inappropriate for many projects since the point of analysis is to look for trends across groups or to identify and categorize a range of issues. The approach that may work best is to make summary statements and then support them with illustrative verbatim comments (hence the need for the transcripts; going back to the tapes is usually far more expensive). The type of person making each comment is identified (e.g., Baltimore primary care physician).

The report itself should contain an introduction describing the program and the objectives of the research study; a methodology section outlining the number of groups, their composition, and when they took place; a section detailing the findings of the research; and a section discussing conclusions and recommendations. The report may also contain an executive summary at the beginning.

In-Depth Interviews

With in-depth interviews, a trained interviewer talks with one research participant at a time. The interviews can take place over the telephone or in person. In-depth interviews are commonly used when a group setting is not feasible (for example, if appropriate participants are scattered across the country or state) or if it would have a chilling effect on discussion. For example, if the research participants are very young children, a one-on-one format is better suited to their attention span and tendency to become shy in groups of children they do not know.

Table 11–2 provides guidance on deciding when to use focus groups and when to use in-depth interviews.

The process of designing, conducting, and analyzing in-depth interview studies is similar to that used for focus groups. Minor differences are described below. For a detailed discussion of the approach to each step, please refer to the focus group section of this chapter.

Designing the Study

Step 1: Determine what you need to know and set research objectives. The average in-depth telephone interview lasts about half an hour; some run 45 minutes. Interviews conducted in person can run longer (up to about an hour), except with young children, in which case they should be kept to the length of a telephone interview. If you cannot adequately address all of the objectives in that amount of time, cut some objectives. As with focus group studies, determining what decisions will be made based on the study can help refine objectives. The conversation should focus on one subject as much as possible; too much bouncing around distracts respondents.

Step 2: Prepare proposed study design. The study design should spell out the research objectives, the total number of interviews to be conducted, the types of people to be interviewed, and how to obtain the names and phone numbers. It should also present a rough timeline and budget.

It is good practice to conduct at least 8 to 10 interviews with each subgroup. As with focus groups, consider conducting some interviews with "doers" (those who already engage in the desired behavior) and "nondoers" (the target audience). This approach can help you identify the determinants of doers' behavior and then find out to what extent these determinants and values can be tapped in the target audience.

In some instances, it may desirable to set up the interviews as dyads, in which the interviewer talks to two people at once. For example, dyads can be useful for discussing some behaviors involving couples.

Table 11–2 Which To Use: Focus Groups or Individual In-Depth Interviews?

Issue To Consider	Use Focus Groups When:	Use Individual In-Depth Interviews When:
Group interaction	Interaction of respondents may stimulate a richer response or new and valuable thoughts.	Group interaction is likely to be limited or nonproductive.
Group/peer pressure	Group/peer pressure will be valuable in challenging the thinking of respondents and illuminating conflicting opinions.	Group/peer pressure would inhibit responses and cloud the meaning of results.
Sensitivity of subject matter	Subject matter is not so sensitive that respondents will temper responses or withhold information.	Subject matter is so sensitive that respondents will be unwilling to talk openly in a group.
Depth of individual responses	The topic is such that most respondents can say all that they know in less than 10 minutes.	The topic is such that a greater depth of response per individual is desirable, as with complex subject matter and very knowledge-able respondents.
Interviewer fatigue	It is desirable to have one interviewer conduct the research; several groups will not create interviewer fatigue or boredom.	It is desirable to have numerous interviewers on the project. One interviewer would become fatigued or bored conducting the interviews.
Stimulus materials	The volume of stimulus material is not extensive.	A large amount of stimulus material must be evaluated.
Continuity of information	A single subject area is being examined in depth and strings of behaviors are less relevant.	It is necessary to understand how attitudes and behav-iors link together on an individual basis.

continues

Table 11-2 continued

Issue To Consider	Use Focus Groups When:	Use Individual In-Depth Interviews When:
Experimentation with interviewer guide	Enough is known to establish a meaningful topic guide.	It may be necessary to develop the interview guide by altering it after each of the initial interviews.
Observation	It is possible and desirable for key decision makers to observe "first-hand" consumer information.	"First-hand" consumer information is not critical or observation is not logistically possible.
Logistics	An acceptable number of target respondents can be assembled in one location.	Respondents are geographically dispersed or are not easily assembled for other reasons.
Cost and timing	Quick turnaround is critical and funds are limited.	Quick turnaround is not critical and budget will permit higher cost.

Source: Reprinted with permission from M. Debus, *Handbook for Excellence in Focus Group Research,* © 1988, The Academy for Educational Development.

Step 3: Prepare data collection instruments. Some in-depth interviewing projects require a recruitment screener (for example, if participants will be recruited from the general population and then come to a central site for interviews). Most telephone in-depth interviews do not require a screener because they are conducted with people known to qualify. Recruitment screeners are discussed in more detail in the focus group section of this chapter.

All interviewing projects require a topic guide, usually one similar to that used for focus groups. Obviously, if the interviews will be conducted by phone, some of the exercises described in the focus group section cannot take place. In-depth interviewing guides are more likely than topic guides to be administered verbatim; when preparing them, read them out loud to make sure they are written in conversational language. Sentences are usually too long and language too abstract the first time through.

Conducting the Interviews

Step 4: Arrange logistics. Vendors may be involved with in-depth interview projects that take place in person. Focus group facilities can also recruit in-depth interview participants for you and usually have interviewing rooms. Interview rooms are smaller, to provide a more intimate setting for the interview, but still provide audiotaping and other amenities (e.g., television monitors if needed).

A professional, staff member, or volunteer with some training can conduct interviews. Chapter 16 will include information on the characteristics of good interviewers and how to train them. Many focus group moderators also conduct in-depth interviews; other qualitative researchers specialize in interviews. If you contract out for the interviewing, the interviewer will most likely prepare the report (unless you want to read a lot of transcripts or listen to hours and hours of tapes). Asking for sample reports will help ensure that you hire someone who does quality work.

Step 5: Conduct the interviews. As with focus groups, if the interviews are being conducted in person at a commercial facility by an outside interviewer, all you must do is show up and watch. After the first two or three interviews, take a look at the guide, and revise it as needed.

If you do the interviewing, you have the option of taping telephone interviews, taking notes, or a combination of both. Taping allows the conversation to flow more naturally (although it's a good idea to take some notes in case something happens with the tape recorder). If you tape interviews, make sure to inform each interviewee that you are going to tape the conversation. Informed consent is particularly important with telephone interviews to avoid violating federal wiretapping laws. If you take notes, it is helpful to write in pencil and go over them the minute you put the phone down. You often can expand on them considerably.

Analyzing the Results

Steps 6 and 7: Analyze data and prepare report. In-depth interview reports can be organized much like focus group reports are. As with focus groups, the approach is usually to make summary statements of findings and then support them with illustrative verbatim comments. If more than one type of person was interviewed, identify the type of person making the comment.

The report should contain an introduction describing the program and the objectives of the research study; a methodology section outlining the number of interviews, their composition, and when they took place; a section detailing the findings of the research; and a section discussing conclusions and recommendations. The report may also contain an executive summary at the beginning.

CONCLUSION

Formative research is central to the marketing approach and plays a critical role in shaping public health initiatives. As Lefebvre and Flora (1988) noted, "in an arena characterized by lower levels of funding, the importance of formative research cannot be overemphasized. Although budget-minded persons might view the additional costs of such research as frivolous, it will prove to be money well spent. Not only can such research suggest changes in program content or delivery that will enhance its reach and/or effectiveness, but it can also circumvent a costly and ill-fated intervention before it receives broad exposure" (p. 305).

Both qualitative and quantitative techniques are used to conduct formative research; each is appropriate for different types of research questions. Quantitative techniques can tell us *how many* people act or feel a certain way; qualitative techniques can tell us *why* and uncover additional issues. Using the two together can help identify the appropriate target audience(s) and then package, position, and frame the social change so that it is consistent with audience members' core values.

REFERENCES

Ajzen, I., & Fishbein, M. (1980). *Understanding attitudes and predicting social behavior.* Englewood Cliffs, NJ: Prentice-Hall.

Andreasen, A.R. (1988). *Cheap but good marketing research.* Homewood, IL: Business One-Irwin.

Andreasen, A.R. (1995). *Marketing social change: Changing behavior to promote health, social development, and the environment.* San Francisco: Jossey-Bass.

Bandura, A. (1986). *Social foundations of thought and action.* Englewood Cliffs, NJ: Prentice-Hall.

Chaffee, S.H., & Roser, C. (1986). Involvement and the consistency of knowledge, attitudes, and behaviors. *Communication Research, 13,* 373–399.

Doner, L., Eisner, E.J, Giusti, R., & Nayfield, S. (1998). Perceptions and attitudes of women at increased risk of breast cancer toward participation in prevention research: Focus group report. Bethesda, MD: National Cancer Institute.

Green, L.W. & McAlister, A. (1984). Macro-interventions to support health behavior: some theoretical perspectives and practical reflections. *Health Education Quarterly, 11,* 322–339.

Grunig, J.E., & Hunt, T. (1984). *Managing public relations.* New York: Holt, Rinehart & Winston.

Harris, J.F. (1995, June 11). Clinton urges "zero tolerance" for young drinking drivers. *The Washington Post,* p. A6.

Hypotenuse Inc. (1994). *Bullet poll: California smoking research.* Verona, NJ: Author.

Kotler, P., & Andreasen, A.R. (1996). *Strategic marketing for non-profit organizations* (2nd ed.). Upper Saddle River, NJ: Prentice-Hall.

Krueger, R.A. (1994). *Focus groups: A practical guide for applied research* (2nd ed.). Thousand Oaks, CA: Sage.

Krueger, R.A., & King, J.A. (1998). *Involving community members in focus groups.* Thousand Oaks, CA: Sage.

Langner, P., & Laidler, J. (1993, December 14). Traffic deaths restart debate: 3 fatalities fuel push for new laws. *The Boston Globe,* pp. 37, 38.

Lefebvre, R.C., Doner, L.D., Johnston, C., Loughrey, K., Balch, G., & Sutton, S.M. (1995). Use of database marketing and consumer-based health communications in message design: An example from the Office of Cancer Communications' "5 A Day for Better Health" program. In E. Maibach

& R.L. Parrott (Eds.), *Designing health messages: Approaches from communication theory and public health practice* (pp. 217–246). Thousand Oaks, CA: Sage.

Lefebvre, R.C., & Flora, J.A. (1988). Social marketing and public health intervention. *Health Education Quarterly, 15,* 299–315.

Macdonald, H., Aguinaga, S., & Glantz, S.A. (1997). The defeat of Philip Morris' "California Uniform Tobacco Control Act." *American Journal of Public Health, 87,* 1989–1996.

Maiman, L.A., & Becker, M.H. (1974). The health belief model: Origins and correlates in psychological theory. *Health Education Monographs, 2,* 384–408.

Marttila & Kiley, Inc. (1994). *A survey of voter attitudes in California.* Boston: Author.

Morgan, D.L., & Krueger, R.A. (1998). *The focus group kit* (Vols. 1–6). Thousand Oaks, CA: Sage.

Mothers Against Drunk Driving. (1991, April 1). *How to compendium.* Irving, TX: Author.

Murphy, S.P. (1994, January 21). Gloucester couple seeks tougher drunken driving law. *The Boston Globe,* pp. 17, 25.

National Cancer Institute (1993, December). *5 a day for better health: NCI media campaign strategy.* Bethesda, MD: Author.

Slater, M.D. (1995). Choosing audience segmentation strategies and methods for health communication. In E. Maibach & R.L. Parrott (Eds.), *Designing health messages: Approaches from communication theory and public health practice* (pp. 186–198). Thousand Oaks, CA: Sage.

Strecher, V.S., DeVellis, B.M., Becker, M.H., & Rosenstock, I.M. (1986). The role of self-efficacy in achieving health behavior change. *Health Education Quarterly, 13,* 73–91.

Wallack, L., Dorfman, L., Jernigan, D., & Themba, M. (1993). *Media advocacy and public health: Power for prevention.* Newbury Park, CA: Sage.

Wong, D.S. (1994a, March 25). Drunken driving bill OK'd by House: Tough rule could allow cars to be forfeited. *The Boston Globe,* pp. 29, 34.

Wong, D.S. (1994b, May 26). Tough bill on drunken driving OK'd: Blood alcohol limit lowered; Weld expected to sign package. *The Boston Globe,* pp. 1, 34.

Building Support for Coordinated School Health: Using Multiple Formative Research Techniques To Shape an Initiative

BACKGROUND

The Council of Chief State School Officers (CCSSO) and the Association of State and Territorial Health Officials (ASTHO) represent, respectively, the top education official and top health official in each U.S. state and territory. The two organizations came together to develop joint materials that their respective constituents can use to help build support for coordinated school health programs. Such programs link, or coordinate, eight components of school health: health education, physical education, nutrition, health services, counseling, psychological and social services, staff wellness, and partnerships between the school and the community and/or parents.

CHALLENGES AND OPPORTUNITIES

A coordinated school health program is a complicated product to market because of the nature of the product and the way it is distributed and implemented. Despite the name, it is not a clearly defined program. Rather, it is a philosophy of ensuring that each aspect of a school contributes to a child's physical, mental, and emotional well-being in a coordinated, reinforcing way. As a result, a coordinated approach can be implemented differently in every school. This is an advantage because it allows schools to customize the approach to suit their local needs, but presents a challenge in that it is complex to explain, obtain resources for, and implement.

Getting the product to the consumer is also complex. Products that require organizational change rather than individual change are inherently more difficult to implement successfully. Changes to school health programs can be particularly difficult because they may not be supported and require many different individuals and departments within an organization to change, and because approval to implement them may require changes at the state, school district, and individual school levels.

An additional challenge for the CCSSO/ASTHO initiative is the broad geographic target audience. Products developed as part of this initiative will be distributed nationally; however, the political, social, and economic environments in which changes are made are different in every state and locality. Indeed, it is sometimes different in every school. Materials developed for national use cannot possibly capture the needs of each community. Therefore, final products need to be customizable.

TARGET AUDIENCES

Although the CCSSO/ASTHO materials are for the chief education and health officials or their designees, the initiative's ultimate target audiences are "easy-to-reach" administrators, teachers, school staff, and parents. "Easy to reach" is defined as being supportive of school health programs and, for parents, being active in activities related to school (e.g., a member or officer of a parent-teacher organization, a volunteer or aide at school, or someone who attends school board meetings).

The rationale for these target audiences is rooted in two complementary theoretical frameworks: diffusion of innovations and stages of change. Both were discussed in more detail in Chapter 10. From a diffusion of innovations perspective, the target audience is parents, teachers, and administrators who are already trying to improve their schools and who are innovators and early adopters—the first people to embrace a new idea. Once members of these groups begin coordinating their schools' approach to health, others are more likely to attempt similar changes. In stages-of-change terms, the target audience encompasses those in contemplation (i.e., they are receptive to the idea of a stronger approach to health and may have considered trying to change aspects of their school's approach, but have no specific plans) and preparation/action (i.e., they may have made a decision to try and change the school's approach and may have taken some steps toward trying to make changes or build support for changes).

ROLE OF FORMATIVE RESEARCH

Formative research was integrated throughout the process of planning and developing the CCSSO/ASTHO materials. The research activities and their major objectives were as follows:

1. Secondary review of other relevant projects and literature: To identify target audiences' likely perceptions of benefits of and barriers to the comprehen-

sive or coordinated approach and to identify striking linkages between children's health and their school performance to support messages about the importance of a strong, coordinated approach to school health.

2. In-depth interviews with administrators, teachers, and parents in school districts that use a coordinated approach to school health: To explore preliminary message concepts, how they define comprehensive or coordinated school health (CSH) and the language they use when they talk about it, benefits of and barriers to approach, and how they would implement CSH elsewhere.

3. Focus groups with administrators, teachers, and parents in districts that do and do not use a coordinated approach to school health: To explore refined message concepts, definitions of CSH and language used, perceived benefits and barriers, and the first steps they would take in trying to implement it. (A sample recruitment screener and moderator's guide are provided in Appendixes 11–B and 11–C.)

4. Nationally representative survey of American adults: To quantify reactions to concepts in the messages.

5. Focus groups with administrators, teachers, and parents: To pretest prototype materials.

The final materials will be pilot-tested in six states for 1 year.

Major Findings

The first round of formative research helped CCSSO and ASTHO to understand how school health programs are currently defined and positioned in the minds of target audience members and provided insights into the types of messages that would frame the need to move toward a coordinated approach to school health in a compelling, relevant way. After initial materials were developed, research helped the project team revise the content of those materials to better meet the needs of the target audience.

The following sections present some of the major findings in chronological order to provide a sense of how research at each stage was used to shape and then refine the messages about comprehensive school health and the materials developed to deliver those messages.

Definitions of School Health

Target audience members tended to have a narrower definition of school health than that used in the eight-component model. Furthermore, there was no common definition of what school health encompassed. Health education was mentioned most often; physical education, school meals, and on-site health services (particularly among participants whose schools had them) also came up quite a bit. A fair number of focus group participants asked if mental health was included in the definition of health. Parents often spoke about an approach to health education, saying they would like to see their children learn more practical skills. After seeing a list of the eight components, research participants generally thought that all were part of a school's approach to health; however, they did not think their schools had all eight, or thought they needed to work on strengthening some of them.

Benefits of a Coordinated Approach to School Health

People from schools that have implemented coordinated school health associated a number of benefits with the approach, including

- impact on important numbers, such as reduced absenteeism and fewer behavioral problems. All groups—parents, teachers, and administrators—said it would be easier to make the case for coordinated school health programs if they had data showing that such programs would make a difference in the numbers by which school districts and individual schools are evaluated.
- improved classroom performance, in the form of higher test scores after the program was implemented, as well as more alert students and more positive attitudes among students;
- teaching real skills students can use rather than rote knowledge;
- bringing everyone together, either by providing a forum for greater parental and/or community involvement, providing an opportunity for the school and other agencies to collaborate, bringing staff together within the school, or providing a program in which students in all areas can participate; and
- for disadvantaged children in particular, getting them ready to learn by meeting their basic needs.

Barriers to Change

Participants whose schools did not have a coordinated approach mentioned the following barriers to implementation:

- Tremendous pressure to "teach to tests," and health isn't a topic on state-level achievement tests.
- Health teachers aren't "part of the team," sometimes figuratively and sometimes literally.
- Health is not stressed in teaching degree programs.
- Parents are not making it a priority, probably because they do not realize how health issues are (or are not) currently addressed in schools.

Message Development: Lessons Learned

After testing a variety of message concepts in the initial in-depth interviews and focus groups, the project team reached the following conclusions:

1. In general, focusing on an immediate problem and presenting a comprehensive or coordinated approach to school health as part of a solution worked best.
2. Tying school health programs to "numbers" that affect funding or by which schools are rated, such as absenteeism and drop-out rates, provided a compelling message to many administrators and teachers. Parents also thought such linkages would help garner support for health programs.
3. Positioning school health programs as providing support and practical skills was believable and likely to be well received by most administrators, teachers, and parents.
4. A lot of teachers, in particular, reacted well to a "whole child" message, but it may not be the best choice for widespread use because some teachers and administrators thought it was "jargon" and some seemed to anticipate negative community reaction to such a message.
5. Positioning a coordinated school health program as unique by saying that it is the *only* approach to addressing multiple health threats was not credible to the target audiences and was viewed as promising too much. While some teachers, in particular, were strong proponents of the comprehensive or coordinated approach and viewed it as the foundation of a successful school, others—and many administrators—viewed it as one component of strengthening a school, not a complete solution.
6. The phrase *comprehensive school health programs* conjured up "expensive" and "daunting." This may be because the word *comprehensive* brings to mind "many changes and many resources," and the word *programs* is interpreted as a separate line-item on a budget. Given the negative reaction to *comprehensive school health programs*, the phrase *a coordinated approach to school health* may be a better term to use.

Based on the results of the research, the final message concepts were as follows. The first two are for teachers and administrators; the second two are for parents.

1. There's a lot of concern these days about absenteeism, drop-out rates, and discipline problems in our schools. But did you know a lot of these problems are health related? A coordinated approach to school health is about more than keeping kids healthy. It's about improving schools by supporting students' capacity to learn.
2. Keeping kids healthy today means focusing on the complete child, from drug and alcohol use to sexuality and stress. A coordinated approach to school health gives students the essential information and practical skills they need so they can deal with the problems they face in and out of school.
3. Being smart isn't all it takes to succeed in today's world. Kids also need to make smart decisions about sex, alcohol, tobacco, drugs, nutrition, and fitness. School health programs help students learn how to make the right choices—for life.

4. For today's kids to succeed, they need to learn to read, write, and understand math. But how much can they learn if they're using alcohol, tobacco, and other drugs; suffering from stress; or having a baby? A coordinated approach to school health gives kids practical skills to deal with today's problems so they have a better chance for success in and out of school.

DEVELOPING AND TESTING INITIAL MATERIALS

The initial materials were designed to broaden target audience members' definition of school health and provide them with information to use when talking with others to build support for a coordinated approach. They used the message concepts above to highlight the importance of changing school health and providing relevant benefits for doing so. The materials included two booklets that illustrated a coordinated approach to school health (one for administrators and teachers and one for parents), a slide presentation, talking points, and a series of questions and answers about school health.

The administrators, teachers, and parents who reviewed the materials thought they were attractive but were pessimistic about being able to make changes and wanted specific advice about how to build support. In addition, they suggested adding case studies and repackaging the information to reduce impressions of coordinated school health as complex and overwhelming.

DEVELOPING AND TESTING REVISED MATERIALS

The project team refined the content of the materials and the way in which they were packaged, turning to the literature on diffusing innovations in organizational settings and social cognitive theory (see Chapter 10) for guidance on addressing the concerns raised by target audience members.

In refining the materials, the goal was to emphasize that schools can work toward a coordinated approach, and that a coordinated approach will reinforce the role of the family. This positioning was chosen to increase perceptions that the innovation (a coordinated approach to school health) could be compatible with existing practices and values and could be implemented piecemeal—and, if necessary, discontinued—while decreasing perceptions that it had to be complex and/or resource intensive, and, consequently, was risky to attempt.

The final materials are a school health starter kit (basically a community action kit), a Powerpoint slide presentation, two posters, assessment resources, case studies, and a booklet to give guidance to the chief state school officers and health officials and their staffs on how to use the other materials. The starter kit is packaged as a foldout spiral-bound kit with pockets on each side. Graduated page sizes are used for each section (i.e., the pages get progressively wider) to create a "hyperlink" feel and ensure easy access to relevant information. The writing style (light and a bit whimsical) and packaging work together to reduce the impression that the subject is overwhelming. The kit incorporates many of the types of messages recommended by Maibach and Cotton (1995) in their staged social cognitive approach to message design to be described in Chapter 12. Specifically, the materials

1. *identify how to effectively overcome barriers to change and encourage people to identify and plan solutions to the obstacles they are most likely to face.* The kit outlines a step-by-step approach to analyzing the current environment, including ways to identify barriers to making changes. It includes questions and answers to prepare people for the objections they are likely to face as they try to build support and a worksheet to help analyze how receptive their environment is to change. Items on the worksheet were drawn from a review of the diffusion of innovations literature (Academy for Educational Development, 1996).

2. *encourage people to set specific goals and instruct them on appropriate ways to set incremental goals.* The kit encourages people to start slowly (rather than trying to change everything at once) and includes a worksheet they can use to identify needed changes and then prioritize them based on how easy or difficult the changes will be to accomplish. Items on the worksheet operationalize many of the innovation characteristics that were presented in Table 10–1 in Chapter 10.

3. *bolster self-efficacy to cope with specific situations that people are likely to encounter in their change efforts.* Formative research indicated that people did not know where or how to start building support for a coordinated approach to school health and consequently had no confidence in their ability to do so. The materials outline an approach that is intended to guide people through the initial steps of building support, allowing them to build their self-efficacy as they go along. Many resources (such as the previously mentioned worksheets, as well as sample letters to the editor, press releases, and a listing of additional sources of information) are included.

4. *model appropriate behaviors* through a series of case studies from schools, districts, and states that have implemented changes consistent with a coordinated approach to health.

REFERENCES

Academy for Educational Development. (1996). *Developing the marketing plan: Insights from the diffusion of innovations literature.* Guidelines Diffusion Project. Washington, DC: Author.

Maibach, E.W., & Cotton, D. (1995). Moving people to behavior change: A staged social cognitive approach to message design. In E. Maibach & R.L. Parrott (Eds.), *Designing health messages: Approaches from communication theory and public health practice* (pp. 41–64). Thousand Oaks, CA: Sage.

Sample Recruitment Screener

Interviewer: _____

Date: _____

Time: _____

Hello. My name is _____, from _____, a research company in _____. We're putting together a series of small discussion groups with school administrators, teachers, and parents from certain school districts. The discussions will focus on health programs in area schools. The groups are being held for the purpose of opinion research only. I'd like to ask you a couple of questions.

1. How supportive would you say you are of having health programs in schools?
   _____ Very supportive   (CONTINUE. ASK Q2.)
   _____ Somewhat supportive   (CONTINUE. ASK Q2.)
   _____ Not very supportive   (THANK AND TERMINATE.)

2. What is your position in or relationship to the school?
   _____ Teacher   (CONTINUE. ASK Q3.)
   _____ Administrator   (CONTINUE. ASK Q5.)
   _____ Parent   (CONTINUE. ASK Q8.)
   _____ None of the above   (THANK AND TERMINATE.)

3. What grade(s) do you teach presently? (RECRUIT A GOOD MIX OF GRADE LEVELS.)
   _____ K through 6th grades   (CONTINUE. ASK Q4.)
   _____ 7th through 8th grades   (CONTINUE. ASK Q4.)
   _____ 9th through 12 grades   (CONTINUE. ASK Q4.)

Courtesy of The Academy for Educational Development, Washington, D.C.

4. What courses do you teach?
   _____ Health education/programs only
   _____ Health education and physical education
   _____ Some health education and some other (specify: _____)
   _____ Other (specify: _____)

   GO TO TEACHER INVITATION.

5. At which school are you employed? _____

   (CHECK QUOTAS. CANNOT HAVE TWO ADMINISTRATORS FROM SAME SCHOOL.)

6. What grade levels are you involved with in your present position?
   _____ K through 6th grades   (CONTINUE. ASK Q7.)
   _____ 7th through 8th grades   (CONTINUE. ASK Q7.)
   _____ 9th through 12 grades   (CONTINUE. ASK Q7.)

7. What is your administrative position? (DO NOT READ)
   _____ Superintendent
   _____ Principal
   _____ Vice principal
   _____ Dean
   _____ School nurse/health provider
   _____ Curriculum coordinator

   GO TO ADMINISTRATOR INVITATION.

8. Do you have any children who are currently attending school in this district?
   _____ Yes   (CONTINUE.)
   _____ No   (THANK AND TERMINATE.)

9. What grade(s) is/are your child(ren) in currently?
   _____ K through 6th grades   (CONTINUE.)
   _____ 7th through 8th grades   (CONTINUE.)
   _____ 9th through 12 grades   (CONTINUE.)

10. Which school(s) does/do your child(ren) attend? _____

    (CHECK QUOTAS. CANNOT HAVE TWO PARENTS OF KIDS IN THE SAME GRADE FROM THE SAME SCHOOL.)

11. In what type of school activities do you participate?
    _____ PTA/PTO officer   (GO TO PARENT INVITATION.)
    _____ PTA/PTO member   (GO TO PARENT INVITATION.)
    _____ Teacher's aide/assistant   (GO TO PARENT INVITATION.)

_____ Volunteer at school functions   (GO TO PARENT INVITATION.)
_____ Attend school board meetings   (GO TO PARENT INVITATION.)
_____ Other (specify: _____)   (GO TO PARENT INVITATION.)
_____ None   (THANK AND TERMINATE.)

INVITATION

Okay, that's all the questions we have for you. We would like to invite you to participate in our discussion group. The group will take place at _____ (time) on _____ (day of week and date). The discussion will take about an hour and a half. For helping us with this research, each participant will receive _____.

The discussion groups will be held at: (NAME, ADDRESS, & TELEPHONE NUMBER OF FACILITY)

We will send you a letter confirming the date and location of the group. Could I please have your name and address?

Name: _____

Address: _____

City: _____ State: _____ ZIP: _____

We will call you a day or so before the group to confirm the time. What is the best time to reach you? What is the best telephone number to reach you at that time? Is there another time and number we can try if we miss you?

Time: _____

Telephone: _____

2nd time: _____

2nd telephone: _____

If anything comes up and you have to cancel, please give us a call at: _____. Because it is such a small group, it is important that you let us know if we will need to replace you. You can call anytime, and if we are not here, please leave a message. Thank you.

Sample Focus Group Moderator's Guide

DEVELOPING MESSAGES TO SUPPORT COMPREHENSIVE SCHOOL HEALTH PROGRAMS (CSHP)

FOCUS GROUPS WITH PARENTS: MODERATOR'S GUIDE

I. WARM-UP, EXPLANATIONS, AND INTRODUCTIONS (10 minutes)

  A. Introduction and Purpose

    1. Good afternoon/evening. My name is _____, and I will be facilitating our discussion tonight. We're here to talk about school health.

    2. Thanks for joining us. All of your comments—both positive and negative—are important.

    3. There are no right or wrong answers, and it's important that I hear what everyone thinks. So please speak up, even if you disagree with someone else.

  B. Procedure

    1. Our discussion tonight will be audiotaped so that I don't lose any of your comments. I'll use the tapes to write a report summarizing what was said. However, the report will not identify any of you by name.

    2. (IF APPROPRIATE:) Behind me is a one-way mirror. Some people who are interested in what you have to say may be sitting behind the glass on and off during our discussion. They aren't in the same room with us because they can be distracting.

    3. This is a group discussion, so please don't wait for me to call on you. Please speak one at a time so the tape recorder can pick up everything.

Courtesy of The Academy for Educational Development, Washington, D.C.

4. We have many topics to discuss in a very limited amount of time, so at times I may change the subject or move ahead. I'll try to come back to earlier points at the end of our session if there's time.

C. Self-Introductions

Let's do a quick round of introductions. Please tell us your name, how many children you have, and what grades they're in.

II. DEFINITION OF SCHOOL HEALTH PROGRAMS (20 minutes)

A. Role of Schools Vis-À-Vis Health

1. Name THE (one) biggest health problem facing students at your child's school today.

2. What role do you think most OTHER *parents* think the school should play relative to health? Do you think the role of a school changes relative to their grade level?

3. How do you think your children's health affects their performance at school? Do you link your children's health to school performance?

B. Think for a minute about the ideal school. What is included in its approach to health? (PROBE: Are there any other components? What about . . . health education? Physical education? Health services? Food service? Counseling? School environment (e.g., caring/supportive, tobacco-free, food sold, violence, safety, indoor air quality)? School, community, or parent/family partnerships? Faculty and staff wellness programs?

C. All of the components on this list are referred to as a comprehensive or coordinated school health program. (SHOW LIST ON EASEL.) How many of you have children in schools that have all or most of these components?

1. What ones does your school do the best job on? What needs improvement?

2. Of these, which are the most important?

3. Which is the least important?

III. BENEFITS OF AND BARRIERS TO CSHP (20 minutes)

A. Benefits of CSHP

1. What do you see as the *major benefits* of an approach like the one on the list?

   PROBES: Would you expect to see an impact on classroom performance? Behavior? Attendance?

2. How about those of you whose children go to schools that use a comprehensive approach? What do you find are the major benefits? (PROBE: What impact, if any, have you seen on academic performance? Behavior? Student health? Interest in health? Has it made a

difference in the community? For example, has the interaction between the school and the community changed? In what way?)

B. Drawbacks

 1. For those of you whose children come from schools with*out* a comprehensive approach, what do you see as the *potential drawbacks* to
 such an approach?

 2. How about those of you who have programs like we described earlier
 in place? What drawbacks have you encountered?

IV. STARTING A CSHP (15 minutes)

A. For those of you whose child attends a school with a comprehensive or
coordinated approach in place: Did you help to get your program started?
Who asked for your help?

 1. Who are the biggest supporters of the current program? How is support demonstrated?

 2. How about the biggest opponents of the current program? How is opposition demonstrated—and how did you address the opposition?

B. For those of you who *do not* have a comprehensive approach in place:
What are the first changes you would try to make? Why would you start
there?

C. For all of you: There are a variety of steps people can take to foster support for comprehensive school health programs. What actions do you
think parents could take? (PROBE: Speak to health teacher? Speak to a
principal or school board member? Invite to a meeting or spend time with
a knowledgeable school district or state official who supports comprehensive or coordinated health programs to learn what the approach
would entail? Discuss at a PTA/PTO meeting?)

V. MESSAGE CONCEPTS (25 minutes)

We're in the process of developing messages that could be used to promote
comprehensive school health programs. I'd like to run a couple of messages
by you and see what you think. It's important for you to know that I didn't
develop these messages.

A. READ EACH MESSAGE AS YOU PASS THEM OUT TO PARTICI-
PANTS. ASK:

 1. What comes to mind when you hear this message?

 2. Now please number the messages so they are ranked from most compelling to least compelling to you. Use a "1" to indicate most compelling, a "2" to indicate next most compelling, etc.

B. READ FIRST MESSAGE. ASK HOW MANY PUT IT ON TOP OF
STACK, PUT IT SECOND, PUT IT LAST. RECORD ON EASEL

BOARD. CONTINUE FOR ALL MESSAGES. ASK FOLLOWING QUESTIONS AS APPROPRIATE FOR EACH MESSAGE.

1. For those of you who put (READ MESSAGE) in first or second place, what was appealing to you about it?
2. Was there anything you disliked about this message? Again, I didn't write these, so please be honest.
3. For those of you who rated this message last, what did you dislike? Could it be changed to make it more appealing to you? How?
4. Have we missed something? Is there something you could think of that would present a stronger, more compelling reason to support CSHP?

VI. MATERIALS (15 minutes)

A. What do you usually want to know about health at school? How do you usually find out?
   1. Are there any materials that you get from your children's schools that describe their schools' approach to health? Could you describe these materials to me? How helpful are they?
   2. Are there any materials that you would like to have, but don't? What would they be?

VII. CLOSING

A. That's the end of my questions. Do you have any final comments?
B. On behalf of the Council of Chief State School Officers and the Association of State and Territorial Health Officials, I'd like to thank you for participating in our discussion today. Your input was extremely valuable. Have a nice day.

APPENDIX 11–D

Information Resources

Claritas (Potential Rating Index by Zip Markets [PRIZM])
(PRIZM: geodemographic clustering system integrating demographics, consumer spending, business, marketing, and geographic data)
1-800-234-5973
http://www.spider.claritas.com
info@claritas.com

Dialog
(Includes Dialog, DataStar, and Profound. Dialog: More than 470 databases, including full-text articles from more than 7,000 journals, magazines, and newspapers; full text of more than 100 U.S. and international newspapers; wire services. DataStar: More than 350 databases of European business and technical information. Profound: More than 20 million articles, reports, and news studies, including market research reports, news wires, newspapers, magazines, and trade journals from more than 190 countries)
http://www.dialog.com

Lexis/Nexis
(Lexis: Archives of federal and state case law, state statutes, state and federal regulations, public records, legal information. Nexis: More than 8,700 national and international newspapers, news wires, magazines, trade journals, and business publications)
P.O. Box 933
Dayton, OH 45401-0933
1-800-227-4908
http://www.nexis.com

Mediamark Research, Inc.

(MRI: Comprehensive demographic, lifestyle, product usage, and media data from annual surveys of more than 20,000 consumers)

708 Third Avenue, 8th Floor
New York, NY 10017
1-800-310-3305
http://www.mediamark.com
info@mediamark.com

ProQuest (UMI)

(Online and CD-ROM databases of newspapers, journals, periodicals, and magazines)

http://www.umi.com

Simmons Market Research Bureau (SMRB)

(Includes Study of Media and Markets, a survey of American consumers' media habits, product purchase behavior and beliefs, opinions, and attitudes; The Hispanic Study; Simmons Teenage Research Study (STARS), The Kids Study, and the Gay & Lesbian Market Study)

309 West 49th Street
New York, NY 10019
1-212-374-8900

Framing the Message: Crafting Communication Strategies

Social change interventions always involve communication in some form. Messages might be delivered to members of the public, health professionals, business leaders, or policy makers, and channels used might be the mass media, a training session, a speech, a letter, a booklet, or a community event, but communication is always integral. Communication provides the opportunity to frame the social change so that it is consistent with the values of target audience members. The starting point for making this happen is developing a strong strategy for communication.

The communication strategy describes how the behavior or issue will be framed and positioned in the consumer's mind. It spells out the target audience(s), the action they should take and how they will benefit, and how to reach them with messages. It is based on a thorough understanding of the audience and their wants, needs, and values coupled with knowledge of the types of appeals likely to work in a given situation. Once a communication strategy has been developed, message concepts are developed to present that positioning to the audience and assess whether it is believable, compelling, and relevant.

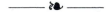

Americans are exposed to a barrage of health information every day. They wake up and hear it on the radio or TV, read it in the newspaper, see it in employer health newsletters (if they have health coverage), and hear more from friends, family members, and health care providers. Many people feel overwhelmed by all of the often-conflicting advice and perspectives.

Communication plays a major role in many public health efforts to bring about social change. Communication can be used to inform, educate, and persuade. It

312

can be used to model simple behaviors or reinforce existing ones. It can call on cultural symbols and icons to frame an issue in a variety of ways. The challenge is to develop and implement communication campaigns that address health behavior and policy objectives by breaking through the clutter and reaching target populations with persuasive, actionable messages that are scientifically sound but audience oriented. This chapter outlines a process for crafting a communication strategy and developing message concepts based on it. The strategy provides the foundation for effective communications by spelling out who the target audience is, what they should do and how they will benefit, and how to reach them. The message concepts translate the strategy into statements that are presented to members of the intended audience—and assessed to determine whether they are believable, relevant, and compelling.

THE COMMUNICATION STRATEGY

A communication strategy frames the issue in a particular way and thus positions the social change in the audience's mind. It must address the following points:

1. Target audience: Who is the person to make the social change?
2. Action: What should people do after exposure to the communication?
3. Key benefit: From the audience's perspective, why should they make the change?
4. Support: What reasons will convince the audience that they will benefit?
5. Openings: How will the audience be reached?
6. Image: How should the action be conveyed?

The audience member might be a "member of the public," a patient, a health professional, a policy maker, a voter, a reporter, or some other type of individual.

The activities conducted to develop an overall strategic plan (described in Chapter 10) start the development of a solid communication strategy. However, target audiences for various communications may have to be refined and/or may require separate communication strategies depending on the action they should take as a result of exposure to the communication.

The communication strategies developed for public health efforts include the same components as their commercial sector counterparts, although some modifications may be necessary to accommodate the marketing of behaviors with no tangible product or service. The consumer-based health communications (CHC) process outlined by Sutton, Balch, and Lefebvre (1995) is an excellent example of modifying the commercial communication strategy development framework specifically to the needs of public health practitioners; it is used as the basis for the approach outlined here.

The Role of Theory

As with development of the overall intervention, the development of communication strategies should be guided by the theories or models of how change is expected to occur. For example, Maibach and Cotton (1995) have developed what they term a "staged social cognitive approach to message design," in which they use the concepts of social cognitive theory to determine the most appropriate types of messages for people in each of the transtheoretical model's stages of change. They recommend the following types of messages to help people move from one stage to the next.

For people in precontemplation (no intention to change behavior in foreseeable future; unaware of risk, will not acknowledge risk, or some other reason):

- Enhance knowledge of and expectations about the consequences—good or bad—of the risk behavior.
- Personalize the risk.
- Emphasize the benefits of the new behavior and encourage a reevaluation of the costs and benefits (or outcome expectancies) that includes the new benefits.

For people in contemplation (considering the need to change behavior but with no specific plan):

- Encourage gaining experience with the new behavior (e.g., through trying the new behavior or trying to refrain from the risk behavior).
- Continue promoting new expectations of positive consequences and reinforce existing positive expectations.
- Consider disputing commonly believed but untrue negative consequences and suggesting ways to minimize bona fide negative consequences, though it is typically easier to promote advantages than to challenge perceived disadvantages.
- Enhance self-efficacy by identifying how to effectively overcome barriers to change.

For people in preparation (making decision to change behavior; may try behavior):

- Encourage people to restructure their environments—and instruct them on how to do so—so that important cues for practicing the new behavior are obvious and supported socially.
- Encourage people to identify and plan solutions to the relevant obstacles they are most likely to face.
- Help people to maintain their motivation by encouraging them to set a long-term goal and instructing them on appropriate ways to set short-term goals to keep them progressing to the long-term goal.

- Increase self-efficacy to cope with specific situations and other obstacles that people are likely to encounter in their change efforts.
- Model social reinforcement of appropriate behaviors.

For people in action (beginning to perform the behavior consistently):

- Encourage refining skills, especially those that will help avoid relapse and that allow productive coping with setbacks to prevent full relapse.
- Bolster self-efficacy for dealing with new obstacles and setbacks in the behavior change process.
- Encourage people to feel good about themselves when they make progress, especially in the face of temptation.
- Make explicit or reiterate the long-term benefits of the behavior change.

Strategic Questions

Crafting a communication strategy should begin with collecting data to answer most or all of the questions shown in Exhibit 12–1. The answers to all of the strategic questions must fit together; changing one answer often necessitates changing others. Each of the questions is discussed in more detail below. As answers are developed, consideration should be given to the issues raised in the Message Content and Construction section at the end of this chapter.

Who Should Be the Target Audience, and What Are They Like?

While many public health agencies have a mandate to serve the public, decisions to target "the general population" do not make for good communications. As Sutton and colleagues (1995) noted, any communication will appeal to some groups more effectively than others, based on executional details (i.e., language used, type of people portrayed, color, music, etc.) if nothing else. It is a far better

---

Exhibit 12–1 Questions To Guide Communication Strategy Development

- Who should be the target audience, and what are they like?
- What is the action they should take—and what are they doing now?
- What are the obstacles that stand between the audience and the desired behavior?
- What is the benefit to the audience of engaging in the behavior?
- What is the support for that benefit—what will make it credible to the audience?
- What are the best openings for reaching the audience—and are the channels available appropriate for conveying the message?
- What image should communications convey?

use of resources to take a proactive approach, carefully identifying the most appropriate audience(s) and then developing program components specifically to address their needs, perceptions, and values. For example, for initiatives seeking to bring about policy change, there are usually at least three audiences: policy makers, some segment of the public, and members of the media. Chapter 10 introduced audience segmentation as a tool for selecting audiences, and Chapter 11 provided information on particular segmentation approaches.

Once each audience has been identified, communication planners should get to know its members. Thinking of the audience as one person, rather than as a group, is useful and leads to more focused, relevant communications. One way to do this is to write a profile of the person based on formative research. Some firms go as far as drawing a picture of a typical audience member. Demographic characteristics (age, marital status, presence of children, ethnicity, political leanings, etc.), are just a starting point. As Sutton and colleagues (1995) wrote, "What's important to this person? What are his or her feelings, attitudes, and beliefs about the behavior change and its benefits and barriers? What can motivate this person to do something different?" (p. 728).

What Is the Action They Should Take—and What Are They Doing Now?

To persuade audience members to take a particular action, communication planners must understand exactly what the audience is willing and able to do. As Roman and Maas (1992) cautioned, "overambition is the pitfall of most strategies" (p. 5). Until we know what people are doing now, we do not know what we are asking them to change—and how great a change we are asking them to make. This information also helps identify the competition and the values underlying both the current and the desired behavior.

Selecting an action is a critical—and difficult—decision to make. Planners should strive to avoid the trap of focusing on a very narrow audience and persuading them to make a complicated behavior change. This sometimes happens with individual health behaviors because there is usually a group of people far from the behavior and therefore most "in need." Often a better strategy—from the viewpoint of both communication success and change in health status or policy—is to address the easier changes first. Targeting the group most willing to make the change often leads to two accomplishments: The audience makes progress toward the social change objective, and social norms are often influenced, thereby creating a climate in which others are more willing to (and indeed may feel pressure to) make changes.

To illustrate, consider a common policy scenario: Voters often divide into those who strongly support the change, those who strongly oppose it, and those who do not feel strongly one way or the other. Often the third group is large enough to decide the vote. If that is the case, focusing on the strong opposition is the wrong approach. It is very unlikely that those people will change their minds. While resources are being wasted trying to reach them, the votes of the middle group—the ones who could ensure passage of the policy—may be lost.

Health Behavior Changes. For campaigns promoting a specific health behavior, the action is a behavior change, but it may not be the behavioral objective per se. Instead, it may be a step toward the desired behavior. For example, the 5 A Day for Better Health media campaign focused on getting target audience members to add two servings of fruits and vegetables each day, rather than to eat five servings. Why? Because they were already eating about three servings, on average, so all they needed to do was eat two more—and they thought "adding two" was much more manageable than "eating five."

How do you select an action? Graeff, Elder, and Booth (1993) suggested first developing a list of "ideal" behaviors. In the context of changing individual health behaviors, they defined ideal behaviors as "the medically prescribed behavioral steps that the target audience should perform in order to prevent or treat the health problem" (p. 65). From this list, they recommended selecting target behaviors, which they defined as "the minimum number of behavioral steps essential for the health practice to be effective" (p. 65). Exhibit 12–2 lists some questions they suggested asking to help with target behavior selection. Although Graeff and colleagues developed these questions to assess behaviors related to individual health practices, they can be modified easily to address other types of social changes.

Once you have a list of target behaviors, a useful next step is to compare the list with a "map" of the target audience's behavior process. As Sutton and colleagues (1995) noted:

> a consumer map can help to identify those points in the process where consumers pull away from the recommended health behavior and toward another behavior. . . . What are they doing now, instead of the desired behavior? That action is the competition—the behavior we want to replace. Answers help formulate the intermediate steps that stand between where the consumer currently is and where the science recommends him or her to be. These intermediate steps are the potential candidates for a communication "action." (p. 729)

Target audience behavior maps can be created by using the qualitative research techniques discussed in Chapter 11.

Finally, when thinking through potential actions, remember that changing lifelong behavior is extraordinarily difficult, particularly when, as is true for many public health messages, people think they have other priorities. They respond best to easy solutions and absolute answers (National Cancer Institute [NCI], 1989). The challenge faced by public health practitioners is succinctly highlighted by

Exhibit 12–2 Questions To Select Target Behaviors

1. *Does the ideal behavior have a demonstrated impact on this specific health problem?* If not, it should not be selected as a target behavior.
2. *Is the ideal behavior feasible for the audience to perform?* An in-depth understanding of the target audience is essential if one is to understand the environmental constraints that will affect adoption.
   - Does the ideal behavior produce negative consequences for the person performing it?
   - Is the ideal behavior incompatible with the person's current behavior or with sociocultural norms or acceptable practices?
   - Does the ideal behavior require an unrealistic rate of frequency?
   - Does the ideal behavior require an unrealistic duration?
   - Does the ideal behavior have too high a cost in time, energy, social status, money, or materials?
   - Is the ideal behavior too complex and not easily divided into a small number of elements or steps?
3. *Are any existing behaviors approximations to the ideal behavior?* Can these behaviors be shaped into an effective health practice through training and skill development? Communication programs are more likely to achieve behavior change if they build on what people are already doing correctly. If existing behaviors are similar to any of the remaining ideal behaviors, they should be included in the list of target behaviors.

Source: Reprinted with permission from J.A. Graeff, J.P. Elder, and E.M. Booth, *Communication for Health and Behavior Change: A Developing Country Perspective,* p. 67, © 1993, Jossey-Bass Inc., Publishers.

advertising professionals Kenneth Roman and Jane Maas in *How To Advertise* (1992, p. 5): "Don't ask people to change deeply ingrained habits; it's much easier to get them to change brands."

Public Health Policy Changes. Selecting an action for public health policy audiences can be clear-cut or challenging, depending on the nature of the initiative. When the time frame is clearly defined and the goal is to get the audience to take some specific action now, not necessarily to continue taking it for the rest of their lives, the action is often obvious. For example, the action for a member of the media might be to frame an issue in a particular way. The action for a voter might be to vote for (or against) a referendum or to call or write a public official to support or oppose a specific policy. The desired action for a food company might be to decrease the amount of salt or fat in its processed foods.

When the time frame is less clearly defined or the behavior changes are more complex or involve more people, the initial action can be difficult to identify and somewhat removed from the ultimate goal. For example, initial efforts to persuade schools to adopt a coordinated approach to school health typically focus on building support among parents and other community members. The action might be asking them to show that support by contacting a school board member.

What Are the Obstacles That Stand between the Audience and the Desired Behavior?

Although this question isn't explicitly addressed in many communication strategy frameworks (see, for example, Sutton et al., 1995; Roman & Maas, 1992), we have included it here because knowing what real or perceived barriers stand in the way of taking action is an invaluable aid to planning realistic actions or activities. Common barriers can include beliefs, pressures, misinformation, and competing ways of framing the public health issue. For example, policy makers may think that constituents do not think a particular public health program is important, may feel pressure to dedicate resources to a different area, or may be receiving messages that the program threatens core values, such as independence or freedom. When the subject is individual behavior change, people can feel enormous pressure relative to health practices; two examples are not using condoms and fixing traditional foods even though they are high in fat.

Two obstacles that health messages about individual behaviors often confront are the lack of a future orientation (the majority of Americans say it is better to live for the present than worry about tomorrow) and the lack of feeling personally susceptible (NCI, 1989). These obstacles are reflected in the finding of Backer, Rogers, and Sopory (1992) that "campaigns are more effective if they emphasize current rewards rather than the avoidance of distant negative consequences" (p. 30). Creating a behavioral map, as discussed earlier, will often identify many of the specific obstacles. The action selected normally provides the target audience with a means of overcoming the obstacle.

For public health policies and promoting public health as an institution, key to understanding obstacles is identifying how the issue is currently being framed on the public agenda. This can be accomplished by analyzing media coverage of the issue and preparing a framing memo that outlines the various ways the issue has been positioned, or framed, by the media. This process was described in Chapter 10; examples are provided in Chapter 10 and later in this chapter.

What Is the Benefit to the Audience of Engaging in the Behavior?

This is a crucial point and an area in which many communication planners make mistakes. "People don't buy products, they buy expectations of benefits" (Roman & Maas, 1992, p. 10). In a review of effective communication campaigns, Backer and colleagues (1992) concluded that "more effective campaigns focus target audiences' attention on immediate, high-probability consequences of healthy behavior" (p. 30). Unfortunately, managers often try to use a long-term population benefit to "sell" the audience, when a short-term personal benefit is more motivating, in part because it is more tightly linked to the audience's core values and needs.

For example, from a public health standpoint, the major benefit of stopping smoking is decreased risk of developing heart disease, various cancers, and a host of other diseases. But from the standpoint of the person deciding whether to try to quit, the major benefit may be ceasing to cough in the morning or no longer smelling like smoke all the time. Similarly, policy makers may not be that motivated by improving the public's health and may not care whether a particular program is funded—but they do care if their constituents are happy. If there is a tangible product or a service involved, another mistake is to confuse attributes with benefits. "Speed in a computer, for example, is an attribute; the benefit is saving time" (Roman & Maas, 1992, p. 10).

The challenge is to identify and focus on one key benefit from the myriad possibilities. Often people have a number of motivations for engaging in a particular behavior. How do you pick one? As we discussed in Chapter 3, understanding the needs and values underlying the current and desired behaviors is critical. Often the greatest need or strongest value provides the most meaningful, compelling benefit. Getting at these basic values can be accomplished in a number of ways. The laddering exercises discussed in Chapter 11, in which qualitative research participants are asked why particular attributes are important, and then why their response is important, are very useful. Another approach that can be used in qualitative or quantitative settings is to ask participants to rate each of a set of adjectives in terms of how well each describes themselves, and then to rate how well each describes people who engage in the desired behavior. What they do—and don't—put in each list speaks volumes about the values they are looking for—and associate with each behavior.

It is important to note that the benefit is "promised" in communications. Often it is never explicitly stated. Rather, it is a conclusion that people draw after exposure to the communication. Sutton and colleagues (1995) recommended using the following sentence to link desired and current behavior with a benefit:

> "If I (action) instead of (current behavior), I will (benefit)."

For example, for the 5 A Day media campaign the action-benefit (or promise, as Sutton and colleagues [1995] label it) statement is: "If I add two servings of fruits and vegetables the easy way instead of making it hard, then I will feel relieved and more in control of my life" (Lefebvre et al., 1995; Sutton et al., 1995). An action-benefit statement for California's anti-Proposition 188 campaign (discussed in Chapter 11) might have been: "If I oppose Proposition 188 instead of supporting it, I will keep Philip Morris from exerting control over my state." This approach is consistent with our discussion in Chapter 3 about positioning the new behavior as superior to the old by showing (implicitly) that maintaining the old behavior will conflict with basic needs and desires.

What Is the Support for That Benefit—What Will Make It Credible to the Audience?

The support is the reason that the benefit outweighs the obstacles. Support is provided through aspects of the message's execution. It can take many forms, such as hard data, demonstrations of how to perform the action, or demonstrations of the valued benefits to the action (e.g., a person feeling more in control after taking steps to improve eating habits). It can be emotional, factual, or both. Aspects of the execution that influence credibility, such as the degree to which models are like target audience members and how they look, talk, dress, and behave, as well as music, colors, background, design, typeface, and paper stock, can all support or detract from the promised benefit (Sutton et al., 1995). In the terms of Sutton and colleagues (1995) earlier sentence, support is the "because":

> *"If I (action) instead of (current behavior),*
> *I will (benefit) because (support)."*

Signorielli (1993) criticized the antidrug "Just say no" campaign of the 1980s, in part, because it lacked support:

> This campaign is problematic because it fails to take the basic principles of adolescent psychology and functioning into consideration. This campaign preaches and tells young people (and the rest of society for that matter) what to do. It does not provide information about why or even how teens, in the face of strong (or not so strong) peer pressure, can "just say no." (p. 155)

Public health communicators often are tempted to use scientific facts as support. They should proceed with caution. Hard data can work, provided they are understandable, relevant, and believable to the target audience. However, practitioners should bear in mind that many members of the public place little credence in scientific data. They recall too many instances when those data later changed or were debunked by yet another new study. In addition, people often do not understand science, particularly intangible concepts such as relative risk, and so personal decisions may be based on faulty reasoning (NCI, 1989). Furthermore, it can be difficult for hard data to compete with an emotional appeal to core human values. This problem is illustrated in the case study on affirmative action presented later in this chapter.

What Are the Best Openings for Reaching the Audience—and Are the Channels Available Appropriate for Conveying the Message?

First, planners must determine the times, places, and situations when the audience will be most attentive to, and able to act on, the message. Then they must assess (1) whether the message lends itself to delivery via the channels that can be used to reach that time and place and (2) whether the program has access to or can reasonably afford those channels.

For example, most mass media are best suited to providing simple information. With the possible exception of print media, they cannot be used effectively to convey complex information—and cannot take the place of one-on-one education and monitoring. Used alone, they can induce behavior change only under limited circumstances. However, they can frame a public health issue, raise awareness of a behavior change, provide cost-effective support and reinforcement for the change, and stimulate discussions of more complex information in the appropriate setting. Chapter 13 will include a discussion of some of the pros and cons of various types of mass media. Bellicha and McGrath (1990) provide examples of how mass media can be put to effective use within a larger social change initiative. They discuss how mass media are used to help educate patients, health professionals, and the public about high blood pressure and cholesterol as part of efforts to reduce morbidity and mortality caused by heart disease.

Thorough target audience research is critical to identifying the best openings. A useful approach is for researchers to try to walk through a day in the audience's shoes. When would they be most receptive to messages about the behavior? As Sutton and colleagues (1995) noted, "times" may be parts of the day, week, or year. Or they could be wake-up time, exercise time, mealtime, commuting time, or office time. "Situations" may be times when a target is thinking about the benefit ("What can I do to make my constituents happy?" "How can I make my community a better place to live?" "What am I going to have for dinner tonight?").

Once planners identify the best openings, they must assess the channels available to the intervention. Which are best at reaching these openings? Likewise, the channels must be assessed against the type of message. Which will be able to deliver the message in the most compelling, understandable manner? Figure 12–1 depicts this balancing act. In general, a combination of interpersonal and mass communication channels leads to a more effective campaign (Backer et al., 1992).

If there is a conflict between the best channels for the message and the best channels for the audience, the preferable resolution is to examine the message and see if it can be modified to better suit the channels. Likewise, if there is a conflict between the channels that will best reach the audience and the channels you can access, is there a way to access the other channels, perhaps through a partner or intermediary?

What Image Should Communications Convey?

Image is often thought of as the personality of the communication and the action. Image is what makes the communication speak to the target audience. Members must think the communication—and by extension, the action—is designed

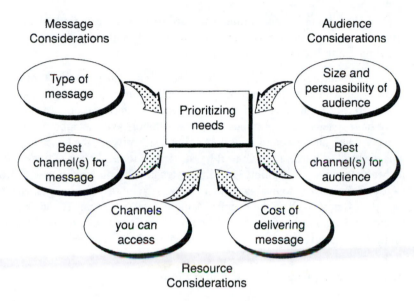

Figure 12–1 Balancing Message, Audience, and Resource Considerations To Select Channels

for "someone like them" or like the people they want to be. The goal is to portray the behavior as something target audience members can see themselves doing and something consistent with their core values. As Sutton and colleagues (1995) noted, "all but the newest behaviors already have an image—a set of expectations and associated feelings among consumers. . . . Developing or changing an action's image involves creating a look and feel for the action that makes it accessible, inviting, distinctive, and compelling" (p. 732).

Image is largely conveyed through how the communication is packaged. The symbols, metaphors, and visuals linked to the behavior or positioning of an issue convey image, as do the types of actors, language, and/or music used. Image taps into what has been termed our *cultural code*, or cultural frame of reference—the associations, expectations, and strategies of interpretation that are shared throughout a culture (Hirschman & Thompson, 1997). As Hirschman and Thompson (1997) noted the following when discussing the role of the cultural code in understanding advertising:

> The cultural code provides a shared understanding of how to read the symbolic meaning embedded in mass media images. From early child-hood, individuals are socialized into a deep knowledge of what mean-ings specific products embody. For example, in U.S. culture, pickup trucks are generally understood to represent rural, blue-collar transpor-

tation, whereas chauffeured limousines are seen as representing urban, affluent transportation. Most consumers within the culture are fluent in reading multiple forms of this code. (p. 45)

Hence, communicators can use a variety of symbols and images as a sort of shorthand and, as Hirschman and Thompson (1997) noted, "can use shared understanding of the code to entice consumers to form certain types of interpretations" (p. 45).

As we have discussed in previous chapters, symbols and metaphors are used extensively when public health issues are framed; identifying the exact symbols and images used to frame a public health issue is key to properly positioning the public health perspective. Exhibit 12–3 illustrates how a framing memo can provide a useful framework to evaluate the metaphors, symbols, and images used to package the offer, as well as the benefits being offered to the target audience by proponents and opponents of a policy, the support used to back up the benefit, and the strength of the core values to which the promised benefit appeals.

Process for Communication Strategy Development

The following steps provide a systematic way of developing the communication strategy and obtaining buy-in from key stakeholders at the same time. Although this process may seem brief, Step 3—conducting additional research—often takes at least 3 to 4 months and sometimes longer, depending on the extent of research conducted. The case studies included in Chapter 11 provide examples of the process in action. Exhibit 12–4 summarizes some potential problems to watch for when developing communication strategies.

1. Develop preliminary answers to the communication strategy questions using the information gathered for the situation analysis. Two worksheets are provided at the end of this chapter to facilitate this process. (See Appendix 12–A.) The first one is designed to help in identifying potential actions; the second one is an aid to working through the costs and benefits associated with each potential action. For public health policy initiatives, the framing memo is a key part of developing a preliminary strategy. Preparing the memo was discussed in Chapter 10; examples are provided in Exhibit 12–3 and Chapter 10.

2. Convene a workshop of experts in the public health issue (often internal and external to the sponsoring organization) and expert communication practitioners. There should be no more than about 10 people total, including internal and external people. During the workshop, work through the strategic questions and determine what additional information is needed to develop answers that work together.

3. Locate additional sources of secondary research and/or conduct primary research. (See Chapter 11 for details.)

Exhibit 12–3 Framing the Affirmative Action Debate

BACKGROUND

Woodruff, Wallack, and Wallis prepared a framing memo to guide the development of more effective strategies for promoting affirmative action programs (Certain Trumpet Program, 1996). They used the Lexis/Nexis database to search nine major newspapers for mentions of "affirmative action," "racial preference," "California Civil Rights Initiative," or "CCRI" in the first three paragraphs of articles. They identified 221 placements that included news articles, editorials, op-ed pieces, and letters to the editor. Each item was coded for its news type, subject matter, and position(s) on affirmative action. From the articles, the authors identified frames in support of and in opposition to affirmative action. They analyzed each frame for its core position, metaphor, symbols, catch phrases, images, and appeal to principle.

The analysis revealed 11 distinct frames on the issue of affirmative action: five pro-affirmative action (Table 12–1) and six anti-affirmative action (Table 12–2).

RESULTS

The analysis revealed that "those seeking to eliminate affirmative action have done an excellent job of using drama to capture and frame the news coverage. They are very adept at personalizing their argument by putting a face on it. A highly qualified young White girl is turned away from a selective public high school; her father leaves a prestigious law practice to seek justice for her. This is the stuff of high news drama" (Certain Trumpet Program, 1996, p. 11). In contrast, "the pro-affirmative action groups have simply not yet captured the necessary drama to put forth their argument. The benefits of affirmative action tend to be framed not in personal but in social terms, which don't have the same impact. The gentle, gradual progress toward a more just society does not pack the dramatic wallop of a single sympathetic individual denied a deserved opportunity because of affirmative action" (p. 11). "Those supporting affirmative action have some difficulty in putting a face on the benefit. While there are some examples of a woman or person of color acknowledging that affirmative action policies opened a door and gave him or her a fair chance, in the world of aggressive American individualism this is not a very interesting argument. When government helps people, the story is less dramatic and compelling than when someone is shut out because of a government policy gone bad" (p. 12).

USE OF SYMBOLS AND IMAGES

Woodruff and colleagues found that both sides of the affirmative action debate effectively used symbols and images of the civil rights movement and appealed to the core values of "fairness, justice, equality, and protecting the American dream. . . ." (p. 12). "However, evocative images of discrimination and civil rights are being used in opposition to affirmative action. These symbols resonate because most Americans support the concept of civil rights; it is a strongly held, shared value. . . . Proponents of

continues

Exhibit 12–3 continued

affirmative action do not effectively highlight the fact that imagery of the civil rights movement is being applied to measures that could un-do the gains of the past" (p. 12).

Woodruff and colleagues also found that proponents of affirmative action failed to invoke the most powerful image of civil justice: Dr. Martin Luther King and his "I have a dream" speech. On the contrary, anti-affirmative action groups adopted Dr. King's message as a call for a color-blind society and as an argument against affirmative action.

Perhaps more problematic, Woodruff and colleagues found that supporters of affirmative action were relying on communitarian rather than individual values, and communitarian values tend to be less salient and influential than individual values:

> Many of the symbols used by the supporters of affirmative action tend to evoke idealistic values that put community above individuals. The call for "open doors" and a "level playing field," the description of affirmative action as "the medicine American must take for the ills of inequality," and the picture of a multicultural "rainbow community" where diverse groups get along: these images all appeal to a concept of the social good that simply may not resonate to the extent that the opposition message does. On the other hand, the image of individual achievers in formerly white field—female firefighters, black doctors—may appeal by putting a face on the successes of affirmative action. (p. 13)

MESSAGE CONSISTENCY AND TYPES OF AREAS

Two other conclusions of the framing memo were quite revealing. First, anti-affirmative action groups delivered a strong and consistent message by relying on a few simple and consistent arguments: 70% of the anti-affirmative action messages used were either *content of one's character* or *reverse discrimination*. In contrast, the pro-affirmative action groups used many different arguments. No single message accounted for more than 10% of all pro-affirmative action arguments used. The authors concluded that "this argumentative overkill by supporters of affirmative action may dissipate the power of these frames" (p. 13).

Second, the anti-affirmative action frames tended to use more emotional appeals, while the pro-affirmative action frames tended to rely more on facts. In other words, the support for the benefit promised by affirmative action groups tended to be scientific documentation, while the anti-affirmative action groups backed up their promised benefit with stronger and more compelling documentation: human emotion.

Based on their findings, Woodruff and colleagues offered six concrete suggestions to affirmative action advocates. They recommended that advocates (1) "simplify their arguments, focusing on one or two frames that are most likely to sway voters"; (2) "create more dramatic stories that put faces on the success of affirmative action efforts"; (3) "counter the 'reverse discrimination' theme by involving

continues

Exhibit 12–3 continued

> white males in message delivery"; (4) "reclaim Dr. Martin Luther King, Jr.'s language and other dramatic symbols of the civil rights movement"; (5) "stress that quotas are already illegal and are not part of current affirmative action programs"; and (6) "emphasize that measures like Prop. 209 are radical approaches that go too far and would eliminate successful, worthwhile programs" (Certain Trumpet Program, 1996, pp. 14, 15)

4. Revise the answers to the strategic questions based on the research.
5. Reconvene the group to review the answers. This is best done interactively and, ideally, in person.
6. Develop *message concepts* based on the communication strategy. A message is the thought or feeling audience members should walk away with after they have been exposed to communications, either through the mass media or directly from materials or events. Messages should stimulate action; for example, an audience member should change his or her mind, vote a different way, or substitute one behavior for another as a result of the message. A message is different from a slogan, a theme line, or a sound bite; each of these is a way of packaging a message to make it accessible to the audience.
7. Test the message concepts with target audience members to explore whether the positioning is in fact relevant, appealing, and motivating to them. A useful format for testing is the following sentence:

I (new action) because (benefit and support).

8. Message concept testing is often conducted using qualitative research techniques, and it provides an opportunity to gather insights into all aspects of the communication strategy. Alternatively, message concepts can be tested through quantitative techniques, such as a public opinion poll. More detail on approaches to message concept testing was provided in Chapter 11. The communication strategy should be revised if needed based on the research results.
9. Prepare a *creative brief*—a one- or two-page summary of the communication strategy that is given to the creative team to use for guidance when developing the program materials. (See Exhibit 12–5 for a sample creative brief from the 5 A Day for Better Health media campaign.)

The creative brief should also be used by anyone else developing program components, to ensure that everything developed reflects the strategy. For example, if the program goal is to increase mammography rates among older women, and components include outreach to women and physician education materials or a continuing medical education module, the individuals developing the physician

Table 12–1 Pro-Affirmative Action Frames

Frame	Core Position	Symbol/Metaphor/ Visual Image	Catch Phrases and Quotes	Source of Problem	Appeal to Principle
Keep the doors open	We must maintain the gains of the civil rights and women's movements to keep opportunities available.	Level playing field Open doors CCRI is a "U-turn toward exclusion" Women in traditionally male jobs Minorities in professional positions Rights are "a valued heirloom women have fought for."	"CCRI would take women back to second-class status. . . . We won't go back." "At PG&E, we don't have preferential treatment and never have. We don't have quotas and never have. But we do have affirmative action, that is affirmatively reaching out and assuring equal opportunity for everyone." "We should mend, not end, affirmative action."	White men trying to slam the door on further progress Fearful White men who are insecure	American Dream—the land of opportunity Maintain/protect civil rights gains
Necessary medicine	Affirmative action is a necessary remedy for historical and continuing discrimination.	Legacy of racism and slavery Symbols of continuing racism: Rodney King beating, power and wealth gulf, glass ceiling	"The reality is that without affirmative action, 230 years of official spoils system based on race, ethnicity and the like will continue." "Prejudice against minorities and White women continues to be the single most important barrier to their advancement." "In order to treat some people equally, we must treat them differently."	Historical racism, sexism, and White male privilege Persistent inequality in housing, education, and jobs	Justice Correcting historical inequities

continues

Table 12–1 continued

Frame	Core Position	Symbol/Metaphor/ Visual Image	Catch Phrases and Quotes	Source of Problem	Appeal to Principle
Political football	Anti-affirmative action forces are playing the politics of divisiveness.	Affirmative action as a wedge issue that divides Democrats Building walls Dirty politics Playing the quota card Political bargaining chip	"Anger has become the emotional gold of American politics."	Cynical, manipulative politicians	Common sense to see through political manipulation
Benefits of diversity	Affirmative action recognizes that the diverse community is of value to all. We must recognize a wider definition of "merit" than mere test scores.	Multicultural society Richness of diverse experience	"Diversity is a 'compelling interest' of educational institutions." All students benefit from a diversity of experiences in the classroom. "The issue is not a person's race-based characteristics; it is experience. And any judge who thinks Black Americans have not had a different experience is blind."	Institutions not ad- equately responding to shift in demographics Fear of difference Failure to understand benefits of diversity	Value of inclusiveness Difference as a strength rather than a weakness
Preference for the privileged	Admissions and hiring processes are already full of preferences for privileged classes.	"Athletics is the largest preferential program in existence." Preferences extended to "musicians and cheer- leaders, athletes of questionable academic potential and dull off- spring of alumni." Back room admissions "Old boys" network	"I needed all the help I could get. . . . I mean, this is America. It's not what you know, it's who you know." "Does it make sense to give consideration to an African- American man to allow him to dribble a basketball but not to become a teacher or doctor?"	Rot at the top Corruption, hypocrisy, influence peddling	Fairness No special privilege for the rich Equality

Source: Adapted with permission from *Framing Memo: The Affirmative Action Debate,* September 1996 Certain Trumpet Program publication, © 1996, The Advocacy Institute.

Table 12-2 Anti-Affirmative Action Frames

Frame	Core Position	Symbol/Metaphor/ Visual Image	Catch Phrases and Quotes	Source of Problem	Appeal to Principle
Content of one's character	People should be judged on their character and merit, not the color of their skin or their gender.	MLK Jr. "I have a dream" speech Color-blind society	Treat people as individuals "It's your ability that counts, not your disability." Reward merit, not skin color/ gender.	Sense of group entitlement Lack of individual initiative	Equality Merit
Reverse discrimination	You can't solve discrimination with more discrimination. Affirmative action lowers standards by admitting the undeserving	Color-blind constitution Qualified White males denied opportunities Level playing field Quotas	"Equal right for all, special privilege for none." "Racial discrimination is not the way to end racial discrimination." Government-sponsored discrimination	Unconstitutional preferences Misguided overcompensation for past wrongs	Fairness
Hurts those it intends to help	Affirmative action is demeaning to minorities and women; people internalize low expectations.	The stigma of being an affirmative action recipient Affirmative action infantilizes/coddles minorities Affirmative action squelches ambition	It's wrong to have "every single minority tarred with the notion that they're less qualified." "Affirmative action is . . . instilling in (minorities) a permanent sense of dependency and inferiority." "You don't want people to think you only go in here because you're Black."	People live up—or down—to society's expectations. Reducing expectations squelches human potential.	Respect for all Equal expectations
No longer needed	Affirmative action is unnecessary because discrimination is no longer a barrier.	Connerly, Thomas, and others who overcame adversity and pulled themselves up by their bootstraps without affirmative action The playing field has been leveled	"Legally sanctioned racism is a thing of the past." "Affirmative action is a strong-arm tactic that has outlived its time." "If I made it, anyone can."	Confusing real racism of the past with isolated slights of today.	Work ethic Honor for the struggles of the past

continues

Table 12-2 continued

Frame	Core Position	Symbol/Metaphor/ Visual Image	Catch Phrases and Quotes	Source of Problem	Appeal to Principle
Divides, doesn't unify	Affirmative action pits groups against each other, and increases racial tension and divisiveness.	Affirmative action leads to the Balkanization of America around racial lines Voluntary resegregation Black against White	"Americans pitted against Americans." Affirmative action "undermines tolerance and mutual respect."	Lack of primary identity as Americans	National unity Patriotism Community cohesiveness
Wrong solution	Focusing on affirmative action diverts us from the real problem	Affirmative action is compared to forced busing as a misguided policy. Racial numbers game	"Affirmative action is an obsession with racial balance as an end in itself." The affirmative action debate is an unfortunate "subterfuge" for a discussion about race, one that "demonizes" African-American men, who have barely benefited from affirmative action programs.	Affirmative action distracts from more effective policies	Courage and commitment to tackle the tough real issues

Source: Adapted with permission from *Framing Memo: The Affirmative Action Debate*, September 1996 Certain Trumpet Program publication, © 1996, The Advocacy Institute.

Exhibit 12–4 Pitfalls To Avoid When Developing Communication Strategies

- Focusing on very small audiences
- Targeting too many or too diverse audiences
- Including multiple actions or framing an issue multiple ways rather than focusing on one
- Focusing on long-term public-health benefits rather than short-term consumer benefits
- Appealing to noncritical values (e.g., good health) rather than core values (freedom, autonomy, control, independence)
- Supporting the message with facts alone when an emotional appeal would be more compelling
- Using mass media to convey complex messages
- Developing strategies for different audiences that conflict or send mixed messages

materials should refer to the creative brief for women and integrate information on the strategies that work best for persuading women to get mammograms into the physician materials. The overall content and approach to the physician materials should be guided by a separate communication strategy to ensure that the materials are meaningful, compelling, and relevant to physicians.

After the communication strategy is finalized, specific message points that provide suggestions for how to take the communication action are often developed. For example, the 5 A Day for Better Health media campaign included many messages telling consumers how they could easily add two servings of fruits and vegetables each day, such as adding a glass of juice at breakfast or microwaving vegetables at dinner. Such message points should be assessed against the strategy and tested when the materials are tested.

Some organizations prepare longer documents that summarize the communication strategy but also provide the rationale for the communication effort and include more detail on target audience research and specific message points. These documents are useful for partner organizations; they provide insights that the partner organizations may not have about communicating with the target audience, and they extend the reach of the sponsoring organization by providing an opportunity for partners to develop materials using the same communication strategy. Good examples of this form of strategy statement are produced by the National Heart, Lung, and Blood Institute (NHLBI) for its public education programs (see, for example, NHLBI, 1994).

Message Content and Construction: Additional Factors To Consider

Constructing health messages is a complex art. The final message a target audience member receives is a combination of the communication strategy, how the

Exhibit 12–5 Creative Brief for the 5 A Day for Better Health Media Campaign

Target audience:
People increasing their fruit and vegetable consumption, but eating less than the minimum of five or more servings each day (particularly people currently eating two to three servings). Audience members tend to be 25- to 55-year-olds who lead busy, hectic lives and are strongly motivated by the need to be in control. They are anxiety ridden about nutrition but do not feel urgency to eat healthier. They think fruits and vegetables taste good and know they should eat more, but think doing so is not easy because preparation takes time and they don't think about it. They lack the knowledge and skills to fit in more servings.

Action:
Add two or more servings of fruits and vegetables a day "the easy way" instead of making it hard.

Benefit:
I will feel more relieved and in control of my life.

Supports:
- Illustrations of how fruits and vegetables can fit into busy lives.
- A great number of studies have shown that a diet rich in fruits and vegetables has a protective effect against cancer.
- Fruits and vegetables taste great.
- People keep hearing the phrase "5 A Day for Better Health."
- This information is coming from the National Cancer Institute, a credible source of health information.

Openings:
- Times when people are preparing shopping lists or shopping, choosing foods at a restaurant or take-out, or are in transition between activities.
- Places such as the dinner table; by the TV; in stores or restaurants; in the car, train, or bus; and in the kitchen.
- Situations when people are hungry, thinking about what to eat, starting to relax, and/or reflecting on their day or planning for tomorrow.

Image:
People who eat five servings of fruit and vegetables each day can be responsible, balanced, and warm.

Source: Data from the National Cancer Institute's "5 A Day for Better Health": NCI Media Campaign Strategy, 1993.

message is executed in the materials, and how it is processed by the sender. This section discusses some of the common types of message appeals used in health communications and provides some insights into how to increase the amount of attention people pay to messages.

Common Types of Appeals

Traditionally, messages have been divided into rational and emotional appeals. Using a rational argument rather than emotion to convey a message is said to be using a *rational appeal*. In contrast, *emotional appeals* are those that attempt to elicit some emotional response—feeling good, laughter, fear, etc.—from the message receiver. As Monahan (1995) noted, more recent "analyses find most messages utilize, or at least are perceived by audiences as utilizing, both rational and affective appeals (Stewart & Furse, 1986)" (p. 83). In fact, most commercial messages probably do contain both types of appeals, because marketers have learned that people make decisions for emotional reasons, but they want rational justifications (the "reason why") for those decisions.

Rational approaches can be further divided into one-sided and two-sided messages. One-sided messages usually present a major benefit, but do not directly address any major drawbacks. Two-sided messages address both drawbacks and benefits. Kotler and Roberto (1989) noted that each type of message is appropriate for different audiences: "Studies have identified that one-sided messages appear to work best with people who are already favorably predisposed to an idea or practice and who have a low level of education but that two-sided messages work best when people are not predisposed to the product and have a higher level of education" (p. 196).

Emotional appeals can be positive or negative. In general, positive appeals are considered to be more effective. Based on interviews with 29 health communication practitioners, Backer and colleagues (1992) concluded that campaigns that emphasize positive behavior change and/or current rewards are more effective than those that emphasize negative consequences of current behavior or avoiding future negative consequences. In commercial advertising, positive emotional appeals are most often used for a simple reason: "Research consistently shows advertisements that arouse positive emotions result in more positive feelings toward the product and greater intent to comply with the message" (Monahan, 1995, pp. 81–82, citing Thorson & Friestad, 1989, as an example).

Positive Emotional Appeals. Monahan (1995) divides positive emotional appeals into two types. *Emotional benefit appeals* combine emotional and rational appeals to portray the benefits the message recipients will reap by complying with the message. Her example is "a campaign that shows healthy people engaging in 'fun' activities with a message that tells the viewer to 'live longer and live healthier by eating more fruits and vegetables'" (p. 83). *Heuristic appeals* try to make recipients feel good about the product through executional detail rather than describing the benefits they could derive from complying with the message. Monahan's example is AT&T's "Reach Out and Touch Someone" campaign.

In general, emotional benefits appeals are more useful than rational appeals are to the public health communicator. Monahan (1995) recommended using such appeals in the form of comparisons, demonstrations, satisfaction, and testimonials when the audience is unfamiliar with an issue, and she noted that emotional benefits appeals are an excellent strategy when the audience is undecided or confused. She also noted that positive appeals can help reframe an issue. She recommended stressing positive rather than negative outcomes and control rather than helplessness as a way to increase compliance.

Monahan (1995) recommended using heuristic appeals when message recipients are familiar with an issue or campaign; however, few public health interventions reach audience members with enough frequency to assume that they attain sufficient familiarity. Finally, Monahan cautioned against using positive appeals in an attempt to change strongly held negative attitudes.

Threat (Fear) Appeals. Public health campaign planners are often tempted to use what are commonly termed "fear appeals" to scare the audience into changing their behavior. There is enormous debate among practitioners and scholars about whether, and under what circumstances, this type of negative appeal is effective. As Donovan and Henley (1997) noted,

> several reviews of the fear literature have reached a consensus that fear appeals can be effective for achieving attitude and behavior change and that more fear is more effective than less fear—except perhaps for low esteem targets, and provided the recommended behavior is efficacious and under volitional control (Sutton, 1982, 1992; Boster & Mongeau, 1984; Job, 1988). Nevertheless, because of conflicting findings, social marketers and health promotion practitioners still disagree on their efficacy. (p. 56)

For example, in their summary of interviews with practitioners, Backer and colleagues (1992) concluded that "arousing fear is rarely successful as a campaign strategy" (p. 30).

A number of researchers have suggested that part of the reason for the apparently conflicting evidence about effectiveness is in the definition of a fear appeal, and that these types of appeals might better be called "threat appeals" (Donovan & Henley, 1997; Hale & Dillard, 1995; LaTour & Rotfeld, 1997; Strong, Anderson, & Dubas, 1993; Witte, 1993). LaTour and Rotfeld (1997) discussed the distinction between threats and fear: "Threats illustrate undesirable consequences from certain behaviors, such as car damage, injury, or death from unsafe driving, or bad breath, illness, or cancer from cigarette smoking. However, fear is an emotional response to threats, and different people fear different things" (p. 45).

They further explained: "A threat is an appeal *to* fear, a communication stimulus that *attempts* to evoke a fear response by showing some type of outcome that the audience (it is hoped) wants to avoid. Fear is an actual emotional response that can impel changes in attitude or behavior intentions (e.g., toward auto safety issues or toward the energy crisis) and consumer actions (e.g., cessation of cigarette smoking or more careful driving habits)" (LaTour & Rotfeld, 1997, p. 46, emphasis in original). They noted that some threat appeals (i.e., appeals intended to arouse fear) may in fact arouse other emotions in some audience members.

Decisions to use a threat appeal should be considered carefully, and the appeal should be tested thoroughly before implementation. Hale and Dillard (1995) provided some suggestions about constructing an effective threat appeal. They said that an effective threat appeal includes

- a severe threat of physical or social harm,
- evidence that the target audience member is personally vulnerable to the threat, and
- solutions that are both easy to perform (i.e., high in personal efficacy; the target audience member thinks he or she has the ability to follow the message recommendation) and effective (i.e., high in response efficacy, or the ability of the message recommendation to eliminate the threat depicted in the message).

They also noted that fear appeals are more effective with older people (and generally are not effective with young people), when exposure to the message is voluntary (such as reading a print ad rather than compulsory attendance at a drug prevention program), and with "copers" (people who do not have trait anxiety, i.e., are not "anxious by nature").

Those interested in using threat appeals may wish to review Hale and Dillard's (1995) chapter on the subject, as well as two meta-analyses that are widely cited: Sutton (1982) and Boster and Mongeau (1984).

Humorous Appeals. Humor is another popular emotional approach that must be used carefully. If used, humor should convey the main message, otherwise people are likely to remember the humor and forget the message (Roman & Maas, 1992; the case study in Chapter 16 [see Exhibit 16–2] will also provide an example of what can happen). The advertising literature is littered with examples of very funny, entertaining ads that didn't sell products. And according to Kotler and Roberto (1989), "humorous messages are more effective when the prevailing communications in the field are not humorous. Second, humor becomes stale if it is repeated too frequently, so it needs to be varied if it is not to become irritating. Third, humor works well as long as the basic message is simple; it is inappropriate for complex messages" (pp. 198–199).

Breaking through Inattention

Parrott (1995) lays out a number of content and linguistic factors that can increase the attention people give to health messages, based on Louis and Sutton's (1991) model of "switching cognitive gears." The following recommendations are based on Parrott's analysis:

- Use novel messages, settings, and media. Rather than a skin cancer brochure that begins with a standard factual approach, such as, "Know the signs of cancer," try a positive emotional appeal, such as, "Safeguard your health by knowing the signs of skin cancer." Or try explicitly stating a motive to pay attention: "You can avoid a serious health problem by knowing the following signs of skin cancer so you can detect any unusual skin conditions." Another possibility is to invoke a sense of personal responsibility: "You can help friends and family detect skin cancer early by knowing the following signs." (Examples are modifications of Parrott's.)
- Present unexpected content or present it in an unexpected place. New recommendations, particularly if they run contrary to past recommendations, are one form of unexpected content. Parrott's example is the recommendation to stay out of the sun, when for years sunlight was promoted as health enhancing. An unexpected place can be anywhere people do not expect to receive health messages.
- Instruct the audience to pay more attention by using phrases such as "now hear this," or, less directly, "Is everyone listening for information about . . . ?"
- Use language that conveys immediacy and personal relevance:
  - Use "your" rather than third person or passive constructions.
  - Use *this, these,* and *here* rather than their more spatially distant counterparts *that, those,* and *there.*
  - Use active present-tense verbs.
  - Avoid qualifiers (e.g., perhaps, may, maybe, possibly, it could be, it might be).

CONCLUSION

Crafting a solid communication strategy is critical to properly framing messages and positioning a social change. The strategy describes the target audience, the action they should take and how they will benefit from it, and the details of how to reach them with messages—the times, places, and situations in which they are receptive and the image to use so that they identify the message as being for them. The strategy should be based on a theory or model of how change is expected to occur.

Developing a solid communication strategy is an iterative process involving extensive formative research. Two of the most difficult decisions involve selecting the action that audience members should take as a result of the communication and determining the benefit to promise them for doing so. Knowing what makes the audience "tick" is crucial to crafting persuasive messages. What does the audience value? How can the social change be positioned as providing that value? Asking and answering a series of strategic questions can help create a communication strategy that is focused, believable, and compelling to the target audience.

Understanding what types of appeals work best in a given situation is also an important part of successful communication strategy development. Positive emotional benefits appeals—those that cause the consumer to connect taking the action with feeling good—have the widest applicability to public health interventions: They can be used when an audience is unfamiliar with or undecided or confused about an issue and can be an excellent strategy for reframing a social change—unless existing attitudes are extremely negative. Humor can be part of an appeal, but it must be used to deliver the main message or recall will suffer. In general, threat appeals appear to work best with older audiences and when exposure to the message will be voluntary rather than compulsory.

Once a communication strategy has been developed, using language that conveys immediacy and personal relevance can help increase the amount of attention paid to the message. Presenting a novel message in unusual or unexpected settings also is effective.

REFERENCES

Backer, T.E., Rogers, E.M., & Sopory, P. (1992). *Designing health communication campaigns: What works?* Thousand Oaks, CA: Sage.

Bellicha, T., & McGrath, J. (1990). Mass media approaches to reducing cardiovascular disease risk. *Public Health Reports, 105,* 245–252.

Boster, F.J., & Mongeau, P. (1984). Fear-arousing persuasive messages. In Bostrom (Ed.), *Communication Yearbook 8* (pp. 330–375). Beverly Hills, CA: Sage.

Certain Trumpet Program. (1996, September). *Framing memo: The affirmative action debate.* Washington, DC: Author.

Donovan, R.J., & Henley, N. (1997). Negative outcomes, threats and threat appeals: widening the conceptual framework for the study of fear and other emotions in social marketing communications. *Social Marketing Quarterly, 4,* 56–67.

Graeff, J.A., Elder, J.P., & Booth, E.M. (1993). *Communication for health and behavior change: A developing country perspective.* San Francisco: Jossey-Bass.

Hale, J.L., & Dillard, J.P. (1995). Fear appeals in health promotion campaigns: too much, too little, or just right? In E. Maibach & R.L. Parrott (Eds.), *Designing health messages: Approaches from communication theory and public health practice* (pp. 65–80). Thousand Oaks, CA: Sage.

Hirschman, E.C., & Thompson, C.J. (1997). Why media matter: Toward a richer understanding of consumers' relationships with advertising and mass media. *Journal of Advertising, 26*(1), 43–60.

Job, R.F.S. (1988). Effective and ineffective use of fear in health promotion campaigns. *American Journal of Public Health, 78,* 163–167.

Kotler, P., & Roberto, E.L. (1989). *Social marketing: Strategies for changing public behavior.* New York: Free Press.

La Tour, M.S., & Rotfeld, H.J. (1997). There are threats and (maybe) fear-caused arousal: Theory and confusions of appeals to fear and fear arousal itself. *Journal of Advertising, 26*(3), 45–58.

Lefebvre, R.C., Doner, L.D., Johnston, C., Loughrey, K., Balch, G., & Sutton, S.M. (1995). Use of database marketing and consumer-based health communications in message design: An example from the Office of Cancer Communications' "5 A Day for Better Health" program. In E. Maibach & R.L. Parrott (Eds.), *Designing health messages: Approaches from communication theory and public health practice* (pp. 217–246). Thousand Oaks, CA: Sage.

Louis, M.R., & Sutton, R.I. (1991). Switching cognitive gears: From habits of mind to active thinking. *Human Relations, 44,* 55–76.

Maibach, E.W., & Cotton, D. (1995). Moving people to behavior change: A staged social cognitive approach to message design. In E. Maibach & R.L. Parrott (Eds.), *Designing health messages: Approaches from communication theory and public health practice* (pp. 41–64). Thousand Oaks, CA: Sage.

Monahan, J.L. (1995). Using positive affect when designing health messages. In E. Maibach & R.L. Parrott (Eds.), *Designing health messages: Approaches from communication theory and public health practice* (pp. 81–98). Thousand Oaks, CA: Sage.

National Cancer Institute. (1989). *Making health communication programs work: A planner's guide* (NIH Pub. No. 89-1493). Bethesda, MD: Author.

National Heart, Lung, and Blood Institute. (1994). *A communications strategy for public education: The National Cholesterol Education Program* (NIH Pub. No. 94-3292). Bethesda, MD: Author.

Parrott, R.L. (1995). Motivations to attend to health messages: Presentation of content and linguistic considerations. In E. Maibach & R.L. Parrott (Eds.), *Designing health messages: Approaches from communication theory and public health practice* (pp. 7–23). Thousand Oaks, CA: Sage.

Roman, K., & Maas, J.M. (1992). *How to advertise* (2nd ed.). New York: St. Martin's Press.

Signorielli, N. (1993). *Mass media images and impact on health: A sourcebook.* Westport, CT: Greenwood Press.

Stewart, D.W., & Furse, D.H. (1986). *Effective television advertising: A study of 1,000 commercials.* Lexington, MA: Lexington Books.

Strong, J.T., Anderson, R.E., & Dubas, K.M. (1993). Marketing threat appeals: A conceptual framework and implications for practitioners. *Journal of Managerial Issues, 5,* 532–546.

Sutton, S.R. (1982). Fear-arousing communications: A critical examination of theory and research. In J.R. Eiser (Ed.), *Social psychology and behavioral medicine* (pp. 303–337). New York: John Wiley.

Sutton, S.R. (1992). Shock tactics and the myth of the inverted U. *British Journal of Addiction, 87,* 517–519.

Sutton, S.M., Balch, G.I., & Lefebvre, R.C. (1995). Strategic questions for consumer-based health communications. *Public Health Reports, 110,* 725–733.

Thorson, E., & Friestad, M. (1989). The effects of emotion on episodic memory for television commercials. In P. Cafferata & A. Tybout (Eds.), *Cognitive and affective responses in advertising* (pp. 305–326). Lexington, MA: Lexington Books.

Witte, K. (1993). Message and conceptual confounds in fear appeals: The role of threat, fear and efficacy. *Southern Communication Journal, 58,* 147–155.

Communication Strategy Development Worksheets

COMMUNICATION STRATEGY DEVELOPMENT

Worksheet 1: Identifying Potential Actions

A clear, specific statement of what the target audience is to do will help much more than a vague reference to a favorable result. Please identify the behavior being replaced by listing the current action and desired action in terms of pointed, specific behavior changes.

Audience	Current Actions	Desired Actions

Source: Copyright © 1998, Lynne Doner.

Worksheet 2: Identifying and Assessing Costs and Benefits Associated with Potential Actions

For each audience-action combination, list the likely costs to the audience of taking the action (include financial, psychological, organizational, social, time, and other costs). Then list the potential benefits they might associate with the action. (Remember that the benefits should be important to the target audience.) Circle the one you think is most important. Finally, assess whether you think the target audience will think the benefit is worth the cost.

Audience and Action	Costs	Benefits	Is Benefit Worth Cost?

Development, Testing, and Implementation

Once a strategic plan has been developed, the components that will comprise the intervention are planned, developed, tested, and implemented. This section of the book discusses that process, which begins with translating the strategic plan into solid tactics and a carefully timed implementation based on the types of social changes that need to be made and the environment in which they will be made. As components are developed, process evaluation mechanisms (such as those discussed in Chapter 17) should be integrated into them.

Since efforts to effect social change usually involve a number of organizations and some form of mass communication, we have included discussions of the many roles other organizations can play and some issues to consider when developing tactics for emerging and traditional mass media.

Chapter 16 will present the methodologies most often used to pretest materials that support social change initiatives and discuss how to plan, conduct, and analyze each type of study. Pretesting tactics prior to implementing them is one of the more important marketing principles to integrate into public health practice.

CHAPTER 13

Translating Strategy into Tactics

The cornerstones of successful implementation are strategically driven tactics, careful timing, and constant monitoring and refinement. The strategic plan must be turned into a concrete plan of action that takes into account the environment in which the activities will be implemented, the available resources, and the complementary activities of other organizations. In addition to readying all products, materials, and services, preparation for implementation includes establishing tracking measures (to be discussed in detail in Chapter 17) and ensuring that all partners, intermediaries, and spokespersons are briefed on the endeavor, so that everyone is "on strategy" when they are delivering messages about the program, whether they are addressing internal or external audiences.

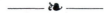

Once the strategic plan (discussed in Chapter 10) has been completed and approved, each component in it must be translated into specific tactics. For example, the strategic plan for an effort to curtail public exposure to secondhand smoke might include outreach to local business owners and briefings of legislators, supported by a mass media component targeting the public and policy makers. The next steps are to (1) decide exactly what activities will constitute "outreach to local business owners," "briefings of legislators," and "a mass media component"; (2) determine what materials or products will be needed to support these activities; and (3) craft a timeline for developing, testing, and implementing these activities. This chapter discusses the steps to take and decisions to make as concrete tactics are selected, developed, and implemented based on the strategic plan.

WHAT IS THE INITIATIVE SUPPOSED TO ACCOMPLISH?

The first step in planning tactics is to revisit the strategic plan and the assumptions underlying it. How is change expected to occur, and what role is envisioned for the initiative in facilitating change? For example, consider the Centers for Disease Control and Prevention's (CDC's) initiative to support implementation of its tobacco control, healthy eating, and physical activity guidelines for school health programs. Each guideline addresses at least six areas: policy, curriculum/instruction, family/community involvement, linkages to other programs, training, and evaluation. The strategic plan (Academy for Educational Development, 1996) was crafted using the diffusion of innovations framework. It assumes that change will occur relatively slowly (because the innovation is complex, involving many changes made by many individuals or groups within a school or school district—some of whom are not adequately trained to implement the changes), that it will be difficult to communicate what changes to make (in part because of the complexity), and that the issue won't be a priority in many school systems.

The planners assumed that the initiative would "work" by supporting each phase of the diffusion process. Accordingly, the strategic plan outlines a three-step approach:

1. Phase 1 involves disseminating the guidelines to professional audiences through journal articles and appearances at appropriate conferences (e.g., school health, physical activity, education, nutrition, and public health) to build awareness of them.
2. Phase 2 continues dissemination efforts (but focuses on a wider range of target audiences: administrators and other policy makers, teachers, parents, community groups, students, and coaches) and supports decisions to adopt the guidelines by providing specific action steps for implementing them.
3. Phase 3 involves supporting the implementation of specific guidelines recommendations by (a) developing and disseminating technical assistance materials and services, (b) training state and local education staff and/or partners to use the materials and services, (c) conducting mass communication and marketing activities to support efforts to implement specific recommendations, and (d) periodically reviewing the literature and field practice to keep the recommendations current.

The expectations of how change will occur and how the initiative will support change have ramifications for the types of tactics likely to be effective and the timing of implementation (e.g., a short-term flurry of activity to support introduction of a new product or service or apply pressure to stimulate policy change, versus a long-term, multi-year effort to promote and reinforce more difficult behavior changes).

ASSESSING RESOURCE AND ORGANIZATIONAL ISSUES

The second step in planning tactics is to identify the resources available to support the initiative and the position that it will occupy within the organization. Green and Kreuter (1991) refer to aspects of this process as administrative and policy diagnosis in the PRECEDE-PROCEED framework. Exactly what transpires at this point depends in part on what has gone before. In general, managers must first assess the resources they will need in terms of time, personnel, and budget and compare that assessment to an assessment of the resources they have available. For more detail, Green and Kreuter (1991) elaborated on some of the steps involved in this process.

Often, one or more of the available resources cannot be adjusted. For example, an initiative may need to accomplish something by a particular date, may not be able to add staff, or may have a fixed budget within which to work. When one of these situations exists, the assessment of resources needed should be adjusted. That is, if something must be accomplished by a particular date, it may require increased staff or budget. If staff cannot be added, budget will have to increase (to contract out some of the work) or the time allotted will have to increase. If the budget cannot be increased, the time frame may stretch out or staff may need to be added. A common solution to a resource deficit (which almost every initiative has) is to identify partners who can handle part of the work.

Consequently, a key part of this step is determining appropriate roles for partners to play. Some roles may be incorporated into the strategic plan; this is a time to flesh out those roles and, if needed, explore the extent to which they are feasible. In addition to determining what roles it makes sense for partners to play from a resource perspective, this is also the time to determine what roles they might be better suited to play because of restrictions on an organization's activities (e.g., an inability to lobby or to produce particular kinds of materials) or internal political issues (for example, there is a mandate to use a particular department for a particular activity, but the people involved do not consider the initiative important or are not as skilled as partner organizations). Chapter 14 will discuss assessing appropriate partner roles.

PLANNING CHANGES IN PRODUCTS AND SERVICES

The products and services that could be developed as part of a social change initiative are diverse, making it difficult to present a meaningful discussion of the issues to consider when the development of a new product or service—or changes to an existing one—is being planned. However, some issues are common to all products and services in terms of their development, distribution, and pricing.

Product Development

Additional formative research is often key to success. Depending on the nature and depth of the information collected during the strategic planning process, this research may begin with a targeted needs assessment among potential users of the new product or service. Using that information, a concept of the product or service can be developed and presented to potential users for their feedback, then refined before production. The needs assessment also provides an opportunity to get a sense of the demand for new or updated products and services, allowing managers to predict resource requirements.

Managing Distribution

All products and services must be distributed in some way to the individuals who will use them. This distribution process can be direct from the provider to the consumer or it can involve some number of intermediaries. When determining how to distribute a product or service, a manager must assess who can best do the job. Factors that feed into this assessment include the type of distribution outlets each possibility provides (clients may prefer or trust one type over another) and the number and locations of outlets.

Training is often an integral component of managing the delivery of messages or services when using interpersonal distribution channels. Initiatives that use interpersonal channels such as physicians, nurses, community groups, or teachers may need to train individuals before distribution can take place successfully. In general, such training is designed to ensure that the people being trained

- understand how to best frame the issues in terms of the benefits to target audience members.
- have the skills required to successfully distribute messages or services. For example, the U.S. Department of Agriculture's Team Nutrition initiative included training of food service personnel so that they could prepare healthier meals and learn ways to support improving students' nutritional knowledge and behavior by linking the cafeteria to the classroom (i.e., by providing students with an opportunity to practice what they learn in the classroom) and to the home (i.e., by including nutritional analyses of school menus). As another example, health care providers may not bring up sensitive topics with patients because they are uncomfortable addressing them. Training can alleviate many of these problems.

Training can take many forms. Sometimes written instruction, for example, in the form of a case study or article that highlights the key points, is sufficient. At other times hands-on practice or role-playing is the best approach.

Pricing

Kotler and Roberto (1989) noted that the financial price of a product or service serves a number of functions. First, the price affects how easy it is for a consumer to obtain the product or service. Low prices make it easy for many people to obtain a product; high prices can be used to "demarket" a product. An example of this is taxes on alcohol and cigarettes designed to increase the cost and therefore decrease demand.

The second function of price is to send a message about a product's quality. As Kotler and Roberto (1989) discussed, "when target adopters have difficulty judging the quality of a social product, they often use price as a standard. A high price may lead target adopters to view the product as having high quality or prestige. . . . Many 'free goods,' such as public health services or legal assistance, do not produce maximum demand because they imply that the product is 'downscale'" (p. 175). The authors provided an example of a new South American hospital that did not charge indigent citizens. Many of the citizens continued to patronize private physicians and street clinics, even though they had to pay for these services. When the hospital started charging a fee, many patients began to use its services.

Setting financial prices involves weighing the provider's cost associated with the product, competitors' prices, and potential consumers' sensitivity to the price (manifest by ability and willingness to purchase at a given price). Kotler and Roberto (1989) noted that if costs are to be recovered, costs serve as a "floor" on price, whereas competitors' prices serve as a ceiling.

In addition to the financial price, managers should try to minimize the time, effort, and psychic costs associated with obtaining a product or service. The most obvious way to do this in terms of distribution is to ensure that the product is nearby and attainable from a source the client is comfortable with. Promotional strategies can also be used to moderate psychic costs. Kotler and Roberto (1989, citing Gemunden, 1985) provide the following examples:

- Minimize perceived *psychological risk* by providing the product in a way that delivers psychological rewards.
- Minimize perceived *social risk,* such as stigma or embarrassment associated with usage, through endorsements of credible sources.
- Minimize perceived *risk of usage* by providing reassuring information on the product or a free trial so consumers can experience how the product does what it promises.
- Minimize perceptions of *physical risk* by obtaining seals of approval from authoritative institutions.

PLANNING PROMOTIONAL ACTIVITIES

Just about every social change campaign includes some form of promotional activities. One of the challenges of structuring an initiative is determining what form those activities should take. Most initiatives include some form of mass media; the following sections discuss the use of it in greater detail.

The Role of the Mass Media

Why are the mass media so important to social change efforts? Because the way they portray the world outside influences the pictures in our heads, to paraphrase Walter Lippmann's famous chapter title (Lippmann, 1922). What we see in newspapers, magazines, television, and the Internet—and hear on the radio—can influence us in two ways: First, it can tell us *what* to think about. Second, it can tell us *how* to think about it.

Much of what we know about the media's influence on *what* we think about comes from communication researchers' studies of the way in which the media set the public agenda. Agenda-setting research began in earnest with McCombs and Shaw's (1972) landmark study of the media's role in the 1968 presidential election. They calculated the media agenda by analyzing the content of the main mass media reporting on the election and measured the public agenda by surveying 100 undecided voters. They found an almost perfect correlation in the rankings of issues on the media agenda and the public agenda.

The mass media can influence *how* we think about issues by the way in which they frame their coverage. As Chapter 6 discussed in more detail, the attributes of an issue that are emphasized in media coverage can have a demonstrable impact on public opinion and behavior. McCombs and Shaw (1993) have noted that "even when multiple attributes of an issue are included on the news agenda, there is likely to be a perceptible set of priorities" (p. 63). The authors noted that many studies have demonstrated that this set of priorities is communicated to the public and reflected in what they deem to be important.

How are health issues and health behaviors portrayed by the media? Wallack and colleagues (Wallack & Dorfman, 1996; Wallack, Dorfman, Jernigan, & Themba, 1993) argue that the media tend to frame health issues in terms of individual health behaviors. Part of the job of social change initiatives is to work to reframe these issues in terms of public policy. However, as Signorielli (1993) wrote in the conclusion of a book discussing mass media images and their impact on health, the way in which media frame health behaviors is problematic as well:

> Much of the research indicates that many if not most of the images in the media are in serious conflict with realistic guidelines for health, nutrition, and medicine. Research on the contributions of these portrayals to

people's conceptions about health and medicine, although scarce, nevertheless indicates that those who spend more time with the media may have beliefs about health-related issues that are in conflict with the things they should do to remain healthy and/or improve the current status of their health. (p. 153)

Some of Signorielli's (1993) observations include the following:

- Characters in prime-time programming are healthy, relatively safe from accidents, hardly ever need glasses (even in old age), and rarely suffer any form of functional impairment.
- Televised characters rarely take precautions to protect themselves, such as wearing seat belts or using condoms. Nor do they act like good environmental citizens: They rarely recycle or use car pools or public transportation.
- Food, nutrition, and weight messages on television are very unhealthy; the diet portrayed is the opposite of dietary recommendations, but hardly anyone on television is even slightly overweight. Some researchers suspect that bulimia and other eating disorders are an adaptation to the conflicting messages. Food is presented as satisfying emotional or social purposes rather than hunger. Snacking (usually on a sweet) is shown as often as sitting down to a meal.
- Smoking and illegal drug use on television are relatively rare (though smokers abound in print advertisements and are usually portrayed as vibrant, healthy, and beautiful), but drinking is common. Characters drink in response to personal crises or tension and to enhance social interactions, but consequences of drinking too much are rarely presented adequately.
- When illness appears on television it takes center stage, is presented as acute, and is readily cured (except on some daytime serial dramas) with no consideration of the costs involved.
- Mentally ill characters are stigmatized, sinister, often violent, and unable to cope successfully with life.
- "Areas in which the media could provide a real service (e.g., providing full details about the dangers of smoking) often are not addressed because of economic and institutional considerations. It is more important to keep advertisers happy than to provide enough accurate information about health" (Signorielli, 1993, p. 153).

Throughout this book, we have noted that people are most strongly motivated by freedom, independence, autonomy, and control. Part of the reason the public—and policy makers—tend to be complacent about health issues is likely that the media, when they portray health problems at all, do not portray them as threatening any of these values. Sick or injured people either die or have virtually instantaneous recoveries (except, as Signorielli [1993] noted, on some daytime serial dramas, where they may linger in a hospital for months). Have a heart attack and wind up in cardiac arrest? Heroic physicians will fix you and you will walk out the door the next day. Have a cold or any other ailment that can be treated with over-the-counter medication? According to the advertisements, taking a pill will make you instantly better (Signorielli, 1993).

It is difficult to measure exactly how much the media influence people's perceptions of a given issue; other variables undoubtedly come into play. For example, there is some evidence that the media influence perceptions more when other alternative sources of information are not available (e.g., a 1975 study by Tipton, Haney, and Baseheart found that agenda setting is less likely to occur in local than in national campaigns; in 1977, Palmgreen and Clarke reported that less agenda setting occurs when members of the public interact on local issues).

Nonetheless, the combination of the inaccurate way in which media (particularly television) portray health behaviors and issues coupled with the media's ability to set the public's agenda by what is or is not covered (and how it is covered) means that planners of social change initiatives are wise to consider the role of mass media in their efforts.

Assessing Mass Media Options

Campaigns that are more effective use multiple media to deliver a single focused message multiple times (Backer, Rogers, & Sopory, 1992; Hornik, 1997). Many early social change campaigns relied primarily on advertisements run by the media as a public service, but using that approach today is unlikely to be effective. Today's successful social change initiatives typically use a sophisticated combination of editorial coverage and advertising, often paying for placement of the latter. Some also include an entertainment education approach. The following sections outline some elements to consider when developing the mix of media activities for a particular initiative.

News Coverage versus Advertising

Many mass communication specialists believe that messages embedded in a medium's editorial content (e.g., in a news story) are perceived by target audience members as more credible than advertising. The major drawback of editorial coverage is the loss of control over message content. A few stations and publications will run a news release or suggested story exactly as written, but reporters often alter the material as they see fit. Key messages can easily become distorted or lost in this process. If editorial coverage is compared with paid advertising placement, lost control over reach and frequency is another drawback.

Compared with editorial placement efforts, advertising allows total control over message content and can include very effective emotional appeals (types of appeals were discussed in Chapter 12). However, the brief and fleeting nature of many advertisements (for example, 30-second TV and radio spots) makes them best suited for reminders or simple messages that require little context or explanation. Only print and some transit advertising provide the space to develop ideas in greater detail.

If placement is paid, advertising provides an efficient means of reaching target audience members at appropriate times, and reaching them as frequently as is desired—or affordable. The cost of placing advertising varies enormously by medium (television is most expensive; radio and newspapers are least expensive). Within a medium, cost again varies widely depending on such factors as how many people are reached by a particular program, station, or publication and who is reached (some target audiences are more desirable and thus advertisers are willing to pay more to reach them). Managers who are considering the use of advertising but are unfamiliar with placement costs might want to invite a media planner from a local advertising agency to speak on the subject. Cost information can also be obtained by requesting rate cards from stations or publications (however, the price of television and radio time, in particular, is volatile and subject to negotiation). A creative media plan can stretch a limited budget and, particularly for a local initiative, may make much more sense than relying on donated placement.

Though donated placement is problematic, many public health interventions rely on it. Although most of the major advertising media run some amount of advertising as a public service, there is tremendous competition among issues and causes for a small amount of public service space. Print media run very few public service announcements (PSAs); magazines run them if they have a "hole" of unsold advertising space and many newspapers don't run them at all. Television stations tend to run PSAs late at night or early in the morning when there are few viewers (and low demand for advertising space). The proliferation of cable and the birth of additional networks have made the monolithic TV audiences of the past all but disappear, further lowering the number of viewers.

Proponents of media advocacy encourage paying for advertising placement (as commercial advertisers do), because doing so provides an opportunity to control reach and frequency as well as content. Many public health program budgets cannot afford advertising placement costs, but there are alternatives to explore, such as media or corporate partners. By cultivating a media partner, an organization can negotiate specific placement in exchange for the partner's exclusive right to sponsor the media component—and garner broader coverage because the media outlet will involve itself in other ways, such as sponsoring contests. Corporate partners can donate some of the advertising space they buy. Because they buy specific spaces (particular television shows, particular times of day on radio, and particular locations within print media), a willing corporate partner can provide a way to execute a particular media placement schedule.

Aside from the increased credibility versus control over content and placement debate, each medium has various characteristics that warrant consideration as plans are developed. Table 13–1 describes some of the major characteristics of mass media channels and the Internet.

Other Sources of Publicity

The following nontraditional "mass" media are often overlooked by program managers but can reach some target audience members through unexpected channels:

- Employer newsletters: Most large employers publish periodic newsletters, and many include a health or wellness column. The newsletter editors often hunt for information to include and might be quite receptive to prewritten articles on topics or upcoming events relevant to their employees.
- Bulletins and newsletters produced by churches, community groups, and civic and homeowners' associations: While unlikely to include a health/ wellness column, they might include mention of an upcoming event in which members could participate (for example, an immunization or screening drive).
- School system newsletters: Many schools send newsletters home to parents periodically and might include upcoming public health activities that would benefit parents (and especially children).

THE DEVELOPMENT AND IMPLEMENTATION PROCESS

The following sections outline a systematic process for selecting and developing the specific tactics to implement the program. Please note that some of the activities described in the next three chapters often take place during this process.

Develop Concepts for Each Program Component

There are usually a million ways to design a program component. For example, in a training module what topics will be covered? In what order? What materials will be used with the module? Do the materials exist or will they need to be created? How many sessions will there be? How long will each session last? Where will sessions take place? Who will conduct the training? Is a train-the-trainer module also required? How long will it take to develop the curriculum and all materials required? How long will it take to train the trainers? When does it make sense to conduct the training?

Table 13–1 Characteristics of Mass Media Channels and the Internet

	Television	Radio	Magazines	Newspapers	Out-of-Home	Internet
Reach	Potentially largest, but audiences are increasingly fragmented.	Various formats offer potential for audience targeting (e.g., teenagers via rock stations).	Can target specific audience segments; audiences are increasingly fragmented.	Can reach broad audiences rapidly. Daily readership in decline. (Sunday readership growing.)	Can target specific neighborhoods; can achieve high frequency with one placement.	Used by approximately 1 in 5 adults; users are predominantly middle to high SES.
Openings for messages (other than ads)	News and talk shows; entertainment programming	News and talk shows; disk jockey chatter	Feature stories; regular columns; letters to editor	News stories; feature stories; regular columns; letters to editor	—	Web sites; list servers; chat rooms
Use of public service announcements (PSAs)	Deregulation ended government oversight of PSA use and public affairs content; weak requirements for "educational" content on broadcast stations.	Deregulation ended government oversight of PSA use and public affairs content.	No requirements for public service/public affairs use; PSAs more difficult to place than on TV or radio.	No requirements for use; few larger papers use PSAs.	No requirements for use; limited PSA space available.	No requirements for use; PSA space available on some sites.
Appropriate messages	Primarily short and simple; viewers usually can't refer back to message.	Primarily short and simple; listeners can't refer back to message.	Can be short and simple or can provide more detail on complex health issues and behaviors.	Can be short and simple or can provide more detail on complex health issues and behaviors.	Outdoor: very short, simple. Inside trains and buses: can provide more detail.	Ads must be short and simple, but can include link to Web site for detailed information.

continues

Table 13–1 continued

	Television	Radio	Magazines	Newspapers	Out-of-Home	Internet
Characteristics of medium	Visual and audio make emotional appeals powerful. Easier to demonstrate a behavior.	Opportunity for direct audience involvement via call-in shows.	Audience can clip, and reread, and contemplate material and share it with others.	Can convey health news/breakthroughs more thoroughly than TV or radio and faster than magazines.	Frequent viewership; retain control of message content.	Permits instantaneous updating; can retain control of message content.
Type of audience interaction	Mostly passive; active possible with call-in shows. Requires attention when aired.	Generally passive; active interaction possible with call-in shows. Requires attention when aired.	Permits active consultation. May pass on. Read at reader's convenience.	Same as magazines, but short life limits rereading and sharing with others.	Passive; attention may be fragmented or complete.	Permits active interaction; audience can easily search out additional information.
Production costs	Ads and video news releases are expensive.	Live copy: very inexpensive. Produced spots: much cheaper than TV.	Ads are inexpensive.	Ads are inexpensive.	Costs are higher than with print.	Depends on site design; distribution is inexpensive.
Editorial placement issues	Requires contacts and may be time-consuming.	Feature placement requires contacts and may be time-consuming.	Long lead time; relatively little control of timing (often determined by editorial calendar).	Newsworthiness is needed for "news" coverage; little control over timing of feature.	—	Few; emphasis is on getting site added as hyperlink on other relevant sites.

Source: Some information adapted from *Making Health Communication Programs Work*, National Cancer Institute, 1989.

Planners of a mass media component would have an equally extensive list of issues to consider: Will there be an official program launch? If so, when? What form will it take—press materials only, press conference, special event? Satellite media tour? Will mass media efforts focus on editorial placement or also include paid or public service advertising? What news hooks might help get coverage of the issue? Will professional media be targeted as well? What spokespeople are available? What products will be developed for editorial coverage: audio, video, or print news releases, columns, story ideas, camera-ready articles, community events? If advertising is being developed, will it be for print, radio, television, outdoor, or transit? How many ads per year will run?

Planners of each prospective component will have to work thorough questions like these, using the answers to fashion a component that makes sense given the program objectives, target audience(s), communication strategy, budget, and implementation time period.

Assess How Components Will Fit Together and Reinforce Each Other

Once planners have developed concepts for each component, they should meet and look at the component in the context of others. How do they fit together? What time sequencing makes sense? What refinements can be made to each so that they work together better? This is a critical step: Components targeted to the same audiences must complement and reinforce each other—what they say and when and where they say it should work together with a goal of reaching audience members in as many places and at as many times as possible within the parameters of the budget.

For components targeting different audiences, a particular sequence may be necessary or may make more sense. For example, in a program to increase children's consumption of grains, fruits, and vegetables, a logical sequencing is to train food service personnel first, so that they know how to prepare appropriate foods and have ideas for cafeteria promotions to increase consumption of these foods. Next, the classroom and mass media components could take place. The food service changes would be in place so that children could act on what they learned at school and through the media. The example of CDC's guidelines for school health programs discussed earlier in this chapter also illustrates a logical sequencing of activities.

Determine General Timing

This step involves looking at the components and drafting a rough timeline. When does it make sense to launch each component? Sometimes it really doesn't matter; components can go into the field as soon as they are ready. But sometimes activities must be coordinated with partners' activities, or certain times of year are more appropriate. For example, social change efforts that include passing or defeating legislation should be timed to correspond with legislative calendars: When the legislature is in session, members can be reached through media in the city where they meet or at their government offices. At other times of the year, members can be approached in their home districts.

Other types of activities may be seasonal for other reasons. For example, the ideal time to distribute classroom materials is over the summer, so that teachers have time to incorporate them into lesson plans. Summer is often a good time for training sessions involving school personnel as well. In contrast, late summer is often a bad time to stage special events because many target audience members will be away on vacation.

For media and community events, it is a good idea to check what else is going on during the time period you are thinking about. Doing so can provide opportunities to "piggyback" onto other events and can help avoid a time period likely to be monopolized by another health issue. Some annual health observances are listed in Appendix 13–A; the National Wellness Association Web site (http://www.wellnessnwi.org) provides an extensive list of national observances with contact information for each listing. Holding an event—or sending information about it—during a time when the publication already has plans to cover the topic can also be useful. Most magazines will provide their editorial calendars so that you can assess their upcoming content and place ads or pitch feature stories accordingly.

Obtain Stakeholder Buy-In

At some point in the process of developing a specific plan of action, it is wise to obtain buy-in from key stakeholders. These stakeholders include individuals with the organization and/or intermediaries who will have a hand in its implementation, as well as individuals whose support is critical to the initiative's success. You can obtain this buy-in by presenting the plan at relevant meetings or by circulating it in written form. It may be more useful to present it, so that you can discuss and clearly understand objections and concerns.

Finalize Budgets and Prepare Detailed Timelines

After laying out the major program components, it is a good idea to develop detailed budgets for each and prepare timelines that include all the steps necessary for successful completion and delivery of each component. These work plans typically detail the activities to be conducted, the materials that will support them, whether these materials exist or need to be produced (and in what quantity), and a timeline specifying each step of development, pretesting, preparation, production, and follow-up required to implement the component.

Once detailed budgets are available, it is a good time to step back and reassess what each component will cost (the total cost is often much higher than the original estimates, but sometimes it is lower than expected). Is the cost reasonable given what the component is expected to accomplish? There are no standard definitions of "reasonable," but there are some questions to ask and steps to take to make sure components do not cost more than necessary. An obvious first step is to obtain multiple cost estimates. To ensure that the estimates are comparable, make sure that each is based on identical assumptions. If one vendor suggests one solution and another goes a different route, ask each one why the proposed solution is superior to the other solution (without naming names, of course). This process often helps identify additional issues or less expensive solutions to consider.

One technique for comparing costs of different components can be borrowed from commercial advertisers, who often compare alternative media placement schedules by calculating the cost per thousand (CPM), or how much it costs for each alternative to reach a thousand people. This calculation can be difficult for many components because reach is unknown and depends on many factors. However, some components have a finite reach (e.g., a training session that includes *x* number of people). In other instances, reach is estimated and implementation will be measured against this estimate to assess success or failure. The same estimate can be used to calculate CPM.

Knowing how much components will cost and how many people they will reach helps you make informed decisions. Will one program component cost much more than another, yet reach far fewer people? If so, is this cost justified? In many instances it may be: The more expensive component may be designed to have a much greater impact on those reached. For example, a 2-hour training session can be expected to have a much more powerful and lasting impact than a 30-second ad. But if impact will be similar, the additional cost may not be justified. Only by taking a broad look at all components can you begin to make these types of assessments.

It is also important to ensure that all components are designed with cost-efficiency in mind. Chapter 15 will provide a range of tips for creating materials that command the most attention but do not rack up unnecessary costs. Making sure that whoever is responsible for approving budgets has a thorough understanding of all the costs involved will also help. In addition to limiting costs by trimming those that are unnecessary or suggesting alternatives that are of equal quality but less expensive, such a person helps avoid cost overruns by ensuring that nothing necessary is left out of the initial budgets.

Finally, it is important to assess to what degree (if any) the timeline is driving up costs, or could drive them up if some preliminary activities happen late. For example, at what point will printers start charging rush charges? Do you run the risk of losing deposits by changing dates for events? Are you going to wind up paying overtime for staff or contractors? It is important that timelines be realistic and have some "float" in them, particularly with large, complex programs—a million things can go wrong and at least a thousand probably will. While timelines shouldn't be developed based on worst-case scenarios at every step, it may help you assess the timeline accordingly if you know what those scenarios are. If you are reviewing timelines for a component with which you are relatively inexperienced, ask the people who will handle each stage what delays could occur and how much time they will take to resolve. Then assess the extent to which the timeline can accommodate likely delays.

The timeline should also be realistic in terms of providing sufficient time to obtain the necessary internal approvals. Asking for expedited approvals now and then may be tolerated, but if you need approval in a rush every time, the approvers will quickly lose patience with you and the initiative.

This is also a good time to prepare a master timeline that clearly identifies all "drop dead" dates. Project management software can be a great help in administering complex interventions. It can be set up to automatically shift the dates of all other activities associated with a project if one activity is late, and it can notify you if the change will make it impossible to meet a deadline.

Develop Program Components and Tracking Mechanisms

Once you have determined that the mix of program components and the timeline are reasonable, the components can be developed and, if necessary, pretested. Providing detailed guidance for developing every conceivable component is beyond the scope of this book. However, Chapter 15 will provide guidance on developing mass communication products and activities, and Chapter 16 will discuss pretesting.

As components are developed, process evaluation mechanisms should be built into them. It is often much more expensive to retroactively collect monitoring data, and doing so makes it much more difficult to refine and improve the initiative. Chapter 17 will provide a range of ideas for process evaluation mechanisms.

Prepare Spokespeople and Other Staff

Anyone who will talk publicly about the initiative is a spokesperson, whether the individual speaks on national television or at an internal meeting. As the time for implementation draws near, it is important to make sure that all spokespeople can frame the issue appropriately and clearly articulate the program's goals, objectives, target audiences, and major activities.

Formal spokespeople should receive thorough briefings and be prepared to deal with questions and criticisms, to minimize the likelihood that they will get blindsided when speaking about the program in a public forum. Two activities can help you prepare spokespeople:

1. Contact other practitioners who have been involved with programs focusing on the same public health problem. Ask them about the usual criticisms or concerns they hear and the responses they provide.

2. Review media coverage in your area and, if possible, attend any gatherings where the topic is likely to be discussed (for example, county or school board meetings). What is the usual angle of attack? How can these statements be defused or (as is sometimes true) shown to be incorrect?

You can use the information gathered from these activities to prepare talking points and "Q&A" (likely questions and their appropriate, on-strategy answers). Spokespersons can better represent the initiative if they review these materials before they speak about it or attend a meeting or event where they are likely to be asked about it. It is a good idea to update the materials regularly as the program evolves and as you develop a better sense of the usual questions about it.

Formal media training can be useful for spokespeople who will speak publicly about the initiative. This process will help them become more comfortable when handling media interviews (or questions from any audience), as well as help them to learn (and, more important, practice) how to make key points, how to respond properly to various types of questions, how to continue to frame the issue appropriately, and how to maintain their composure in stressful situations. Speaking publicly about a program or service can be a mine field, particularly if reporters are present. The bullet points below were drawn from advice to hospital spokespeople who will be interviewed by the media (Lewton, 1991), but they apply equally to any public discussion of a program or service and illustrate a few of the many potential pitfalls. When answering questions during an interview or in other public settings apply these principles:

- Don't answer hypothetical questions.
- Don't accept unfamiliar facts or statistics, or assumptions with which you do not agree. Don't even repeat them—you could end up quoted using exactly those words.
- Don't argue or get angry with a reporter, especially on camera.
- If you need a break to think and regroup, take one. If necessary, have a coughing fit and ask for a glass of water.

Because it is by nature adversarial, it is best if someone from outside your organization conducts media training sessions with spokespeople. Many public relations agencies and some independent practitioners provide media training sessions, but they can vary widely in quality. It is good practice to ask for references and check them before hiring someone for this important task.

Brief Partners, Intermediaries, and Stakeholders

Prior to rolling out a new campaign or making changes to existing products or services, it is vitally important that all partners, intermediaries, and stakeholders be briefed on the upcoming activities. Failing to do so can engender bad feelings from all three entities because it puts people in a position of not knowing what is going on. It can also jeopardize the chances for success.

It is a good idea to tailor the form and nature of the briefing to each entity's involvement in the program. Partners should know, in a general sense, all of the activities that are taking place and the specifics related to the when, where, and how of any component that might involve them, even if their involvement will be tangential. This knowledge helps them complement your activities and ensures that they can respond to questions about them. For joint activities, such briefings probably will focus on details and may take place at a meeting. For separate activities, briefings can be in the form of a memo, phone call, or face-to-face meeting. If partners are playing a role in the activity, it is best to provide the briefing in writing, even if it is a conference report prepared after the meeting that summarizes the decisions made about logistics.

The extent to which intermediaries are briefed depends on the role they are playing and how closely they are involved with the activity. For example, when public service advertisements are distributed to the mass media, the "briefing" normally takes the form of a letter, enclosed with the ads, that describes them, provides some background on the initiative, and makes a case for the importance of playing or displaying the ads to increase the initiative's ability to serve the media's audience. (Chapter 15 will discuss the specifics in more detail.) In contrast, intermediaries who are jointly planning an activity with you may brief you on many of the details. Updating the intermediary on other aspects of the program provides a framework and context for the role the intermediary is playing.

When briefing intermediaries, consider both those who are directly involved with your initiative and those who may have to deal with its results even if they are not serving as a direct conduit to the target audience. The following is an example of what can go wrong if you neglect the latter. A few years ago, one of the institutes at the National Institutes of Health had been testing a new drug regimen to combat a deadly disease. The regimen was so successful in clinical trials that the institute discontinued the trials and announced the treatment so that people in the control group and others across the country could benefit. For various reasons, the letter to physicians discussing the treatment was sent out after the news appeared in the popular media. Physicians found themselves besieged by patients asking about a drug therapy they knew nothing about. The delayed notification of this key intermediary—physicians—meant that patients had to wait before they could talk to their physicians about whether the product would work for them. It also alienated the physicians because they were made to seem less knowledgeable than their patients.

It is also important to brief internal and external stakeholders to make sure that they have an accurate picture of the initiative. Without a briefing, they may piece together what you are doing based on some informal communiqués from people who are less knowledgeable and provide faulty descriptions—or who deliberately take one real or imaginary element of a program and blow it out of proportion. Internal stakeholders may begin to question the need for your program (and may consider diverting the resources it requires). External stakeholders may openly oppose the program, pressuring your organization to discontinue it before it is even in place. Up-front briefings can go a long way toward minimizing such problems.

For example, some school districts working to provide comprehensive school health programs deliberately seek out stakeholders who may be concerned about some aspects of health education or health services, such as how sex education will be taught or whether condoms will be available in school clinics. By briefing these stakeholders before a program is put in place—and, ideally, involving them in the planning process—the administration can make sure that they have a clear picture of what the program really involves. While such an approach will not resolve all opposition, an up-front, open discussion can defuse criticism by making sure judgments of reasonable stakeholders are based on facts and providing an opportunity for them to voice concerns—and time for program planners to address many of these concerns prior to implementation.

Implement, Monitor, and Refine as Needed

The quickest route to failure is to promote a new product or service, get people excited and ready to try it, and then fail to deliver it. All program components need to be ready for implementation before you implement. Often, materials or services are delayed. The best alternative at that point is to delay the launch of your program until they are ready.

Once implementation has begun, close monitoring is essential to success. This can be accomplished by regularly reviewing tracking and monitoring data, as will be discussed in Chapter 17, and comparing progress to what you had planned. What is working? What isn't? What new opportunities are presenting themselves? The review provides an opportunity to plan a course of action and make the changes. The planning, implementation, and refinement cycle is never finished—strong managers always look for, and are open to, ways to improve the initiative.

CONCLUSION

We cannot say it better than Green and Kreuter (1991):

> In the final analysis, textbooks can offer little on implementation that will improve upon a good plan, an adequate budget, good organizational and policy support, good training and supervision of staff, and good monitoring in the process evaluation stage, discussed in Chapter [17]. The key to success in implementation beyond these six ingredients is

experience, sensitivity to people's needs, flexibility in the face of changing circumstances, an eye fixed on long-term goals, and a sense of humor. (p. 205)

REFERENCES

Academy for Educational Development. (1996). *Guidelines for school health programs: Strategic plan for dissemination and implementation.* Washington, DC: Author.

Backer, T.E., Rogers, E.M., & Sopory, P. (1992). *Designing health communication campaigns: What works?* Thousand Oaks, CA: Sage.

Gemunden, H.G. (1985). Perceived risk and information search: A systematic meta-analysis of the empirical evidence. *International Journal of Research in Marketing, 2,* 79–100.

Green, L.W., & Kreuter, M.W. (1991). *Health promotion planning: An educational and environmental approach* (2nd ed.). Mountain View, CA: Mayfield.

Hornik, R. (1997). Public health education and communication as policy instruments for bringing about changes in behavior. In M.E. Goldberg, M. Fishbein, & S.E. Middlestadt (Eds.), *Social marketing: Theoretical and practical perspectives* (pp. 45–58). Mahway, NJ: Lawrence Erlbaum Associates.

Kotler, P., & Roberto, E.L. (1989). *Social marketing: Strategies for changing public behavior.* New York: Free Press.

Lewton, K.L. (1991). *Public relations in health care: A guide for professionals.* Chicago: American Hospital Publishing.

Lippmann, W. (1922). *Public opinion.* New York: Harcourt Brace.

McCombs, M.E., & Shaw, D.L. (1972). The agenda-setting function of mass media. *Public Opinion Quarterly, 36,* 176–185.

McCombs, M.E., & Shaw, D.L. (1993). The evolution of agenda-setting research: Twenty-five years in the marketplace of ideas. *Journal of Communication, 43*(2), 58–67.

Palmgreen, P., & Clarke, P. (1977). Agenda-setting with local and national issues. *Communication Research, 4,* 435–452.

Signorielli, N. (1993). *Mass media images and impact on health: A sourcebook.* Westport, CT: Greenwood Press.

Tipton, L., Haney, R.D., & Baseheart, J.R. (1975). Media agenda-setting in city and state election campaigns. *Journalism Quarterly, 52,* 15–22.

Wallack, L., & Dorfman, L. (1996). Media advocacy: A strategy for advancing policy and promoting health. *Health Education Quarterly, 23,* 293–317.

Wallack, L., Dorfman, L., Jernigan, D., & Themba, M. (1993). *Media advocacy and public health: Power for prevention.* Newbury Park, CA: Sage.

Selected National Health Observances (by Month)

JANUARY

- March of Dimes Birth Defects Prevention Month
- National Volunteer Blood Donor Month

FEBRUARY

- American Heart Month
- National Children's Dental Health Month
- National Child Passenger Safety Awareness Week

MARCH

- National Nutrition Month
- National Poison Prevention Month

APRIL

- National Alcohol Awareness Month
- National Cancer Control Month
- National Child Abuse Prevention Month
- National Public Health Week
- National Infant Immunization Week

Source: Data from National Wellness Association web site (http://www.wellnessni.org).

MAY

- Arthritis Awareness Month
- Asthma and Allergy Awareness Month
- National High Blood Pressure Education Month
- National Mental Health Month
- Older Americans Month

JUNE

- National Safety Month

JULY

- National Special Recreation Week

SEPTEMBER

- Baby Safety Awareness Month
- Leukemia Society Month
- National Cholesterol Education Awareness Month

OCTOBER

- Family Health Month
- National Breast Cancer Awareness Month
- Talk About Prescriptions Month
- National Adult Immunization Awareness Week

NOVEMBER

- National Alzheimer's Disease Awareness Month
- National Diabetes Month
- National Epilepsy Awareness Month
- Great American Smokeout

DECEMBER

- Safe Toys and Gifts Month
- National Drunk and Drugged Driving Awareness Month
- World AIDS Day

CHAPTER 14

Working with Partners

Working with other organizations is an important part of most social change efforts. Building and maintaining effective relationships with other organizations often is critical to achieving desired outcomes. "Partners" can include cosponsors of a program, the media, and a variety of intermediaries that are used to reach target audiences. Working with partners on a social change initiative presents unique opportunities and challenges. This chapter discusses different types of partner involvement and makes suggestions for managing partner relationships.

THE ROLE OF PARTNERS

Partners are often necessary to successfully bring about change. They can provide additional resources, additional reach to audience members, greater credibility with their constituencies, and expertise that your organization does not possess. Partners can play many roles ranging in scope from low involvement—setting out your materials in their waiting room—to involvement on par with, or greater than, the role your organization is playing. Partners might conceptualize, develop, and implement entire components of a program. In some instances, it may be their program, and they want your organization to play a small role.

But building strong partnerships takes time and involves compromise. This chapter discusses some of the many forms partnerships can take and provides suggestions for developing successful ones.

TYPES OF PARTNERS

Partners come in many varieties. They might be

- other public agencies
- health voluntaries, such as the American Cancer Society, the American Heart Association, or the American Diabetes Association
- professional associations
- other consumer organizations, both national and local
- local consumer-based organizations
- foundations, both those specific to particular diseases and those with a more general focus
- the media: specific networks, stations, or publications, or associations, such as the National Association of Broadcasters
- associations of, or foundations set up and supported by, producers of particular products
- individual for-profit manufacturers
- local businesses, such as grocery stores, restaurants, and department stores
- national businesses

Just as partners come in many varieties, partnerships come in many forms. Sometimes it is desirable to assemble coalition*s* of organizations with a shared vision and common goal; generally, each coalition member makes a contribution to the effort based on the organization's capabilities and resources. At other times, it is enough to gather supporters; this approach is a good way to demonstrate (and obtain) widespread support on a particular set of recommendations or guidelines. Often the supporters don't have to do anything except show up for a few meetings and review some documents.

For other situations, two organizations may partner for a specific project or a large-scale program. These partnerships can be relatively simple and narrow in scope, or they can be quite elaborate. An example of the latter is the national 5 A Day for Better Health program. The program began in 1988 with a grant from the National Cancer Institute (NCI) to the California Department of Health and Human Services for a cooperative program between public health groups and private industry. When NCI and the produce industry decided to make the program national in scope, the produce industry established the Produce for Better Health Foundation, an independent, nonprofit consumer education foundation, to fund its part of the effort and centralize contact. (In effect, they created a coalition of growers and retailers.) The foundation then became NCI's partner.

Finally, many public health initiatives work through a number of intermediaries to reach their target audiences. The role of the intermediaries is to deliver messages (or materials or services) to the target populations. The mass media are an important intermediary that most programs work with from time to time. For some national agencies, state health departments are the key intermediaries. For professional associations, their members become intermediaries because they are the ones who will actually deliver the message to the target audience. And for community interventions, community-based organizations are critical intermediaries.

SUGGESTIONS FOR DEVELOPING SUCCESSFUL PARTNERSHIPS

Exhibit 14–1 presents some general suggestions that apply to all types of potential partners; each suggestion is described in further detail below.

Identify Benefits to Partners

Understanding the benefit to a potential partner is important when an organization is actively seeking partners, but it is also important to keep in mind when working with them. Sometimes a partner's actions, positions, or requests may not make sense until you step back and think about it from your partner's position and what your partner is looking for in the relationship. Potential benefits to partners include

- providing a means of furthering their organization's mission to service particular publics.

Exhibit 14–1 Suggestions for Developing Successful Partnerships

- Think of potential partners as target audiences: What is the benefit to them of helping you?
- Consider the partner's impact on the initiative's credibility.
- Find out what your organization can legally and ethically do before exploring possibilities with partners:
  - What partners are appropriate?
  - What can you ask partners to do?
  - What can you do for partners in return?
  - What activities can partners undertake that your organization cannot?
- Develop clear ideas of the roles you want partners to play—and an understanding of what roles they should not have (from your organization's perspective).
- Be flexible—losing prospective partners can limit a program's effectiveness.
- Put agreements in writing.
- Understand the challenges of working with partners.

- enhancing credibility or stature in the community and with target audiences.
- increasing sales (most often for private sector partners).

Consider Impact on Credibility

Partners can be critical for establishing credibility with particular audiences, particularly if the sponsoring organization is unknown or not trusted by target audience members. For example, a government agency trying to reach out to intravenous drug users might be far more successful working through a trusted community-based organization than trying to reach the audience directly.

The other side of impact on credibility is, of course, if a partner would have a negative impact on credibility. This issue often arises when a nonprofit organization or government agency is considering partnering with a private firm. For example, a pharmaceutical company might be interested in sponsoring aspects of a state or local chronic disease initiative, or might want a nonprofit or government agency to partner with it on a particular project. Often such partnerships can proceed without damaging the credibility of the initiative or the nonprofit/government partners, but it is a good idea to think through how the partnership—and the motives of the partners—might be perceived.

Identify Legal and Ethical Restrictions

It is important to find out what your organization can legally and ethically do before exploring possibilities with partners. For example, public sector organizations often have to follow myriad laws and regulations regarding relationships with other organizations. Nonprofit organizations have some limits on their activities if they receive federal funding, or may have limits on how they can spend certain types of grants. Knowing what you can and cannot do before starting to create partnerships helps shape ideas and saves time, headaches, hard feelings, and sometimes money. There are basically four questions to answer: What partners are appropriate? What can you ask partners to do? What can you do for partners in return? What activities can partners undertake that your organization cannot?

What partners are appropriate? It is best to avoid even the appearance of impropriety. Appropriate partners are those with whom your organization can work publicly without appearing to compromise its integrity. Situations in which to be particularly cautious include the following:

- Regulatory agencies must be very careful about working with any organizations they regulate; such relationships can be construed (by the organizations themselves, their competitors, or members of governing bodies) as meaning that the agency will "look the other way" on any regulatory infractions committed by the partner. Worse yet, large agencies can find themselves in the embarrassing position of having one department partnering with an organization that is under severe sanctions by another department.

- Organizations that issue grants and contracts must be careful about partnering with organizations that are or could become recipients of such awards. Again, competitors or other stakeholders may assume that working with the funding agent provides partners with an unfair advantage for upcoming grants and procurement. And, depending on the subject of the social change initiative, it is possible that partner organizations would gain an unfair advantage, by having access to information that other competitors did not have.

In addition to the advice provided by your organization's legal counsel, ask yourself this question: "If I woke up tomorrow and read about the partnership in the newspaper, what negative angles would the article cover?" If the answer is that there aren't any, are you sure that you have thought it through? The media—and legislators with an ax to grind—can find intrigue and misspent public funds in the most innocuous of relationships. If there are truly no negatives, great. If there are negatives, but you think they are outweighed by the positives, it would be prudent to spend some time planning how the organization would respond to criticism. Writing talking points and Q&A (questions and answers) that address potential criticisms of the partnership in advance of such criticism is good preparation.

What can you ask partners to do? Before exploring any options with partners, it's a good idea to find out if there are any restrictions on the types of things partners can do to support the program, and the ways in which they can indicate their involvement. For example, it is usually fine for private companies to print copies of materials for public agencies—but not if the company's sponsorship will be identified by brand name. If you are going to work on a joint project, such as a classroom or community kit, what are the limitations on visible sponsorship? To what extent (if at all) can brand-name products be featured? To what extent can a public agency be represented on the materials? Understanding these restrictions is critical, particularly in public-private partnerships. Often, the main benefit to a private company of working with the public agency is publicizing that relationship. Most commercial organizations believe the imprimatur of the public agency improves the stature of their company and their products with their target audiences. If they can't stamp the public agency's name next to theirs, and their name on products developed as part of the partnership, they may have little incentive to be a partner.

Another issue here is how much control each partner can maintain over the other's activities. For example, if a partner is developing a classroom kit that will feature the program logo, can you approve the contents? For public agencies, the legal answer is often no; you can make suggestions and provide technical assistance, but if the partner is developing it, they control it. Be careful about depending on them to do the right thing.

What can you do for partners in return? The answer to this question may vary somewhat depending on the type of partner—public agency, nonprofit, or for-profit organization—and their existing relationship with your organization. Some of the restrictions here are fairly obvious. For example, most public agencies cannot endorse or appear to endorse particular commercial products. As an extension of this, most public officials must be diligent about ensuring that their presence is not construed as an endorsement of the other organization or their products or services.

On the other hand, providing technical assistance is usually fine—unless the partner is going to sell the resulting product for profit. Then it can become a problem. Asking about specific examples, and as many "what ifs?" as you can think of, is the best way to uncover everything you need to know up front, rather than finding out after the materials are developed that they cannot be distributed as planned. Joint projects can get tricky, particularly if the organization is asking for you to fund part of its work. However, sometimes this can be accomplished through a cooperative agreement, where the roles and contributions of both partners are spelled out.

What activities can partners undertake that your organization cannot? Most public agencies, particularly federal agencies, have myriad restrictions on how they can spend money. Nonprofits often piece together money from a variety of sources, and each source may impose different restrictions. Sometimes partner organizations have far fewer restrictions on their activities and therefore can accomplish things that your organization cannot—or can accomplish them faster. The possibilities range from relatively simple tasks, such as providing food for a luncheon or producing high-quality printed products in a short time frame, to far more complex ones such as controlling copyrights.

The copyright issue can be an important one, particularly if you envision developing a strong program identity. Many organizations may want to associate with an initiative by featuring the program logo or symbol on their products or materials. You may want to control who uses the logo and how it is used; for example, it would make sense to restrict use of the logo to partners who are making a contribution to the program (either a monetary one or through in-kind services or materials). Or if it is a logo to appear on products to indicate, for example, those that are "healthy," you would want to clearly define what constitutes healthy and make sure that the logo or symbol did not appear on products not meeting this definition. Nongovernmental entities control their logos by copyrighting them.

The Food Guide Pyramid developed by the U.S. Department of Agriculture provides an illustrative example of what can happen when there is no copyright. The pyramid is probably one of the most widely used symbols the government has ever produced. Walk down nearly any aisle in the supermarket and you are bound to find it on something, particularly members of the breads, rice, pasta, and cereals group. You will find the original official version. And you will find dozens of permutations of it. Most manufacturers include it as a way of saying, "The government says you should eat this." Actually, the government has said no such thing. Yet, since the pyramid is not copyrighted, the government has no way to control its use. Federal government agencies can only copyright material under very limited circumstances; most of what they publish enters the public domain and can be used by anyone in any way. From the taxpayers' standpoint, this makes sense: taxpayers paid for the work, so they ought to be able to use it. From the standpoint of the government, inability to copyright makes monitoring the use of program logos and symbols very complicated.

Develop Appropriate Roles

As discussed in Chapter 10, your strategic plan should outline some of the roles you expect partners to play. For example, there may be components of the initiative that should be developed by a partner organization because it has greater expertise in the subject matter and more credibility with the target audience. Similarly, the work plans developed for specific tactics will usually include concrete recommendations for specific intermediaries or types of intermediaries to use.

But sometimes the program conceptualization includes the involvement of various types of partners without specifying exactly who they will be. Having a list of things prepared that other organizations can do—and another list that reminds you of what they cannot do—saves time and keeps you from losing potential partners while you try to figure out what role they could play. It also helps you retain control of the initiative and ensure that it stays on strategy—because, of course, all of the items on the list will be appropriate for the objectives the program is trying to accomplish. Without a list, it is easy to get caught up in the frenzy of developing a new program and approve an idea that sounds really wonderful but will not help accomplish any program objectives.

Ideally the list should be divided into low-, medium-, and high-involvement activities, so that you can tailor suggestions to the level of commitment the partner wants to make. Major partners may wind up involving themselves in an entirely different way, but the list serves three purposes: (1) It provides them with some initial ideas to work from, (2) it shows them you are organized and ready to go, and (3) it keeps your program on track.

Be Flexible

Partnership opportunities often arise quickly, particularly as an initiative is gaining momentum. Your program should be flexible enough to incorporate new ideas (as long as they are on strategy) or help from unexpected quarters. One of the challenges of working with partners is marrying their ideas and their mission with yours. If an idea truly will not fit, try to suggest a modification that will.

Put Agreements in Writing

Agreements can be formal or informal, but they should always be in writing. If an intermediary agrees to distribute 1,000 brochures at its next community event, a quick memo or e-mail can confirm the date of the meeting and how the intermediary will get the brochures. Elaborate cosponsored projects or programs normally have a memorandum of understanding outlining the roles and responsibilities of each partner. Some partnerships may be governed by formal cooperative agreements, particularly when funding flows from one partner to the other. Written agreements safeguard against subsequent misunderstandings by providing a record of what was supposed to happen. They serve as memory for current staff and are invaluable in cases of staff turnover. Plus, they help you manage the program by reminding you of who is doing what and when, so that you can ensure that they have everything they need to perform.

Understand the Challenges

As NCI (1989) noted, working with other organizations can

- be time consuming—to locate, convince them to work with you, gain internal approvals, and undergo planning and/or training
- require altering your program—every organization has different priorities and perspectives, and other organizations may want to make minor—or major—program changes to accommodate their structure or needs.
- result in loss of "ownership" and control—because other organizations may change the time schedule, functions, or even the messages, and take credit for their part (or all) of the program.

COALITIONS

Coalitions are groups of organizations that come together to address a common goal. They are most often run by a committee comprised of representatives from each (or many) coalition's members. Coalitions are characterized by two-way relationships: Each member has a say in how the program or its components are developed, and each makes contributions to the program. Many of these same factors characterize a relationship between two organizations that jointly sponsor a program or project, so this section can be of use for assessing prospective partners as well as prospective coalition members.

Coalitions are often formed at the community level, but the scope of coalitions can be international, national, regional, statewide, or local. As noted earlier, one of the partners in the national 5 A Day for Better Health program, the Produce for Better Health Foundation, is in effect a coalition. Federal agencies often assemble or participate in coalitions; for example, the National Heart, Lung, and Blood Institute (NHLBI) has been instrumental in forming coalitions for the National High Blood Pressure Education Program and the National Cholesterol Education Program among others (Bellicha & McGrath, 1990). Each program has a coordinating committee made up of representatives from many organizations, and NHLBI staff serve as the coalition staff. Statewide and local coalitions, such as those assembled to support Project LEAN (Low-fat Eating for America Now), also come together for a variety of purposes.

Coalitions take an enormous amount of time and energy to establish. Exhibit 14–2 lists some questions to ask before establishing a coalition, to help ensure that the coalition approach is the best approach to take.

If you have worked through the list of questions and want to proceed with establishing a coalition or partnership, here are some tips for recruiting and selecting coalition members or partners. They are adapted from information provided in the idea kit commissioned by the Henry J. Kaiser Family Foundation* to support development of Project LEAN's coalitions.

Exhibit 14–2 Questions To Ask before Establishing a Coalition

If your group may take a leading role in establishing a coalition, answer the following questions to determine whether this is the best choice:
- Is there an organization already in place that could effectively and more efficiently address this problem?
- Would this problem be more effectively or permanently solved with the joint ownership and responsibility of others or can our organization be just as effective working on its own?
- Are there gaps in community services that would be met best through collaborative relationships?
- Is this problem perceived as a priority by other organizations?
- Are we willing to relinquish control of the project to a coalition or do we just want advice? (A coalition may be willing to concede lead responsibility to one agency after agreeing on goals and overall strategy.)
- Do funding sources or our own agency constraints make it impossible to give up or share control of the project?

Courtesy of Henry J. Kaiser Family Foundation, Menlo Park, CA.

---

*Courtesy of Henry J. Kaiser Family Foundation, Menlo Park, CA.

- Identify the skills and expertise coalition members will need.
- Look for possible members. Potential organizations (or individuals) should possess at least one of the following attributes:
  - −Interest in and commitment to the issue
  - −Credibility in the community (as formal or informal leaders)
  - −Contacts with other potential members or allies
  - −Familiarity and experience with the political system
  - −Materials or expertise in program development, promotion, implementation, or evaluation
  - −Financial resources or fund-raising ability

  A good way to identify prospective members and make sure that you are not missing anyone important is the "snowball" method: Conduct interviews with people who represent organizations, factions, or constituencies you know are respected in the community. Explain why you are creating the coalition and how you expect it to benefit the community. At the end of the interview, ask the person for names of other organizations or individuals who could potentially contribute to solving the problem. If you are putting together a local or statewide coalition, make sure to include grass-roots leadership. You will know you have identified everyone when the people you interview start providing you with the same names you have heard.
- Take time to get to know potential members, and be cautious before issuing invitations. Make sure that there is a good match between their abilities and the needs of the coalition. Make sure they understand that you are recruiting them not as individuals but as representatives of their organization or constituencies. Assess how committed they are to working cooperatively with others. Think about how they will fit into the mix of members and how they will affect the image of the coalition. Members should not consist entirely of agencies, gatekeepers, and political power holders; grass-roots community leaders and people who have time to work on specific projects and other issues are also important.
- When you issue invitations, be very clear about how much organizational involvement you expect, which could range from public endorsement by their board to the contribution of resources or the appointment of a representative to the board of the coalition.
- Put together participation agreements for all members. The agreements should spell out time limits for membership and any other conditions for involvement in the coalition (for example, if membership is organizational rather than individual, if the individual leaves the organization he or she will no longer be a member of the coalition). Depending on your environment, participation agreements could be an informal memo from you to all members about "keeping everyone informed," or a more formal contract for each member.

Once a coalition has been established, the first order of business is to develop a leadership structure and operating procedures. This process should include the following (many of these suggestions also were adapted from information provided in the idea kit commissioned by the Henry J. Kaiser Family Foundation to support development of Project LEAN's coalitions):*

- *Leadership.* Who will hold leadership roles and how will these people be selected? The chair needs to have the ability to set agendas and conduct meetings efficiently while fostering communication and a strong sense of the coalition's direction. If the membership will elect a chair, members should have enough time to get acquainted so that people with strong leadership skills can emerge. One way to proceed is to appoint an interim facilitator (preferably one who is not interested in the position of chair).
- *Coalition/staff relationships.* Who has the authority to oversee the project's development and operation? In many coalitions, it is the coalition members, not the staff (who are often provided by the organization that established the coalition). Staff often must balance providing technical assistance to members so that members can best carry out their roles with the members' role of decision making.
- *Bylaws or rules of operation.* How often will the coalition meet? How long will meetings last? How will decisions be made—consensus or majority rule? What constitutes a quorum? How will the work get done—by the full coalition or through task forces or committees? Who has the authority to speak on behalf of the coalition? How are coalition members appointed? What are attendance rules, and what happens to members who do not attend and participate? Establishing procedures to address these issues at the outset, rather than dealing with them reflexively when a situation occurs, will make the coalition run more smoothly and should keep members from feeling that they were treated unfairly when issues arise.
- *Mission statement and goals and objectives.* A clear, agreed-on mission is very important to the success of the coalition; every member should contribute to preparing the mission statement. All members should also be involved in developing goals and objectives that are clear, specific, and attainable, and in creating a work plan that emphasizes collaborative linkages among members. These activities are important in vesting members in the coalition and giving them ownership of it.
- *Coalition versus individual recognition.* The coalition should find ways to publicly recognize individual contributions without losing opportunities to advance the goals of the coalition. Recognition often becomes a sticking

---

*Courtesy of Henry J. Kaiser Family Foundation, Menlo Park, CA.

point in coalitions, because member organizations want credit for their contributions. One way to deal with the issue is to ensure that press releases mention the organizations taking the lead on any particular activity; another easy way to provide recognition is to include the names of organizations who developed or printed particular materials on those materials (though less prominently than the coalition name).

- *Guidelines for using logos, theme lines, or symbols.* If a coalition has many members or if it plans to allow other organizations to use its logos or symbols in some way, draw up licensing agreements that spell out what can and cannot be done with logos and other program materials. If possible, coalitions should copyright logos, symbols, and theme lines so that they can control how they are used.

INTERMEDIARIES

In contrast to coalitions, which address a common goal, intermediaries are organizations that may have different goals but are willing to help you accomplish a particular aspect of your initiative by reaching their constituency for you. Some coalition members may also play the role of an intermediary by serving as a conduit to their constituency. Relationships with intermediaries can be thought of as one-way compared with those among coalition members: Intermediaries have a strong voice in how a particular message is delivered to their population, but they do not shape the overall program goals, objectives, or strategies.

It is important to think of intermediaries as another target audience for the initiative. They are gatekeepers standing between you and your target population: They must believe that messages or products will work and are appropriate for their constituency, or they will not deliver them.

Many types of intermediaries may be involved in your program; common ones include the mass media, professional associations, and consumer organizations (who can access their members). Exhibit 14–3 lists steps to help ensure that your attempts to involve intermediaries in program delivery are successful. Most of these suggestions apply to intermediaries with whom your organization works closely, although some also apply to more distant intermediaries such as the mass media. Chapter 15 will provide a thorough discussion of issues to keep in mind when working with the media.

Exhibit 14–3 Steps for Involving Intermediaries in Your Program

1. Choose organizations, agencies, or individuals who can reach and influence your target audience(s).
2. Involve representatives of the organizations you want to work with as early as possible in program planning.
3. Give people at these organizations plenty of advance notice so that they can build their activities into their schedule, and make sure they are comfortable with the role they are to play.
4. Allow them to personalize and adapt program materials to fit their situations, and give them a feeling of "ownership" (as long as they stay on strategy).
5. Ask them what they need to implement their part of the program. Beyond the question of funding, consider other assistance, training, information, or tools that would enable them to function successfully.
6. If necessary, gently remind them that they have responsibility for their activities, but remember that you may need them more than they need you.
7. Provide them with new local, regional, and/or national contacts or linkages that they will perceive as valuable for their ongoing activities.
8. Provide them with your program rationale, strategies, and messages—in ready-to-use form. Remember that strategic planning, creative messages, and quality production are the most difficult aspects of a communication program to develop, and may be the most valuable product you can offer to a community organization.
9. Don't ask for too much at once. Make requests as small, manageable, and discrete as possible, and provide them with a feedback/tracking mechanism.
10. Assess progress through the feedback/tracking mechanism, and help make adjustments to respond to the organizations' needs and to keep the program on track.
11. Remember to provide moral support, frequent thank-yous, and other rewards (e.g., letters or certificates of appreciation).
12. Provide them with a final report of what was accomplished, and meet to discuss follow-up activities and resources they might find useful. Make sure that they know they are a part of the program's success.

Source: Adapted from *Making Health Communication Programs Work: A Planner's Guide,* 1989, National Cancer Institute, Bethesda, Maryland.

CONCLUSION

Other organizations may be involved in public health initiatives as supporters, intermediaries, coalition members, or full partners. The keys to successfully working with other organizations are prior planning, careful consideration, and flexibility. The first step of involving them in an initiative is to assess what type of involvement would best further the initiative's goals. Before approaching other organizations, it is important to clearly understand what roles they can play and what responsibilities you must retain. When they "sign on," carefully articulate—and agree on—the role each will have. Finally, it is good practice to establish procedures governing how the partnership will accomplish its goals at the beginning of the relationship, to ensure smoother and more efficient operations throughout it.

REFERENCES

Bellicha, T., & McGrath, J. (1990). Mass media approaches to reducing cardiovascular disease risk. *Public Health Reports, 105*(3), 245–252.

Henry J. Kaiser Family Foundation (n.d.). *Project LEAN idea kit for state and community programs to reduce dietary fat.* Menlo Park, CA: Author.

National Cancer Institute. (1989). *Making health communication programs work: A planner's guide* (NIH Pub. No. 89-1493). Bethesda, MD: Author.

CHAPTER 15

Mass Communication: Design and Implementation Issues

Some form of mass communication plays a role in most social change initiatives. It can be used to frame a policy discussion or support individual behavior change. This chapter presents some issues to consider as tactics such as publications, press materials, video news releases, World Wide Web sites, and advertising are developed and implemented.

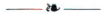

Once a strategic plan has been developed, the program components most suited for effective implementation of the effort are chosen and developed, as discussed in Chapter 13. Because some form of mass communication is almost always a part of one or more components, this chapter focuses on some of the most common methods of communicating with large numbers of people: print publications and the electronic and mass media. Entire books have been written on how to develop and implement many of the tactics discussed here; our intent is to provide readers with an introduction to some of the practical issues involved with designing and using each type of tactic and some suggestions for assessing potential products in terms of their utility, cost, and contribution to the initiative's objectives.

USE OF MASS COMMUNICATION

As Kotler and Roberto (1989) noted, the distinctive function of mass communication "is to inform and persuade, within a given period, the largest possible number of target adopters about how the social product fits into their needs and how it fits better than alternative products" (p. 191). This is true whether the product is a new policy designed to address the underlying social conditions contributing to the problem or whether it is a change in an individual's health behavior. Other investigators have commented on the importance of reaching target audience members through as many channels as possible as often as possible (see, e.g., Backer, Rogers, & Sopory, 1992; Hornik, 1997).

Public health initiatives can use mass communication tactics in a variety of ways. Perhaps most important, they can be used to frame the public discussion of an issue in terms of the core values being threatened. They can also be used to increase knowledge, promote specific behaviors, provide audience members with sources of direct service delivery, and repeat and reinforce the messages target audience members receive in other forums.

PLANNING DEVELOPMENT TIME

Many practitioners have observed that campaign planners are often unrealistic about the amount of time required to develop, test, and produce the many elements that comprise a multifaceted intervention. The following outline of the steps involved in developing materials can be used as a quick check when assessing plans and timelines for completeness and realism.

1. Determine types and quantities of materials to be developed based on the audience and the message. Determine how each material will be distributed.
2. Develop and submit initial concepts (designs and copy points) for each material. Often two or three potential concepts are developed.
3. Prepare prototype materials for pretesting. Print prototypes look like final versions but include "for position only" artwork, rather than final artwork. Headlines and subheads are included, but "Greek" text (gibberish) is often used in place of body copy on lengthy documents. Prototypes for video products are usually storyboards incorporating a script; audio prototypes usually take the form of scratch tapes (quick recordings, often made by amateurs, rather than the talent that will record the final version).
4. Pretest and submit the prototypes for peer or professional review in accordance with processes to be described in Chapter 16.
5. Before or simultaneous with pretesting, obtain commitments from directors, talent, photographers, and so forth. If existing artwork, audio, or video material will be incorporated, obtain necessary permissions and releases.
6. Revise designs and copy to incorporate pretest recommendations.
7. If necessary, prepare and submit a clearance package that includes all necessary forms, pretest results, and revised prototype materials; revise the designs and copy to address the clearance comments.
8. Obtain final preproduction approval.
9. Produce rough cuts of audio and video materials and camera-ready versions of print materials; obtain approvals.

10. Make final edits, and obtain final approval.
11. Oversee production of the quantities required. For print materials, this step involves checking blue lines or chromalins and conducting press checks. For audio and video products, it involves coordinating dubbing.

ASSESSING PROPOSED MATERIALS AND ACTIVITIES

Subsequent sections of this chapter present issues to consider when assessing specific materials and activities. This section outlines some general questions that can help you assess the utility of any proposed material or activity.

- *Is the content accurate and on strategy?* The communication strategy (discussed in Chapter 12) was created to ensure that each product contains the appropriate messages and speaks to the audience in language they will understand. It is good practice to check the content of all materials and activities prior to production to ensure they are scientifically accurate, consistent with public health goals and principles, and consistent with the communication strategy. Especially when outside creative teams are used or materials undergo extensive edits prior to production, accuracy sometimes slips away.
- *Is this the best solution for the least cost?* Compared with most commercial marketing budgets, public health efforts have minuscule amounts of funding, so every material and every activity needs to work hard.
- *Does it complement and reinforce other aspects of the social change effort?* Materials and activities that reinforce each other in tone, in look, and in content are more effective because each additional time an audience member is reached, the new contact can build off of the identity established before.
- *If it needs to be, is it easily reproducible and customizable by partners or collaborating organizations?* By considering customization and reproduction costs when materials and activities are designed, it is easier to ensure the final products can be used as they are intended to be used. For example, if it is likely that intermediaries will photocopy a brochure, designing it on standard-size paper (8.5×11" or 8.5×14") and using inks that are dark enough to facilitate photocopying ensure that people will be able to read the copies. Designing materials and activities that will be used by intermediaries or partners to allow for customization can increase their use and enhance their credibility with the intended target audiences.

ESTABLISHING IDENTITY

Establishing a consistent graphic identity helps build recognition for the social change effort and its messages. Materials that are visually similar to those people have seen earlier will be more familiar to them and will more easily build on the messages delivered in the previous materials. Consistent use of campaign or program names, logos, and theme lines can contribute to this identity, as can identifying three or four standard typefaces and two or three basic colors or shades within one color family (Lewton, 1991). If brochures or other publications are developed, use of the same paper stocks, formats, and layout elements can also contribute to this identity.

Graphic standards help ensure that a consistent image is conveyed by all campaign materials, which is particularly helpful in situations where many organizations may be developing materials (e.g., to support the work of a coalition) or when materials must be developed very quickly in order to respond to competing information (such as in the heat of a legislative or referendum battle). Establishing graphic standards early on also streamlines the review process by confining it to the content and unique elements of each new item. Those working under tight time deadlines or in committee situations appreciate the ability to avoid sparking a new debate about typefaces, color, and where the logo goes each time a new product is presented. Finally, providing creative teams or graphic artists with the standards can limit costs by avoiding situations where they have to start over because the initial proposal was inconsistent with other materials or with the program's image.

When establishing standards, it is helpful to consider other materials developed by your organization and determine if the materials for the new initiative need to be consistent with them. For example, sometimes it is desirable to use similar colors. Large organizations may have existing graphic standards (particularly relating to reproduction costs) that will also apply to the materials for your initiative.

PRINT MATERIALS

Throughout the life of a social change initiative, many types of print publications and materials may be used. For example, brochures, newsletters, manuals, and posters often play a role, as well as a host of other collateral materials, such as folders for meetings or press kits, calendars, letterhead, and envelopes.

Brochures can have many functions in a social change intervention. They may be designed for partners to show them roles they can play, or they may be designed for any of a number of target audiences: members of the public, patients, health care professionals, or business leaders. Brochures provide an opportunity to give people a detailed explanation or information on multiple skills in a form they can take with them. They can be referred to many times and are often shared with others in the target group, thereby increasing the reach of the message. Depending on the topic, longer booklets can be designed for any of these reasons also. There are many keys to effective brochure design, but ensuring that the cover states the positioning or promises a benefit to the reader and that the headings and captions convey the main points is a good beginning.

Sometimes ongoing publications, such as newsletters, are a useful way of maintaining momentum in a program. Newsletters can serve a variety of purposes in a campaign. They can be sent to partners and other interested organizations to keep them abreast of current activities, legal and legislative developments, and recent media coverage. They can play a technology transfer role, providing partners or others implementing a social change initiative with ideas and case studies on activities they could undertake. A variation on the newsletter format can also be used to keep in periodic contact with the media and provide them with story ideas, informational graphics, and camera-ready art.

Other printed materials may be designed for other purposes (such as training sessions, packaging or signage for other campaign products or services, or support for a special event). These all provide an opportunity to convey key campaign messages (through the use of a theme line or initiative name if nothing else), and they will all convey an image. Using the graphics standards discussed earlier in this chapter can help ensure all printed material communicates the right image for the initiative.

When selecting designs and formats, it is useful to consider the purpose of the piece, how it will be distributed, how it will be reproduced, the image to be conveyed, and how much various choices will cost.

Purpose and Use

Will the material be used once and then tossed away? Is it something that needs to last? If a material will have a short life (i.e., posters to be used in conjunction with a 1-day event), using lightweight (and inexpensive) paper stock probably makes sense. If, on the other hand, it is a booklet or newsletter that people could keep and refer to over a long period, a heavier (but more expensive) stock will ensure that the item holds up over time.

Distribution and Reproduction

Lewton (1991) offered a number of suggestions for reducing mailing costs. For material that will be mailed, mailing costs can be minimized by using standard-size envelopes (odd sizes cost extra postage) or self-mailers (the latter also eliminate the cost associated with purchasing envelopes and assembling their contents) and mailing using bulk-rate permits, rather than first-class postage. Reviewing and updating mailing lists regularly can also help control costs by eliminating duplications and dead wood.

Reproduction costs can be minimized in many ways. One of the first steps is to determine whether a particular item should be printed or photocopied. Often if 2,000 or more copies are needed, printing is less expensive (even for black-and-white reproductions). Some other methods of stretching a budget include printing lengthy documents such as manuals or reports on both sides of the page (saving paper and mailing costs), or printing newsletter mastheads or folders in color (and in large quantities to reduce the cost per piece) and then printing or photocopying onto them in black or some other single color when they are actually used (Lewton, 1991).

Image and Cost

Many aspects of a printed piece convey image: size, type of paper stock (i.e., matte or glossy, heavy or light, recycled or not), use of color (particularly the number of colors used) and photos, special effects (i.e., die cuts, foil stamping, embossing), and the graphic standards (typeface, layouts) discussed earlier in this chapter. Many of the choices that affect image also affect cost and some affect reproducibility. For example, set-up charges for special effects can be substantial and are the same for small or large press runs. If a publication or collateral material (such as a poster or tabletop card) is intended to serve as a model that will be customized and printed in relatively small quantities by collaborating organizations, avoiding special effects set-up charges will reduce printing costs significantly.

The following questions may help you assess proposed print materials:

- *Will the reader get the key messages by reading the headlines, subheads, and captions?* These elements are all many people read.
- *How easy is it to read the material?* Color, type size and style, and line justification can all affect readability. Black, dark blue, and other dark-colored inks on light backgrounds are easiest to read. Reverse type (light type on a dark background) is very hard to read, as is type that has been printed over a photo or illustration. All capital letters are more difficult to read than a mixture of upper case and lower case. Serif typefaces are easier to read than sans serif. (This sentence, and most of this book, is in a serif typeface; the tables are sans serif.) Ideally, type size should be 12 points or larger and definitely no smaller than 10 points. Type that is set *ragged right* (ending wherever the words end, rather than adding spaces or hyphenation to fill each line) is easier to read. The way in which the text is laid out on the page also affects readability. Layouts that are simple and open are more inviting than those with densely packed text, as are those that break up large amounts of text with visuals.
- *Is the writing style appropriate for the audience?* In general, text that is as simple, short, and jargon-free as possible is best. However, some professional audiences interpret simple language as an indication that a publication is designed for laypeople, so a balance must be struck.
- *What type of artwork is used: illustrations or photos?* In general, photography is more effective than illustrations, and one strong, large photo is more

effective than a series of smaller photos (Lewton, 1991; Roman & Maas, 1992). It is also less expensive than shooting multiple photos or buying the rights to multiple stock photos. However, color photography is more difficult to reproduce well. If illustrations are used, drawings should be professional quality so they do not detract from credibility.

- *If photos or illustrations are used, are captions included?* Photo captions are read almost twice as often as body copy (Roman & Maas, 1992), so they provide an ideal venue for making key points.
- *Is sufficient identifying information included?* Date of publication or publication number (in tiny type at the bottom or on the back) can save endless headaches when people call to request a copy of a material; often requests will come years after the publication was first produced. Depending on the design and purpose, most print materials also include some or all of the following: the organization's name, complete mailing address, phone number, and e-mail or Web site address.

For materials that will be printed rather than photocopied:

- *How many colors are used, and are they all necessary?* Color can be very powerful, and it can be very expensive. Every additional ink color used increases the cost.
- *Are there any special effects that are increasing cost?* For example, bleeds (printing to the edge of the paper, rather than leaving a margin), die cuts, embossing, and special folding all add costs.
- *Do the materials make full use of standard size press sheets?* Some odd-sized publications may not take up the whole sheet, resulting in wasted paper.
- *Can the same paper stock be used for several materials so quantity discounts can be obtained?* Along the same lines, is there a comparable paper stock that is less expensive?

Once a material's design and content have been approved and it is being readied for printing, a few final checks can prevent a lot of headaches. For example, it is a good idea to have someone other than the writer read all copy, checking it for typographical and other errors before it is sent to the printer. Once the printer is ready to go, ordering proofs and checking them carefully often reveals mistakes. When the job is on the press, having someone there to do a press check is a final step that can detect errors and ensure a high-quality product.

ELECTRONIC MEDIA

In the last decade, computer technology has improved to the point where ever-larger numbers of people rely on it to obtain and transmit information. In many ways, electronic media in the form of the Internet and CD-ROM technology represent a new, hybrid channel of communication that combines elements of both interpersonal and mass communication, as Cassell, Jackson, and Cheuvront (1998) noted when describing Internet-based resources. They pointed out that Internet-based resources are likely to be superior to mass media in their ability to persuade, because "the capacity of these resources to provide immediate, transactional feedback suggests that they can be used to realize health behavior change in a manner that is similar to that of interpersonal channels, while their resemblance to forms of mass media suggests an ability to do so on a larger scale than previously considered possible" (p. 74).

Hypermedia

The advent of *hypermedia* applications (computer-based documents that can be accessed "nonlinearly"; i.e., the user can hop around from section to section) permits people to process information in new ways. As Jaffe (1997) noted, "computer-based multimedia, including hypermedia, present the potential of combining all known visual and audio communication media formats" (p. 238). Computerized media can combine the video and audio capabilities of television and radio with the flexibility of print by permitting the user to determine the order in which information will be accessed and the amount of time spent on particular sections of information. Researchers do not yet understand all of the ramifications of these new information processing possibilities.

Hypermedia applications can be distributed on a CD-ROM (or, in some instances, a floppy disk) or run on an Internet World Wide Web site. They can range from simple hypertext documents (such as the help text for most Windows-based application software) to complex multimedia extravaganzas. Hypermedia applications are new enough that it is difficult to provide recommendations for developing or assessing them. Jaffe (1997) noted that they may provide an opportunity to increase self-efficacy (a person's confidence in his or her ability to perform an action) because "learners can easily repeat all or part of a sequence at will, which increases the opportunities for symbolic modeling and cognitive rehearsal, two factors theorized to enhance self-efficacy" (p. 241). At the same time, he noted that if people have difficulty finding the information they seek, either due to poor design or user disposition, their self-efficacy may decrease.

The Internet and the World Wide Web

The Internet is a powerful tool for communications, and the number of people who use it is expanding almost as quickly as the technology that drives it; the annual growth rate is estimated to be 100% (Cassell et al., 1998). The Internet provides a number of fast, inexpensive communication options for social change initiatives. A World Wide Web site can provide information to all interested parties. List servers and e-mail provide nearly instantaneous access to partners or advocates, facilitating fast responses to questions and requests.

However, before relying too heavily on the Internet to reach a particular target audience, it is important to understand who it reaches and who it does not reach. According to 1997 data from Mediamark Research, Inc. (MRI), slightly fewer than 1 in 5 American adults reported using the Internet in the past 30 days (type of usage, e.g., World Wide Web, e-mail, newsgroups, etc., was not specified). Compared with all American adults, those who use the Internet are much more likely to be highly educated and affluent: 84% have attended or graduated from college, compared with 48% of the population overall, and 69% have household incomes of $50,000 or more, compared with 39% of the general population. These differences may be due in part to age: As might be expected, Internet users tend to be younger. In fact, just 8% said they were age 55 or older, compared with 28% of the total adult population (MRI, 1997).

Cassell and colleagues (1998) argued that the Internet can also be used to reach people who do not have access to computers: "Members of a target audience need not know how to use a computer—or even have access to one—to have access to video, audio, and text-based information supplied through the Internet. . . . Public health interventions that use Internet-based technologies could be delivered in familiar intervention sites, such as clinics, schools, community centers, workplace settings, and the home" (p. 76).

Web Site Design

An Internet Web site often forms the core of an organization's on-line identity. The site can serve a variety of functions. It can provide information on a social change initiative and the steps visitors can take in support of the initiative. It can serve as a distribution channel, providing a means of downloading materials that can then be printed or used in other ways (e.g., brochures, presentations). It can be a gateway to other information by including links to other relevant sites or a system for ordering materials.

Earlier in this chapter we recommended establishing a graphic identity and graphic standards for an initiative's printed materials. The same recommendations hold true for Web sites: Paying some up-front attention to site design can improve readability and use, as well as speed approval of additions to the site. A Web site's graphic identity can be established by using the same colors, fonts, backgrounds, and signature icons throughout the site.

Color, Fonts, and Backgrounds. To reduce eye fatigue (which occurs when the eyes have to refocus constantly), experts recommend limiting screens to four nonneutral colors and avoiding complementary colors and red-blue combinations. When assigning colors to various screen elements, keep in mind that users assume objects of the same color are related. Dark type (black or dark blue) on plain, light-colored backgrounds is easiest to read. In general, blue, red, and purple should not be used for text other than hyperlinks (otherwise those text elements may be confused with default hyperlinks). Selecting one or two font families and sticking with them provides a consistent look without creating clutter. As with printed publications, type in all capital letters is more difficult to read. Finally, although background patterns are a popular way to establish a site's identity, care should be taken in their use because strong background patterns can render text unreadable.

Site Layout. The best layout for a particular site depends on its content. However, there are some technical aspects of site design that can determine the degree to which the site is friendly (or unfriendly) to use. For example, including a search capability or index on the home page is a good way to help users locate the information they want. Such a feature is particularly helpful on large sites that include many different topics.

Organizing the site contents in a user-friendly manner is critical. In particular, sites that regularly add menu items run the risk of becoming disorganized and unwieldy over time. A general rule of thumb is to limit lists to seven choices, breaking longer lists into smaller groups. Frequent visitors will appreciate a "last updated" date next to menu items; this feature lets them avoid waiting for a screen to load only to discover there is no new information. Adding hyperlinks to partner sites and resources provides site users with access to more information and increases the perceived value of your site.

Including a means to contact the organization sponsoring the site is also important. People may have comments on the site itself (ensuring that each Web page has a clear, brief title will help them comment and help you understand what they are talking about), or they may have questions about the initiative or want to know if more information is available on a particular topic. It is a good idea to provide both electronic and traditional addresses and telephone numbers, because some people will access the site to find out how to contact the organization through traditional means. Similarly, if the site includes suggestions on actions to take (such as contacting a policy maker), information should be provided on how to contact the appropriate parties (e.g., name, address, phone number).

Images and Photos. Part of the Web's appeal is the ability to bring ideas to life and simplify complex information using illustrations and photographs. Adding many images to Web pages is tempting because it is an opportunity to use all those full-color images an organization could never afford to print. However, they have their own hefty price in response time. Every image added to a Web page increases the time it takes for the page to appear on someone's screen. While a target audience member is waiting for your organization's page to appear, he or she may get bored and decide to go somewhere else.

By using images sparingly and paying attention to how they are constructed, you can harness the visual power of the Web while minimizing response time. In general, Web designers recommend that graphic elements be kept small (less than 30K) and that animation be avoided unless it is truly necessary, because continuous animation tires the eyes. Using progressive JPEG format (raster image format defined by Joint Photographic Experts Group) for photographs and interlaced GIF (Graphics Interchange Format) format for line art will make images appear to load faster.

Testing the Site

One of the most important steps in Web site design is testing the site after it is constructed. Sites are often built and tested using state-of-the-art setups: large monitors, the most current versions of software, and, most important, the fastest modes of access. If your site is intended to provide information to members of the public, looking at it through their eyes (and their computers) can help you make sure it does its job as effectively as possible. Some aspects of the site to consider when testing it out include the following:

- *How long do pages take to load using a slow modem over a dial-up line?* Users are typically unwilling to wait more than 20 or 30 seconds. Some of the techniques mentioned earlier in this section can make the wait seem shorter (because images are materializing on the screen). Putting up brief descriptions that users can click on to proceed before the images load is another way to retain user interest and let them make progress—and to let them know what is on the screen if they have graphics turned off.
- *What do pages look like when viewed with different browsers or lower end graphics settings?* For example, do the pages still make sense if they are viewed with a text-only browser or one with deactivated graphics? What happens if the monitor is set to 16 or 256 colors rather than millions of colors (if the monitor cannot display some of the colors used, whatever is in those colors can "disappear") or if the screen resolution differs from that of the screen the site was developed on?
- *How "user-friendly" is the menu structure?* The goal is to strike a balance: If users have to wade through huge lists, they may get frustrated and quit looking before they find what they need. On the other hand, if they have to navigate through a series of menus, each with two or three choices, they may also get frustrated and stop before they reach their destination. Every screen they have to wait through increases the chance that they will get bored and go elsewhere.

- *If your pages are part of a larger site, what steps would users have to take in order to find the pages relevant to the initiative?* Most look for content, not departments. Many large organizations create Web sites that are arranged according to their organizational structure. This schema may work for their employees, but it has the effect of burying information on social change initiatives unless a search option is part of the site's home page.

MASS MEDIA

The traditional mass media—newspapers, magazines, radio, and television—provide a wealth of opportunities to deliver social change messages, and an important forum in which to do so. As discussed in Chapter 13, research on media effects and agenda setting has illustrated the important role the mass media can play in determining what we think about and how we perceive health-related issues and behavior. Planners of public health initiatives can use news coverage, advertisements, entertainment programming, or a combination of all three to reach their audiences through the mass media.

The mix of advertising and editorial coverage appropriate for a particular initiative depends on many factors. Program goals, communication objectives, the media environment, competition, and available resources all play a part. Chapter 13 included information to help you make those decisions. The following sections outline issues to consider once those decisions have been made and news, advertising, or entertainment products are being developed.

News Coverage

We use the phrase *news coverage* to refer to any newspaper, magazine, radio, or television content that is not an advertisement and, for television and radio, not an entertainment program. Public relations professionals often refer to this type of placement as *editorial* coverage because it encompasses all the content under the control of an editor, such as news and feature stories, columns, editorials, op-ed pieces, and letters to the editor. However, the term *editorial coverage* can be confusing to noncommunication professionals.

To successfully obtain news coverage of an initiative, it is important to understand

- how to build relationships with members of the media.
- how "newsworthiness" is determined.
- how to frame a topic to increase its newsworthiness and at the same time deliver the public health message.
- the characteristics of the various options for placement in each medium.

Building Relationships with the Media

The first step of effectively using the mass media is building relationships with the reporters, editors, and producers who determine what stories get covered. Many people are understandably uneasy about interacting with members of the media, but learning how to do so effectively can facilitate accomplishment of an initiative's goals. If your organization has a separate press office or public information department (and you are not part of it), a first step in planning media efforts is to determine what contact you can have with the media independent of that office and what support they can provide. This office may not be able to handle all of your media relations needs, either because of other responsibilities or because they have limited experience in "pitching" the media (trying to get them to cover a particular story).

The best way to begin building relationships with the media is by finding out who covers what. Read some recent issues of newspapers and magazines or watch or listen to recent shows to get a sense of what is covered and how it is covered. If you are working regionally or nationally, a number of media directories can help you identify media to target. One of the most popular is *Bacon's* (http://www.baconsinfo.com). Purchasing a set of the directories can be quite expensive (there are separate volumes for newspapers/magazines, radio/TV/cable, medical/health media, and editorial calendars), but local libraries often have copies. It is important to use the most current copies possible because reporters and editors change positions frequently. In addition to providing you with reporter and editor names and contact information, the directories provide statistics on circulation and audience size, information on the editorial profiles of publications and programs, and types of press materials accepted.

One of the goals of building relationships with reporters is to position yourself (and your initiative) as an important, reliable source of information so that the reporters will call you when they are running a story on your topic. Once you have developed a media list, you can send a package introducing yourself, your initiative, and why it is important to your community (or region or the nation, as appropriate). When reporters call, it is important to understand the parameters within which they work. In particular,

- be ready. Know how you want to frame the topic and have short, pithy "sound bites" developed to support this positioning.
- be sensitive to deadlines. If reporters call wanting additional information, ask what their deadline is and then make sure you get them whatever they need before then.
- be available. Make a list of who can talk to the press, and make sure someone on that list is always available. Make sure everyone else in the office knows who those people are.

- Be aware of the "rules" of talking to reporters: Never say anything to a reporter that you do not want to see in print or broadcast. With some reporters, it is possible to go "off the record" (i.e., say something that cannot be published or cannot be attributed to you as the source), but it is wise to do so only after you are sure you can trust the reporter.

Framing the Topic

In order to successfully gain coverage of a social change initiative, it is important to understand the goals of journalists, producers, and editors. In general, they want to appeal to the broadest number of audience members possible, and they want to tell a compelling story that is relevant to their audience and in the public's interest. Television producers need a visual aspect to the story as well. Therefore, it is incumbent on promoters of social change to frame the issues so that they are easily understood and have broad appeal. One way to ensure the latter is to frame the issue in terms of freedom, autonomy, independence, or control. Chapters 3, 6, and 12 discussed the process of framing an issue in more detail.

The following quote from an interview with Edwin Chen, at the time a science writer for *The Los Angeles Times*, on the role he has played in health communication campaigns illustrates the journalist's perspective:

> The U.S. surgeon general might say that smoking is bad or eating fatty food is detrimental for health, and heart disease prevention might be featured in a campaign by a government agency. But the *L.A. Times* does not see itself involved as a partner with, or part of, such education campaigns for health. The job of the *L.A. Times* is to cover the news. The newspaper might handle campaign press releases and promotional materials or report on the statements of different media campaign officials as long as such material is considered *newsworthy.* . . .
>
> Editorial decisions are made to do certain stories, projects, or a series about some specific issue. . . . For example, the paper might write news stories on how to lose weight or measures to reduce the likelihood of AIDS transmission, but it does not see itself as part of a campaign to combat AIDS or other health problems. . . . The newspaper also seeks to inform its readers about what the government and government officials, other agencies, and concerned people are doing or not doing in combating AIDS or other health issues. (As cited in Backer et al., 1992, p. 58, emphasis in original)

Signorielli (1993) described the characteristics that define news:

> Timeliness (news must be new); proximity (it happens close by or has psychological proximity); prominence (importance of the people); consequence (something that may have an impact on the lives of people in

the audience); conflict (clashing of opposing interests); and human interest (stories that arouse emotion). News also must be inoffensive, fit into existing constructs (typically stereotypes), have a window of credibility, and be able to be packaged in small discrete chunks or bites (the 20-second sound bite) (Dominick, 1990; Meyer, 1990). It also must attract and maintain an audience. (p. xi)

Exhibit 15–1, compiled by Wallack, Dorfman, Jernigan, and Themba (1993), lists some common questions journalists may ask themselves to determine whether a story is newsworthy.

As Wallack and colleagues (1993) noted, "media attention on health tends to be framed in terms of personal, individual issues that revolve around life-style, disease, and medical breakthroughs" (p. 56). Journalists often frame their stories from the vantage point of the individual's plight. Wallack and colleagues argued that this perspective creates problems when the goal is to stimulate policy changes, because it leads to an emphasis on what individuals should do to avoid a problem, rather than a discussion of changes that need to be made to address the underlying social or environmental conditions. One of the examples they cited is a crime story that focuses on what individuals can do to improve their safety (in reaction to a woman being kidnapped, raped, and murdered), rather than on what could be changed to improve the safety of the environment (e.g., better lighting, more secu-

---

Exhibit 15–1 Elements of Newsworthy Stories

- Breakthrough—What is new or different about this story?
- Controversy—Are there adversaries or other tensions in this story?
- Injustice—Are there basic inequalities or unfair circumstances?
- Irony—What is ironic, unusual, or inconsistent about this story?
- Local peg—Why is this story important or meaningful to local residents?
- Personal angle—Who is the face of the victim in this story? Who has the authentic voice on the issue?
- Celebrity—Is there a celebrity already involved with or willing to lend his or her name to the issue?
- Milestone—Is this story an important historical marker?
- Anniversary—Can this story be associated with a local, national, or topical historical event?
- Seasonal—Can this story be attached to a holiday or seasonal event?

Source: L. Wallack, L. Dorfman, D. Jernigan, and M. Themba, *Media Advocacy and Public Health,* p. 98, copyright © 1993 by Sage Publications, Inc. Reprinted by Permission of Sage Publications, Inc.

rity). Chapters 6 and 12 discuss how to work toward framing the content of coverage so that it better addresses the social issues rather than personal problems.

Tactics To Increase Coverage

Supporters of public health initiatives can employ a number of tactics to increase the likelihood that their voices will be heard. One popular approach is to create news, for example, by convening a press conference, special event, or demonstration. More details on press conferences and special events are provided later in this chapter. Demonstrations can take many forms. For example, Wallack and colleagues (1993) discussed how tobacco-control advocates used an embargo on Chilean grapes to gain access to the media: The grapes were embargoed after cyanide was found on them. At press conferences, advocates stacked several bushels of grapes next to a pack of cigarettes to illustrate the quantity of grapes needed to equal the cyanide in one pack of cigarettes and the difference in government policy on fruit versus cigarettes.

Another approach is to sponsor a study that frames the issue in a striking way. The Center for Science in the Public Interest (CSPI) has mastered this technique. Its studies often generate enormous media coverage and stimulate product changes because it successfully creates news that applies pressure to decision makers. For example, after its analysis of the nutrient content of movie popcorn was reported in the media, many major movie chains began using oils lower in saturated fat or offering air-popped options. This study illustrates the key components of CSPI's approach: Frame a critically important public health issue (the fat content of the American diet) in terms of a product many people use (broad appeal), at least some of whom probably select it because it is supposed to be "healthier" (irony and loss of control) and, instead of presenting numbers that people do not really understand (e.g., percentage of calories from fat or grams of fat), equate the fat to that found in a given number of Big Macs.

The latter part of the CSPI approach is something referred to as *social facts* or *social math*—the art of making numbers, especially large numbers, meaningful. Social math can be a valuable tool: It can help persuade a journalist to cover a story by increasing the perceived news value or providing a new angle, and it can make the story more compelling. Wallack and colleagues (1993), citing Pertschuk and Wilbur, described three approaches to making large numbers meaningful: localization, relativity, and effects of public policy. Localization involves taking a large national number (like tobacco causes 400,000 deaths in the United States each year) and applying it to a particular state or community. Relativity is what the preceding CSPI example used: Compare the number with something that audience members can easily identify. A variation is to make numbers smaller and more familiar. Wallack and colleagues wrote, "You might want to remember that $1 billion a year translates into roughly $2.7 million per day, $114,000 per hour, and $1,900 per minute" (p. 109).

Another important tactic is to summarize an issue's positioning in compelling sound bites, what Wallack and colleagues (1993) referred to as *media bites* and described as "short, concise summaries of your issue or position that can be conveyed in a few sentences or less than 10 seconds" (p. 112). Sound bites often make their points through ironic analogy, much as CSPI does when it reports the amount of fat in a food in number of Big Macs.

Coverage Opportunities in Each Medium

Newspapers, magazines, radio, and television all structure their news coverage somewhat differently and hence provide opportunities for different types of coverage. The following sections introduce some of the characteristics to weigh as tactics are planned.

Newspapers and Magazines. Newspapers and magazines both offer three main ways of reaching target audience members (other than through advertising): news coverage, a feature story, or a letter to the editor. Newspapers also offer the *op-ed* (opposite the editorial page) option. Beyond these basic similarities, each medium has important differences in terms of lead times, ratios of news stories to feature stories, and geographic area of interest. For the most part, newspaper reporters are writing tomorrow's story today, and with the exception of some special feature sections, newspapers contain mostly news. In contrast, magazine reporters and editors are writing July's story in January, February, or March, according to an editorial calendar determined long before that. Weekly news magazines (e.g., *Time, Newsweek, U.S. News and World Report*) fall between the extremes of daily newspapers and monthly magazines in terms of news-to-feature ratios and closing deadlines.

In newspapers, news coverage is often considered the most desirable because the news section of the paper tends to be the most read (especially by policy makers). In contrast, health-related feature stories often wind up in what used to be called the women's pages, although there are times when newspapers run feature stories that take more of a social justice perspective (particularly series) in the news section. Letters to the editor and op-ed pieces are useful because the writer retains control over the message (and op-ed pieces are widely read by policy makers), but they are often run in response to previous coverage of a specific issue. Wallack and colleagues (1993) recommended meeting with the newspaper's editorial board as an important way to ensure that the paper at least considers the perspective of the initiative. They noted that sometimes such meetings can result in an editorial supporting an initiative's position; at other times such a meeting may at least moderate the newspaper's criticism of the position.

Radio. Many practitioners think that radio is underutilized by social change initiatives (Backer et al., 1992; Wallack et al., 1993). Radio coverage of an initiative can include news programs, call-in shows, or a station's special promotion. News coverage often results from a written press release or an audio news release (a prerecorded story or interview that the station can run). Some initiatives make their experts available for interviews by station reporters during specific times, often in conjunction with an event; this process is often referred to as an *armchair media tour*.

Call-in shows are a chance to hear community reactions to a proposed social change, but also provide an opportunity for callers (or the host of the show) to disseminate messages that are decidedly off strategy. Before attempting to place a speaker on a call-in show or accepting an invitation to appear, it is wise to listen to a few shows to get a sense of the host and the audience.

Television. Television provides a number of openings to reach audiences with social change messages: news programs, talk shows, and entertainment programming. Entertainment programming is discussed in more detail in the Entertainment–Education section of this chapter.

For television news, the competition for high ratings is intensely competitive in most markets; therefore, what gets on the news is usually what producers think will be most shocking or intriguing when used on news promos throughout the day. Because television "wraps every story in pictures" (Wallack et al., 1993, p. 56) and news segments are short, stories must be visually striking and simple.

Television talk shows run the gamut from completely news-oriented to completely entertainment-oriented programs. Morning shows, such as *Good Morning, America* and its national and local equivalents, sometimes provide a forum to frame an issue (particularly if there is controversy about how it should be framed) or raise awareness of an event, such as the launch of a new initiative, or a specific week or day (such as the Great American Smokeout). Appearing on talk shows requires contacts with the producers; a celebrity spokesperson or a very newsworthy development coupled with an articulate, photogenic expert; and luck: The segment will get bumped if something the producers think is more important comes along.

News-Generating Tactics

The following sections discuss some of the basic building blocks that are used to generate media coverage.

Press Conferences. Managers of public health initiatives often reach for press conferences as a way to make their initiative a news story instead of a feature story. Press conferences can be useful, for example, as a tool for framing an issue, as discussed in Chapters 6 and 12. However, the decision to hold a press conference should be carefully thought through, because there are a number of potential drawbacks. Press conferences can be expensive, particularly when they are held in conjunction with a special event designed specifically for the media in an effort to increase turnout. There is a very real risk that no (or few) members of the media will show up. One breaking news story can ruin months of careful planning and preparation. Even without a major story stealing your thunder, reporters get paid to cover news. Although the launch of your new public education program may be very important to you, it may not be considered newsworthy.

If a press conference is held, Lewton (1991) provided what she described as "a number of tried-and-true press conference rules. These include using schoolroom-style tables and chairs, having visuals and handouts available, sending [media] kits and/or tapes to reporters who did not attend, having the conference somewhere easy for media to get to and limiting the conference to 30 minutes" (p. 201). Speakers should be the highest level, most visible individuals you can find. To attract television coverage, there needs to be something visually interesting at the press conference. Providing footage (or *b-roll*) of activities relevant to the initiative can also help increase television coverage. Such footage can be distributed on tape at the conference and sent to stations not attending, or the time and coordinates for a satellite uplink of it can be provided.

Handouts generally consist of, at a minimum, a folder containing the press conference agenda, speakers' remarks, speakers' biographies, a press release discussing the conference and reason for it, and a backgrounder (2- to 5-page description) on the initiative. Program logos and publicity photos are often included as camera-ready prints or slides. Setting up and staffing a sign-in table outside the room where the conference is held ensures that you know who attended. Inviting other people to the press conference guards against the room looking empty to the speakers if few members of the media appear.

Press Kits. The heart of many efforts to gain editorial coverage is the press kit. It can appear in numerous incarnations, from very simple to very elaborate, employing many different gimmicks. In efforts to generate ongoing coverage and establish a dialogue with reporters, it may appear as a newsletter rather than a kit.

The contents of the kit are determined in part by the reason it is sent. If it is in conjunction with an event (such as a press conference), the kit will generally include the event agenda; a news release covering who, what, when, where, why, and how; and background information on the program. It also often includes biographies of the speakers. If the kit is sent separate from any event, it often includes a news release or cover letter, sample story ideas, and artwork or photographs (or b-roll for television producers). Including slides or camera-ready slicks of the initiative's logo and those of sponsoring organization(s) is also a good idea.

For news releases and any sample stories that you include, use the inverted-pyramid structure that journalists normally use. The most important information should be at the beginning of the story, followed by progressively less important information. By using this structure if the story needs to be shortened to fit in the available space, it does not have to be rewritten.

For print media, quizzes and "top 10" lists can communicate key messages in a format many editors like and are disinclined to alter. Startling or unusual data presented in a graphically interested fashion are also useful, and many editors like to include mentions of materials that their readers can order.

Video News Releases. Materials that can be produced to support efforts to obtain coverage on television news shows include *video news releases* (VNRs) and b-roll (raw footage that producers can integrate into a reporter's story). A VNR is typically about 90 to 120 seconds long and designed as a stand-alone news story. VNRs to support public health initiatives frequently include an interview with someone authoritative, such as a physician, and often a target audience member as well. They can also include footage of the initiative "in action," for example, shots of a new clinic department or an event that took place as part of the initiative.

A standard VNR package consists of

1. the full narrated story (ideally with the announcer track on a separate audio channel from the natural sound to facilitate customization).
2. all supers or chyrons on separate slates in the order in which they would be used. (This allows stations to customize the VNR by using the typefaces they standardly use for any labels that will appear on the screen.)
3. 3 to 5 minutes of b-roll.

Practitioners recommend also including each element of the produced story (e.g., separate shots of expert interviewees answering each question) so that news outlets can localize the story and build it to suit the available time slot. For example, an interview segment can be localized by shooting a station reporter asking the same questions that the VNR reporter asked and then editing the interview segment together so that it appears the station reporter actually conducted the interview.

There are a host of technical factors to consider when designing and producing VNRs; the help of a producer skilled in broadcast news production is a must. The description of the production process outlined in the television advertising section of this chapter is also applicable to VNR production, although VNRs should be shot in broadcast news style. When selecting who will appear in a VNR and reviewing a rough cut, it may be helpful to keep in mind the following nonverbal elements that Kotler and Roberto (1989) identified as influencing communication effectiveness:*

Source: Adapted with the permission of The Free Press, a Division of Simon & Schuster from SOCIAL MARKETING: Strategies for Changing Public Behavior by Philip Kotler and Eduardo L. Roberto. Copyright © 1989 by The Free Press.

- *Vocal expression.* Messages should be articulated with a consistent and force-ful volume and by spoken voices that are neither "throaty" nor "breathy."
- *Facial expressions.* Facial cues can convey any of the seven primary emo-tions: happiness, surprise, fear, sadness, anger, disgust/contempt, and interest (citing Ekman, Friesen, & Ancoli, 1980).
- *Body movement.* Media figures who are given to more gestures and facial activity and who display a body-open position are more likable and persua-sive. Those who use more hand shrugging and more facial control are more suspect (citing Druckman, Rozelle, & Baxter, 1982).
- *Eye contact.* Media figures who sustain eye contact with their audience have a persuasive effect. However, sustained eye contact in the context of an ag-gressive message can have a negative effect.
- *Spatial distance.* The projection of intimate space is suited to intimate situa-tions and nonintimate space is suited to nonintimate situations. The violations of norms of personal space may render a message ineffective.
- *Physical appearance.* A physically attractive media figure is more persuasive than is an unattractive one. However, under some circumstances physical at-tractiveness can overwhelm a message so the viewer will recall an attractive communicator rather than the message that was conveyed.

VNRs can be distributed on videotape or they can be distributed via satellite by services such as Medialink. Prior to distribution, they can be encoded with an electronic marker and then tracked using electronic monitoring systems such as SIGMA (from Nielsen Media Research) and VeriCheck (from Competitive Media Reporting). Chapter 17 will discuss the type of tracking data available in more detail.

Entertainment–Education

Entertainment–education refers to the process of embedding social change messages in entertainment media (i.e., movies, television programs other than news, some radio programs, comic books). In an analysis of what "works" when designing health communication campaigns, Backer and colleagues (1992) noted that public attention can be achieved by embedding a message in an entertainment program, and that more effective campaigns utilize educational messages in enter-tainment contexts. They discussed the following examples of how the entertain-ment–education approach has been used:

- In 1989–90 the Harvard Alcohol Project got the concept of a "designated driver" incorporated into episodes of 35 prime-time television series. A sub-sequent evaluation by Winston (1990) showed a resulting increased use of the designated driver idea by the U.S. public.

- Johns Hopkins University has commissioned songs by popular recording artists in Latin America, the Philippines, and West Africa to deliver family planning messages. The 1988 song "Cuando Estmos Juntos" ("When We Are Together") recorded by Latin American singers Tatiana and Johnny was so popular in Mexico that it was played an average of 15 times a day over a period of several months. Backer and colleagues (1992) noted that "this massive, repeated exposure led to knowledge, attitude, and overt behavioral effects concerning sexual abstinence and contraception among the target audience of Mexican teenagers" (p. 169).

Other examples include

- *Once a Year. . . . for a Lifetime,* two half-hour programs (one in English and one in Spanish) that told the story of women whose lives were touched in different ways by breast cancer and educated about mammography and breast exams. The programs were produced by The Revlon/UCLA Women's Cancer Research Program in cooperation with the National Cancer Institute and distributed in part by the National Association of Broadcasters, which offered them free of charge to member stations.
- print and CD-ROM materials, such as comic books, novellas, and interactive "games" that teach about health.

As these examples illustrate, the entertainment–education approach can involve developing custom products or working with others who develop programming and materials to incorporate health messages. In the United States, developing custom print and CD-ROM (or Internet) products may be helpful to many initiatives, particularly for some audiences (e.g., comic books or a comic-strip format for young people, novellas when working with Latin American audiences, CD-ROMs for young people or the technologically inclined). To use an entertainment–education strategy with television, working with producers and writers of existing television programming is probably the most useful (and affordable) approach for most initiatives. Backer and colleagues (1992) noted that this approach is increasingly used by so-called "Hollywood lobbyists" who "seek to persuade U.S. television programs to give attention to their causes: alcoholism, AIDS prevention, mental health, the environment, gay and lesbian rights, and teenage contraception" (p. 169).

There are a number of reasons to include an entertainment–education approach as part of a social change effort. First, as was discussed in more detail in Chapter 13, the media help people structure their perceptions of reality, and when it comes to health behavior the entertainment media often do not provide accurate depictions of the consequences of health behaviors or good examples of appropriate behaviors. Second, many practitioners stress the importance of reaching audience members multiple times through multiple channels. Entertainment vehicles provide an additional way of reaching audience members and a means of reaching people who might not pay attention to a health program or product. Third, influencing existing programming is generally less expensive than developing custom programming and thus is more affordable for initiatives with limited resources.

Entertainment–education approaches can support a social change effort in many different ways. For example, they can be used to

- model skills and appropriate behaviors. Simple behaviors can be portrayed, such as wearing seat belts, seating young children in the back seats of cars or in safety seats, taking blood pressure medication, or scheduling a mammogram. Entertainment vehicles also provide a forum for illustrating more complex skills, such as the negotiation or refusal skills needed to manage sexual encounters (although it may be difficult to convince script writers to incorporate such topics into their story lines).
- educate about realistic consequences of health-related actions and medical conditions. For example, include concern about becoming pregnant or contracting the human immunodeficiency virus (HIV) in story lines that include unprotected sexual encounters or add characters with chronic conditions such as asthma or more serious illnesses such as breast cancer.
- influence social norms by portraying acceptable behavior, as the Harvard Alcohol Project previously described did. This influence can take the form of highlighting appropriate behavior or commenting on unacceptable behavior. However, when approaching writers or producers with suggested story lines, it should be kept in mind that television shows have sponsors and therefore are unlikely to highlight any behavior that might make advertisers unhappy. As an example, Backer and colleagues (1992) noted that the Harvard Alcohol Project addressed drunk driving, not alcohol consumption per se.

The idea of using entertainment media to "market" a behavior, product, or service has been around a long time. As Hirschman and Thompson (1997) noted, "the emergence of standard mass media formats such as soap operas, situation comedies, and game shows was intimately tied to advertising interests (Fox, 1985). Plot lines of soap operas, for example, were often written in conjunction with sponsors" (pp. 43–44). Commercial marketers also use entertainment media to convey a particular image for a brand and reinforce awareness through product placement in movies and television programs and tie-ins between products and entertainment programming. Backer and colleagues (1992) suggested that some product placement ideas could be incorporated into entertainment–education approaches; for example, encouraging set designers and production designers to use prevention-oriented posters as part of their set decorations.

Advertising

Advertising is at once a flexible and constrained method of communicating with an audience. It can be used by a social change initiative in many ways ranging from helping to frame an issue to modeling simple behaviors. Because print, out-of-home, radio, and television ads have unique considerations, each is discussed separately here. However, there are some basic principles that can be used to guide the development of all advertising, regardless of medium and whether placement will be paid or provided as a public service.

- Advertising provides an opportunity to communicate using the powerful cultural frames of reference created by the mass media. But as advertising researchers have noted, "the relative success of an advertisement depends not only on the rational merits of the message being promoted, but also on how well it appropriates desirable mass media images, styles, and cultural icons to its promotional purposes" (Hirschman & Thompson, 1997, p. 44; citing Jhally, 1987; McCracken, 1989; Scott, 1990; Sherry, 1987).
- Advertising messages should be consistent across media and consistent with messages delivered through other channels.
- The goal of advertising should be to sell, not entertain. As was discussed in Chapter 12, humor can be dangerous because sometimes people remember the joke but forget the product. Roman and Maas (1992) noted that there is no correlation between entertainment value and sales.
- As the saying goes, "Sell the sizzle, not the steak." The sizzle is the benefit to the consumer, not the product, service, behavior, or sponsoring organization.
- Celebrity spokespeople should be used with care; generally, it is not a good idea to build an entire campaign around a particular celebrity. Celebrity spokespeople can be effective if target audience members believe their involvement is authentic (i.e., the topic has personal relevance to them—they actually have the health condition or truly believe the social change is important; they are not just doing it because they are getting paid for it), and for campaigns relying on donated airtime, they can be an effective way to increase airplay. However, they can also overwhelm the message (people remember them but forget the product or service being advertised). Equally important, celebrities can do something embarrassing to your organization, such as hawking an "unhealthy" product or getting arrested for drunk driving, indecent exposure, or spouse abuse.
- With many health behaviors, it may be tempting to "scare" the target audience into the desired behavior. However, messages that involve threat appeals must provide a resolution and be carefully tested prior to use. Chapter 12 discussed the use of threat or fear appeals in more detail.

- The first few seconds of a radio or TV ad and the headline and visual of a print ad are critical: You must capture the audience's attention then, or you are not going to do so.

Print

Of all the advertising media, newspaper or magazine ads are the ones most likely to be tackled by "do-it-yourselfers," in part because the production process is more likely to be familiar. Creating great print advertising is much harder than it looks. The following tips, compiled from personal experience and from Roman and Maas (1992), are intended to help you assess print ads and get the maximum amount of use from them. Some of the suggestions for publications earlier in this chapter can also help you ensure print ads are effective.

- Writing print ads requires special expertise that other writers, even excellent ones, are unlikely to possess. Using an advertising copywriter is a good investment.
- When assessing a print ad, try to react to the whole message and assess whether it is on strategy. Once you have done that, the specifics can be examined.
- Ask to see the ad pasted in a likely editorial environment. Readers will never see it by itself, mounted on a board, and printed on glossy paper, so it is best not to assess it that way. Because print production is going electronic, the rough ad will look pretty much like the final ad, except stock photography ("for position only") will be used in lieu of custom photos.
- Illustrations are critical. As Roman and Maas (1992) noted, ideally, they will make the reader ask, "What's going on here?" In general, photographs are more compelling than artwork. Many small pictures are best avoided; they lead to cluttered layouts, and production costs more because you have to purchase the rights to each picture.
- As a general rule, a reader should be able to "get" the message from reading the headline alone because it is often all that is read. "Headlines make ads work. The best headlines appeal to people's self-interest or give news. Long headlines that say something out-pull short headlines that say nothing. Remember that every headline has one job: it must stop the reader with a believable promise" (copywriter John Caples, quoted in Roman & Maas, 1992, p. 45).
- Appropriate copy length depends on the message and the layout. Some argue that copy should always be short, but some very successful print ads have used a lot of copy. Body copy, especially long body copy, often causes much gnashing of teeth as everyone works to get it just right. It is more important to have an ad that works than to have perfect body copy in a weak execution.
- Remember that the ad may be reproduced in a range of sizes. What looks good and is readable on a full page may be lost if the ad is reduced to fit in a

small space in a magazine or newspaper. Initiatives with small budgets may need to design ads that will work in all sizes; those with more resources may want to consider Roman and Maas's (1992) recommendation to redesign the ad for various size spaces, for example, by cropping the photos used in smaller ads to suggest what appears in the larger versions.

- Black-and-white ads are usually distributed as camera-ready "slicks," but can also be distributed on a computer disk. Color ads can be distributed as slides or on computer disk (in a common graphics format). Many publications prefer ads distributed on disk because they can easily crop and scale the image to fit the available space.

Out-of-Home

The phrase *out-of-home* refers to two very distinct types of advertising: outdoor (billboards, posters, dioramas) and transit (ads appearing in buses and subway trains). Outdoor ads need to communicate instantly. Transit ads provide an opportunity for more complex messages; the Transit Advertising Association says the average ride is 22.7 minutes (Roman & Maas, 1992).

- "Posters are the art of brevity. Cut out all extraneous words and pictures; concentrate on essentials" (Roman & Maas, 1992, p. 54). The goal is to convey one very simple message. Billboards should have a maximum of seven words of copy; Roman and Maas argued that the best billboards use no copy at all (although that approach probably works much better for branded products than for behaviors).
- Transit ads that appear on the outside of buses and in train stations should follow the same rules as outdoor ads. Transit ads that are inside buses or trains provide an opportunity for more detail (remember, they provide an opportunity to talk to bored, captive commuters for an average of almost 23 minutes). They can also include tear-off pads to deliver coupons, messages, or "send-for-more-info" request forms.

Radio

Many health communicators think that radio is underused in health initiatives; radio commercials are inexpensive and quick to produce. Radio provides an opportunity to stretch the listener's imagination by using voices and sound to evoke pictures. Because of this characteristic, radio is, in many ways, an intensely personal medium. Radio can be a very targeted medium: There are over 140 different radio formats (e.g., all-news, classical, many kinds of country, many kinds of rock, etc.) in the United States (Roman & Maas, 1992). Radio ads can take the form of scripts for an announcer to read or recorded spots of 15, 30, or 60 seconds. Announcer scripts are more flexible; most can be used with all radio formats (types of stations). Prerecorded spots are appropriate for some formats but not others.

When evaluating a proposed radio spot, Roman and Maas (1992) recommended listening to it (have the copywriter read it or record it) so that you evaluate it the way listeners will hear it (they cannot go back and reread anything they do not understand). The following are some other issues to consider:

- Does it focus on one idea? Radio listeners have too many distractions to grasp or remember more.
- Does the ad tell target audience members why it is for them early in the spot?
- Does the ad reinforce messages delivered through other media?
- How will the spot work with the station format(s) targeted?

Television

Television ads are the most complicated and expensive to produce. They are also the most complicated to assess prior to production, because it is difficult for most people to make the leap from the concept to picturing the final product. As Roman and Maas (1992) put it, "the challenge is to look at a piece of paper with tiny illustrations and a few words and be able to visualize an involving, dramatic piece of film" (p. 15). Concepts for television ads are usually presented as a *storyboard*, which is basically a comic strip with a written description of what the viewer will see and hear underneath. Each frame illustrates the action of the ad.

Television ads usually use one of four approaches. *Demonstrations* can be used to model a skill or show a product advantage. *Testimonials* are endorsements from ordinary people, experts, or celebrities. They can help make a claim believable and are particularly useful when a behavior or product advantage cannot be visualized. *Slice-of-life* involves actors telling a story. Roman and Maas (1992) provided the following tips for creating effective slice-of-life ads: Concentrate on a single benefit, set up a human problem that the product or behavior solves (they noted that the classic slice-of-life always features a doubter who is converted), use an "authority figure" that is relevant to the product or behavior to deliver the message, use a demonstration to make claims more believable, and use a serious tone of voice (humor tends to lower effectiveness). The fourth approach, *animation,* can be especially effective when talking to children, but can also be a solution to other problems, such as simplifying complex ideas (often in demonstrations) or treating abstract (or even distasteful) subjects.

The following tips for evaluating storyboards and designing television ads were compiled from Roman and Maas (1992) and the National Cancer Institute (1989).

- *"Does it deliver the strategy as the central idea*? If it doesn't, *turn it down"* (Roman & Maas, 1992, p. 15).
- Look at the pictures first: Do they tell the story? As Roman and Maas (1992) put it, "television is a *visual* medium; that's why the people in the audience are called *viewers*. They react to and remember what they *see*" (p. 16).
- Is there a "key visual," or one frame that visually sums up the message?

- Does the commercial grab the viewer's attention in the first 5 seconds?
- Is the ad focused and single-minded? It must identify the issue or behavior, the consumer benefit, and the reason the viewer should believe the benefit in a 30-second ad. Sixty-second ads should not add points; they should tell the same story but with more time and detail. They provide an opportunity to repeat the message.
- Does the ad emphasize the solution as well as the problem?
- Does every word count? Thirty-second commercials usually allow no more than 65 words. If you want to add words, what words will you delete in their place?
- Is the message sent via both senses, sight and hearing? For instance, if the action is to call or write, does the ad show the phone number or address on the screen for at least 5 seconds and reinforce it orally?

Often, the answers to the next questions can be found in the research conducted to support development of the communication strategy. If not, it is a good idea to ensure that they are addressed during a pretest.

- Is the message presenter, whether an authority, celebrity, or member of the target audience, seen as a credible source of information?
- Is the message, and its language and style, considered relevant and appropriate by the intended audience?
- If music is used, does it aid, rather than subtract from, recall? Often two versions of the spot (one with the music and one without it) can be tested against each other to answer this question.

Because the process of producing a television ad is likely to be unfamiliar to many readers, Exhibit 15–2 presents the three phases of the production process and discusses the decisions that must be made at each step.

Public Service Placement

Successfully obtaining public service placement of advertisements requires building a relationship with the people who decide what public service ads a station or publication will run. Newspapers and magazines have no obligation to accept public service advertising. Many newspapers do not; many magazines run them only if they have unfilled advertising space. Because radio and television stations lease the airwaves from the public, they are regulated by the Federal Communications Commission and are supposed to serve the needs of their communities. Broadcasting deregulation in the early 1980s seriously weakened community service requirements, but nonetheless radio and television stations remain the largest users of public service advertising. Part of the job of each station's community affairs director is to determine what public service advertisements to use.

Exhibit 15–2 The Phases of Producing a Television Ad

1. *Preproduction decisions.*
   - *Talent—national actor, local/regional actor, real person?* There's no right answer, but generally the more important a role the actor plays in the spot, the more you need an actor with experience doing TV spots (it's nothing like stage or movie acting). If the actor is an extra or has a nonspeaking part, less experience is needed. A lousy actor can ruin even the best script—and voice, physical presence, and the ability to work with the camera are critical. Using "real people" can lend a touch of authenticity to a spot, but *very few* amateurs can handle the demands of saying it right in 6.5 seconds. If it's important that the copy be read as written, a professional actor is almost a necessity. Many clients take an active role in selecting the talent—either viewing a tape of auditions or actually attending the casting session—rather than letting a director or the agency pick the talent.
   - *Studio or location?* Again, no right answer. Location looks more realistic for "slice of life" spots, but it's much more difficult to control lighting, background noise, and so on, and location shoots can be more expensive than studio shoots.
   - *Film or videotape?* Videotape is cheaper and easier to do; film generally looks better (less harsh lighting, richer color, a better-quality appearance). Consider the budget and the "look" desired, and make the best choice, but if the cheaper choice can't produce a high-quality look, don't do TV spots. Pick a medium that can be afforded.
   - *Production company and director—Hollywood or Pittsburgh?* There's a lot of hype about how a Los Angeles director or a New York director is critical, but there are dozens of extremely competent, creative directors working with highly professional production companies in cities between the two coasts. Consider budget ("big-time" directors charge more per day and may have to travel a day to get to your city), and look at the reels (sample tapes of spots the director has done). You want creativity and a solid track record of satisfied clients.
   - *"Little details" that can ruin a spot—wardrobe, set, and props.* What the actors wear conveys an image—right down to earrings ("those look like rich lady earrings"). Don't count on the talent or the production company to come up with the right wardrobe—it's pretty expensive to stand around on a set while a production assistant goes out to find a different sweater. The same caution applies to props and set decor—the more specific you can be, the fewer the problems that will occur on the day of the shoot.
2. *The shoot.* The following are four principles staff members should observe:
   - *Be there.* Although many national clients are content to let the agency represent them when the commercials are being shot, they usually have budgets that allow them to reshoot spots if there's a problem.

continues

Exhibit 15–2 continued

> - *Be patient.* Shooting a 30-second spot can take 8 to 10 hours—or more. All of those little details—camera angles, lights, special effects, prop placement, and so on—can make the difference between a spot that looks professional and one that looks amateurish.
> - *Ask a lot of questions, so you learn and understand what's going on, but follow protocol on that set.* Some directors are happy to talk with you during the shoot; others want to stay focused on the talent and the camera and would rather have you talk with the producer or someone from the agency or crew.
> - *Be assertive.* If you see or hear something that bothers you—the way the talent reads a line, lights that cast ugly shadows, whatever—speak up. Listen to the explanations (there may be a good reason), but if it really bothers you, make sure the director understands why and is willing to discuss a compromise or alternative.
>
> 3. *Postproduction.* How a spot is edited—each scene selected and sequenced together—and finally produced (music, logos, special effects added) can have as much impact on the finished product as the talent does. Again, it's advisable to be present and have input into these decisions. The more costly alternative is to look at the completed spot and discover something that has to be changed.
>
> *Source:* Reprinted with permission from *Public Relations in Health Care: A Guide for Professionals* by Kathleen Larey Lewton, M.H.A., A.P.R. published by American Hospital Publishing, 1991. All rights reserved.

There are services that will handle public service placement for an initiative, but the cost can be high and often it is to an initiative's advantage for staff to build their own relationships with the community affairs directors. In order to do so, it is important to understand the environment in which community affairs directors work. McGrath (1995) outlined the following aspects of the community affairs directors' realities, based on presentations and discussions at four annual meetings of the National Broadcast Association for Community Affairs:

- Their activities are expected to generate or enhance revenues for the station.
- They strive to find a unique position for their station in their market.
- They work in a pressure-cooker environment and are always in a time crunch.
- They are more receptive to people and organizations they know on a personal basis.
- They are committed to their communities and to the organizations working to make these communities a better place to live.

McGrath (1995) made the following recommendations for working with community affairs directors, based on Grunig and Ripper's (1992) situational theory:

1. Help the community affairs director recognize the issue as a problem in the community. For example, provide information on how many people are affected and what the consequences are in terms of individual or family suffering, cost, reduced wages or purchasing power in the community, and so forth.
2. Identify and resolve the constraints the community affairs director faces. Three common constraints are a perception that the issue does not affect enough people; a perception that there are other, more serious issues; or the station is promoting another issue this year. McGrath's (1995) suggestions for resolving the first two constraints are to note, respectively, that although the number of people affected may be small, there is profound impact on individuals and their families; and other, more pressing issues can continue to be addressed while adding this issue into the mix. If a station is focused on promoting a different issue, he suggested identifying similarities between the issues or seeking a portion of time for other issues.
3. Increase the community affairs director's level of involvement with the issue. For example, he or she can be asked to review a script before production, to address a meeting, or to respond to a brief questionnaire about perceptions of conditions in his or her community.

Meetings and Conferences

Establishing a speaker's bureau provides an additional way to spread program messages and to increase the visibility of the organization and its contribution to the community. Basically, a speaker's bureau is a service for placing initiative spokespersons at events. It can be primarily reactive (e.g., responding to requests for speakers from community groups) or it can be a proactive component of the initiative, designed to spread program messages by seeking out appropriate venues for speakers. The latter form of a speaker's bureau can be designed to address groups within the general public or professional audiences.

Lewton (1991) advised setting up a system to efficiently book speakers by developing a three-part form that includes all details (group name; expected audience size and composition; date, time, location, and directions; audiovisual equipment needed; length, nature, and style of presentation; group's expectation of topic; and names and phone numbers for the group contact person and the speaker). Copies of the form should be given to the speaker and the contact person for the group the speaker will address. (One copy should be retained by the speaker's bureau coordinator.) Lewton also advised providing each contact person with a confidential evaluation form so that the performance of individual speakers can be monitored and addressed if necessary. In addition, the evaluation form provides an opportunity to improve future talks by assessing how relevant the information was to the group and what additional information they would like to have had presented.

Whether a speaker's bureau is proactive or reactive, it is a good idea to develop a standard presentation on the initiative (or, more broadly, the topic addressed by the initiative). Such a presentation normally consists of a slide show and accompanying talking points for the speaker as well as some type of handout for audience members. For coalitions or organizations with many members, this standard presentation can be duplicated and used by all members.

If slides are developed,

- be careful not to cram too much information into each slide.
- be aware that yellow lettering on a royal or dark blue background is most readable; combinations of red and blue tend to be the least readable.
- try out some sample slides to see if they are readable from a distance and in varying light conditions; many people use type that is much too small.
- use the right number of slides for the presentation. People should not feel like the slides are going so fast they do not have time to read them, but the slides should not sit up on the screen forever, either.

Special Events

A variety of events can be used to support implementation of the program and draw attention to the issue. Many public health initiatives are launched with some type of special event, often designed to increase media coverage. At other times, special events are used to generate media coverage of specific activities or to get target audience members involved. Some common events for health topics include conferences for professional audiences, health screenings (often at partner sites, such as a worksite, a shopping mall, or other areas where people congregate), or exhibits in conjunction with events sponsored by partners or intermediaries. If the initiative includes providing some type of service, sometimes a tour (for press or for potential users of the service) of new facilities is a good way to attract attention.

Special events require a great deal of planning, preparation, and resources. The first step is to delineate what you want to accomplish with the event and then determine what shape the event should take. Next, a date should be selected based on when other program components will take place, the amount of time needed to plan the event (as much as 4 months can be required), and the timing of other community, regional, or national activities that might impact the attention the event receives. It is generally wise to avoid 3-day weekends, holidays, and major vacation times (i.e., late December, school holidays in spring, and August).

In addition to the date, think carefully about the time of day for the event (assuming it is not predetermined because it is taking place in conjunction with something already scheduled, like a baseball game) and try to find out what time is best for the people you want to have attend.

As the event is taking form, remember to attend to important details, such as ensuring that food, if served, is healthful. Plan for some sort of material that participants can take away that reinforces the message. The material does not have to be elaborate, but it should be something participants would want to keep. Items such as refrigerator magnets, buttons, pens, pencils, or (for children) balloons or stickers can all be used to deliver short messages.

CONCLUSION

A broad range of activities can be used to draw attention to a public health initiative, including obtaining coverage in the mass media, establishing a presence on the Internet, speaking at various forums, creating special events, and advertising. The tactics used in a specific situation depend on the communication objectives, the audience(s) to be reached, the message(s) to be delivered, and the available time and resources.

REFERENCES

Backer, T.E., Rogers, E.M., & Sopory, P. (1992). *Designing health communication campaigns: What works?* Thousand Oaks, CA: Sage.

Cassell, M.M., Jackson, C., & Cheuvront, B. (1998). Health communication on the Internet: An effective channel for health behavior change? *Journal of Health Communication, 3,* 71–79.

Dominick, J.R. (1990). *The dynamics of mass communication* (3rd ed.). New York: McGraw-Hill.

Druckman, D., Rozelle, R.M., & Baxter, J.C. (1982). *Nonverbal communication: Survey, theory and research.* Beverly Hills, CA: Sage.

Ekman, P., Friesen, W.V., & Ancoli, S. (1980). Facial signs of emotional experience. *Journal of Personality and Social Psychology, 39,* 1125–1134.

Fox, S. (1985). *The mirror makers: A history of American advertising and its creators.* New York: Vintage.

Grunig, J., & Ripper, F. (1992). Strategic management, public, and issues. In J. Grunig (Ed.), *Excellence in public relations and communications management* (pp. 117–157). Hillsdale, NJ: Lawrence Erlbaum Associates.

Hirschman, E.C., & Thompson, C.J. (1997). Why media matter: Toward a richer understanding of consumers' relationships with advertising and mass media. *Journal of Advertising, 26*(1), 43–60.

Hornik, R. (1997). Public health education and communication as policy instruments for bringing about changes in behavior. In M.E. Goldberg, M. Fishbein, & S.E. Middlestadt, *Social marketing: Theoretical and practical perspectives* (pp. 45–58). Mahwah, NJ: Lawrence Erlbaum Associates.

Jaffe, J.M. (1997). Media interactivity and self-efficacy: An examination of hypermedia first aid instruction. *Journal of Health Communication, 2,* 235–251.

Jhally, S. (1987). *The codes of advertising.* New York: St. Martin's Press.

Kotler, P., & Roberto, E.L. (1989). *Social marketing: Strategies for changing public behavior.* New York: Free Press.

Lewton, K.L. (1991). *Public relations in health care: A guide for professionals.* Chicago: American Hospital Publishing.

McCracken, G. (1989). *Culture and consumption: New approaches to the symbolic character of goods and activities.* Bloomington: Indiana University Press.

McGrath, J. (1995). The gatekeeping process: The right combinations to unlock the gates. In E. Maibach & R.L. Parrott (Eds.), *Designing health messages: Approaches from communication theory and public health practice* (pp. 199–216). Thousand Oaks, CA: Sage.

Mediamark Research, Inc. (1997). *CyberStats, Fall 97.* Available: http://www.mediamark.com.

Meyer, P. (1990). News media responsiveness to public health. In C. Atkin & L. Wallack (Eds.), *Mass communication and public health* (pp. 52–59). Newbury Park, CA: Sage.

National Cancer Institute. (1989). *Making health communication programs work: A planner's guide* (NIH Publication No. 89-1493). Bethesda, MD: Author.

Roman, K., & Maas, J.M. (1992). *How to advertise* (2nd ed.). New York: St. Martin's Press.

Scott, L. (1990). Understanding jingles and needledrop: A rhetorical approach to music in advertising. *Journal of Consumer Research, 17,* 223–226.

Sherry, J.F. (1987). Advertising as a magic system. In J. Umiker-Sebeok (Ed.), *Marketing and semiotics: New directions for the study of signs for sale* (pp. 441–452). Berlin: Mouton de Gruyter.

Signorielli, N. (1993). *Mass media images and impact on health: A sourcebook.* Westport, CT: Greenwood Press.

Wallack, L., Dorfman, L., Jernigan, D., & Themba, M. (1993). *Media advocacy and public health: Power for prevention.* Newbury Park, CA: Sage.

Winston, J.A. (1990). *The designated driver campaign developed nationally by the Harvard Alcohol Project.* Cambridge, MA: Harvard University School of Public Health.

CHAPTER 16

Pretesting Messages
and Materials

Pretesting involves assessing how target audiences react to messages and prototype materials and identifying what needs to be changed before final production or implementation. It assesses whether messages are clear and compelling to audience members, identifies any unintended messages, and identifies other aspects of materials that may require modification. Common methodologies for pretesting include central-site interviews, focus groups, in-depth interviews, and professional review.

——————— ॐ ———————

THE ROLE OF PRETESTING

This chapter focuses on pretesting messages and materials. Other program components, such as new products or services or entire interventions, can also be pretested. Some of the methodologies discussed here may be helpful, or pilot tests (to be discussed in Chapter 18) may be employed.

Regardless of methodology, the goal of pretesting messages and materials is to assess message appeal, recall and comprehension, sources of confusion or offense, and motivation to act. Although materials pretests will not tell us exactly how materials will perform, they will identify any "red flags" in terms of unintended interpretations and executional details that need changing (typeface, type size, colors, music, voices, timing, etc.). Pretesting ensures that the final versions of materials contain messages that are clear, effective, true to the strategy, and easily understood by the intended audience and that they do not generate any unintended reactions. Pretesting also can help "sell" the materials internally by providing information on target audience reactions to counter criticism from non–target audience members.

415

PRETESTING MESSAGES: A CONTINUATION OF COMMUNICATION STRATEGY DEVELOPMENT

At times it is desirable to pretest messages before materials containing them are developed. Perhaps exploratory research conducted to inform communication strategy development was inconclusive as to which type of appeal would work best, or perhaps all message concepts were refined following exploratory research and need to be pretested with a wider audience before resources are expended on materials development. In such situations, the messages alone can be pretested, either via central-site interviews or an omnibus survey. (Both methodologies are discussed in detail later in this chapter.) It is unwise to explore reactions to the message and test materials at the same time, because it is extremely difficult (and often impossible) to determine what the participants are reacting to—the message or the execution of it.

When messages are tested, they are usually presented as statements, often in the form *"I (action) because (benefit)."* Respondents' reactions can be assessed a number of ways:

- Ask them to sort the messages from most compelling to least compelling. (This approach works best if the respondents are interviewed in person.)
- Ask them to indicate how much they agree or disagree with each statement (using a scale of responses).
- Ask them to rate each statement on dimensions such as believability, relevance, and importance to them (again, using scaled responses).

 If interviews are conducted in person, one useful way to pretest messages is to prepare each message as a separate brochure title or headline and ask participants which they would be most likely to pick up and why. If such a process is used, everything about the brochure covers should be identical except the message—the same type, colors, graphics, and so on, should be used.

PRETESTING MATERIALS

Materials that are often pretested include brochures or booklets; print, radio, or television advertisements; or longer audiotapes or videotapes. Sometimes only one version of the material will be tested; at other times, different approaches that convey the same basic message may be tested against each other. Materials being pretested can be in various stages of readiness; the most common formats are discussed here. Exhibit 16–1 lists some topics commonly covered in pretests; the exact wording of questions addressing each topic depends on the method used for the pretest. For example, see Appendix 16–A, which provides a sample mall-intercept questionnaire covering many of these topics.

Exhibit 16–1 Topics Commonly Included in Materials Pretests

GENERAL TOPICS

- What is the main idea of the (ad, booklet, etc.)?
- What, if anything, did you particularly like?
- What, if anything, did you particularly dislike?
- Was anything offensive? (What? Who would it offend?)
- Was anything hard to understand? (What?)
- Was anything hard to believe? (What? Why?)
- Who is this (ad, booklet, publication, etc.) for? Who would get the most out of it?

TOPICS FOR PUBLICATIONS

- How was the length of the publication—was it too short, about right, or too long? Are there particular sections that should be longer or shorter?
- Were there topics you expected to see covered that were not? Were topics covered that you think are unnecessary?
- Do you have any additional questions about the subject of the publication that were not answered?
- What do you think about how the publication is laid out? How easy or hard was it to find information? What do you think about the amount of white space used?
- What do you think about the type? Was it too large, about right, or too small? How easy or hard was it to read?
- What do you think about the language used? How easy or hard was it to understand?
- What do you think about the (photos or style of illustration)? How easy or hard was it to understand the diagrams? Are there places where diagrams or illustrations would clarify the text? Are there places where they are unnecessary?
- What do you think about the use of color? What types of people do these colors appeal to? (Certain colors have different meanings in different cultures; probe for cultural sensitivity if necessary.)
- Are there any other changes that you would make to improve the publication?
- Where would you expect to get the publication?
- For professional audiences: How would you use this publication in your work?

Brochures and booklets can be tested in near-final form, with all graphics included and all type in the proper places, or in manuscript form.

With today's desktop publishing capabilities, *posters and print ads* are most often tested in a form that looks finished to consumers. Headlines and text are final (unless changes need to be made as a result of the pretest), and the layout and typeface(s) used are those planned for the finished ad. If an ad includes photographs, stock photos that are similar to those planned for the final ad are generally used. Greek text (characters that look like words but really are not) may be used in ads with lots of body copy, or text.

If different headlines or tag lines are being tested against each other, all other elements of the ad, poster, or brochure (layout, typeface, type size, etc.) should be identical if possible. Print ads or posters are usually mounted on black poster or matte board for testing. If the final version will be in color, they are printed on a color-capable printer; otherwise, they are printed in black and white. Ads can be inserted into a magazine that respondents then flip through, but this process is more expensive and rarely done for social change efforts.

Radio ads and other audio products are most often tested in the form of scratch tapes, in which recordings are made by amateurs (often someone on the program or agency staff), rather than by the talent that will be used in the final version. These tapes do not have music or sound effects included unless they are critical to comprehension.

Videos and television ads can be presented as storyboards (similar to a cartoon strip, with separate frames depicting each scene and the script typed or written underneath), animatics (basically the storyboard is videotaped; the dialogue is also taped, and each scene changes to match the dialogue), or prefinished products (scenes are videotaped and the actual audio track is included, although final music may not be included).

The form in which video products are tested depends largely on the available budget and, to a lesser degree, on the characteristics of the final product. Each format is progressively more expensive. Storyboards almost always test much worse than the other versions because they are not as visually interesting and are often more difficult to follow. Additionally, if the interviewers read the script, each will read it differently, resulting in a less consistent test. Animatics are often used if the visuals include text, because it is difficult for someone to read the type and the script at the same time.

Prefinished products are obviously the best format to test because they are closer to what the final version will be like, but they are prohibitively expensive and rarely tested unless there is some reason they must be tested in that format (i.e., if there is no other way to truly communicate what the final product will be like). If a prefinished version is tested, one way to assess memorability of and attention to ads is to embed the material being tested in a few minutes of other advertising and then begin the test by asking the respondents what ads they remember seeing. An alternative is to use theater-style testing, discussed later in this chapter.

COMMON PRETESTING METHODOLOGIES

A number of methodologies can be appropriate for pretesting depending on what is being tested, the type of target audience, and the type of results needed.

These include central-site interviews, omnibus surveys, theater-style testing, in-depth interviews, focus groups, and professional or field review. The same basic process is followed for each type of study.

Step 1: Prepare a proposed study design (specifying study objectives, methodology, number and characteristics of participants, sampling method, rotation order, question topics, etc.).

Step 2: Prepare instruments (questionnaires for central-site interviews, recruitment screeners and topic guides for in-depth interviews or focus groups, and review forms or questionnaires for professional review).

Step 3: Arrange facilities if necessary (i.e., interviewing locations, meeting rooms).

Step 4: Conduct fieldwork.

Step 5: Analyze the resulting data using appropriate methods.

Step 6: Prepare a report containing a description of the methodology, a summary of findings, and recommendations for changes to the message concepts or materials, as appropriate.

Each methodology is described in more detail in the following sections. Pros and cons of the method are discussed, and considerations unique to the method for each step of the pretesting process are presented.

Central-Site Interviews

Central-site interviews are simply interviews conducted in a place where target audience members gather. Because these interviews frequently take place in shopping malls, this methodology is often referred to as *mall-intercept interview,* due to the way interviewers "intercept" shoppers as they walk around the mall, ask them a couple of questions to see if they meet the target audience description, and then expose them to the materials to be tested and ask them a series of questions about the materials.

With appropriate permission, a central-site interviewing methodology can be used at other places target audience members gather, such as clinics, meetings, fairs or other community events, or exhibit halls. The same methodology can be used to test materials among non–target audience members to make sure they do not offend, confuse, or upset such groups.

Central-site interviews can be thought of as a quasi-quantitative methodology. They are similar to quantitative studies in their design and administration: Most questions are closed ended, the interview itself typically lasts 10 to 20 minutes, and results are reported in percentages (i.e., 60% of the respondents understood the ad's main message).

However, the type of sampling used precludes being able to project the results to the population from which participants are drawn. Central-site interviews usually use convenience samples—the group of people interviewed is composed of those most accessible and willing to participate—rather than scientifically random samples where each member of a population has an equal chance of participating. Additionally, central-site interviews often involve quotas, or a preset number of interviews completed with people in certain categories. For example, a central-site interviewing study might be conducted with 100 men and 100 women, divided equally among predefined low-, middle-, and high-income categories. Once a quota has been reached, no further interviews with participants in those categories will be conducted.

When To Use

Central-site interviews are appropriate when you want to know how a target audience is reacting but do not need great detail on why they react that way. The methodology is generally not appropriate for exploratory work that requires probing by highly trained interviewers. Central-site interviews are commonly used to test messages and to test print, radio, and television advertising. They can also be used to test posters, brochure covers, or pamphlets. They are generally not a good forum for testing longer print materials because of the length of the interview that would be required. Sometimes only one item is tested; at other times, alternative executions may be tested against each other or executions in different media will be tested at the same time. The case study in Exhibit 16–2 discusses a central-site interviewing project.

Process

Step 1: Determine number of interviews, characteristics of the sample, and location(s) where interviews will be conducted. At least 60, and ideally 100, interviews should be conducted with each group of interest. For example, if you are interested only in overall reactions, then you can conduct 100 interviews. If you are interested in how women react compared with men, you will need to interview 60 to 100 women and 60 to 100 men. If you are interested in how different racial or ethnic groups react, you will need 60 to 100 interviews with each group of interest.

Each interviewee should also have specific characteristics based on the target audience definition. For example, if most target audience members are low income, or are the main food shopper in the household, interviewees should also have these characteristics. However, care must be taken not to set out specifications so narrow that few people will meet the criteria; this will increase both the time and the cost of the project enormously. Also, it is important to think about the environment in which the screening will take place when selecting characteristics that will be assessed using screening questions. Consider what would happen if mall-intercept interviews were being used to test a human immunodeficiency virus (HIV)-prevention ad targeting promiscuous young adults. An interviewer can-

Exhibit 16–2 Using Pretesting To Refine Television PSAs

BACKGROUND

The U.S. Department of Agriculture's Team Nutrition initiative was designed to improve the health and education of children by promoting healthful food choices through the media, schools, families, and the community. Media activities included television public service advertisements (PSAs) targeting young children.

Initial strategy development for the program included conducting mini focus groups with children in grades 3 to 5 and in-depth interviews with children in grades K to 2. The research revealed that children had difficulty recognizing foods that were high in fat or that contained grains, and that they did not immediately think of the latter as "healthy." Younger children also tended to have difficulty recognizing vegetables. Reactions to advertising concepts shown during the interviews and focus groups emphasized the literal interpretations children make and the need to be precise in communicating with these age groups.

Based on the consumer research findings, four 30-second television PSAs were developed and pretested. Three of the ads focused on eating the correct proportions of foods (based on the Food Guide Pyramid). Each ad tied a desired behavior change to a different benefit that children had mentioned during the qualitative research. The fourth PSA emphasized reading labels to eat less fat and illustrated a consequence: feeling bad from eating too much fat. All four used a humorous approach and featured the characters Pumbaa and Timon from the Disney movie *The Lion King*. Three of the PSAs used humor to deliver the main message; one used humor elsewhere in the spot.*

This case study is drawn from a paper that summarizes the initial qualitative research and the pretests (Doner, 1995). Objectives of the pretests were twofold:

1. To determine the key messages being communicated in the four TV PSAs.
2. To explore children's knowledge of foods containing fats and grains.

METHOD

The PSAs were tested in sets of two via mall-intercept interviews with children and adults. They were produced in animatic form (a videotape featuring accurate voices with video footage showing drawings of key action sequences) for the testing. The first pretest included children in grades K through 6 (divided approximately equally between those in grades K through 2 and those in grades 3 through 6) and parents of children in those grades. The second pretest was conducted with children in the same grades, but not with parents.

The following procedure was used for each pretest: (1) Potential respondents were intercepted in a shopping mall and a screening questionnaire was administered to the parent/guardian to qualify respondents with regard to the grade level of the child and to ensure a reasonable representation of various income and ethnic groups. (2) Each respondent was exposed to two back-to-back showings of the first PSA; the order in

---

*The PSAs were developed and produced by Disney as part of a cooperative agreement with the U.S. Department of Agriculture.   *continues*

Exhibit 16–2 continued

which the PSAs were shown was rotated from respondent to respondent. (3) The questionnaire for the first PSA was administered. (4) Each respondent was exposed to the second PSA. (5) The questionnaire for the second PSA was administered.

As with most central-site interviews, this research has two major limitations. First, the results cannot be projected to all children in these grades or to their parents, because the facilities where the interviews were conducted were all located in urban/suburban locations within large metropolitan areas. Additionally, respondents formed a convenience sample, in that not all members of the population had an equal chance of being selected—only those who went to the shopping malls on the days the interviewing took place. Second, respondents saw the commercials in a forced viewing situation with little or no distraction. For all of the information to be adequately communicated, multiple exposures in a normal viewing situation may be necessary.

RESULTS

- Key messages were most memorable when humor was used to communicate them. For the three PSAs that tied the key message to humor, the key message was among the most often recalled elements of the ad. In contrast, respondents were most likely to remember the humorous aspects—rather than the message—of the one spot that did not tie the key message to humor.
- The PSAs were effective in communicating the relative proportion of each food to eat. After viewing any of the three PSAs dealing with proportions, a majority of respondents thought that the lead character should eat a lot of fruits, vegetables, and grains, and some meat and dairy products.
- Overindulgence or gluttony was not communicated. Prior to the pretest, there had been some concern that children would think they should eat large quantities after seeing the PSAs (i.e., because one character dumps a wheelbarrow full of vegetables and a truckload of grains into the other character). When asked if the PSA said the character could eat whatever he wanted or if he should watch what he eats, the great majority of respondents said he should watch what he eats.
- Confirming the previous findings, children's ability to correctly name foods with fat in them appeared fairly limited, particularly among those in grades K through 2. Similarly, awareness of grains among children in the latter group appeared to be limited to cereal and bread, lagging significantly behind the awareness of their older schoolmates.
- The PSAs appeared to be age-appropriate: although each age group (K–2 and 3–6) preferred different PSAs, the majority of children thought each PSA was appropriate for their age group as well as younger or older children (although respondents from grades 3 through 6 were not sure someone older would like it).

As a result of the pretesting and comments received during the clearance process, one PSA was not produced because it did not appear to communicate clearly to children and because the joke overwhelmed the nutrition message. Two were produced basically as presented during testing. One was revised to place more emphasis on the benefit at the end and less on an earlier scene.

continues

Exhibit 16–2 continued

CONCLUSIONS

Testing the PSAs prior to final production identified an ad that was not communicating adequately and allowed revisions to be made to others to improve clarity of the final product. On a more global level, the testing also highlighted the importance of using humor carefully: Because it is likely to be what is most memorable about a communication, it should accent the main message. Finally, the testing replicated findings from the strategy development phase relative to children's understanding of the grains food group and their ability to find fat in food. It underscored the need to teach children the skills to make food choices based on grain or fat content.

not very well walk up to a potential respondent and ask, "How old are you?" and then "About how many sex partners have you had in the past month?"

The location where the central-site interviews will take place also must be decided. National campaigns often conduct interviews in two or more locations across the country, usually selecting places that are likely to have above-average concentrations of the type of people to be interviewed. If material is to be pretested with a professional audience, sometimes it is possible to hold the pretest in conjunction with a conference or meeting. In addition to geographic suitability, the location must also provide whatever logistical support may be needed. Can the respondents answer questions relatively free from distraction? If audiotapes or videotapes are to be played, is there a place to do so without disturbing others?

Step 2: Design the questionnaire and prepare materials. The first part of the questionnaire usually consists of two to four screening questions that are used to determine whether or not a potential respondent meets the criteria for being included in the project. The remainder of the questionnaire is the actual pretest.

A sample central-site interviewing questionnaire that illustrates the typical questions to include is shown in Appendix 16–A. As you can see, many questions are asked open ended—the respondent can give any answer—but likely responses are shown on the questionnaire, a process called *precoding*. This process speeds interviewing time by allowing the interviewer to circle the response rather than writing out each answer. Questions about the main idea, the call to action, sources of confusion, and likes and dislikes are often divided into "first mention" and "all other mentions." Separating the responses in this fashion allows the analyst to identify those responses that were most prominent—and therefore most likely to be remembered—in each category.

For questions that involve a preset scale of responses, interviewees are often handed a card with the response categories listed. If multiple materials are being tested at the same time, the order in which participants are exposed to the materials should be rotated to minimize order effects (differences in reactions to subsequent materials caused by exposure to previous materials). To facilitate rotation, separate mini-questionnaires are usually developed for each material.

At the same time, materials to be pretested must be prepared and reproduced in sufficient quantities. Each interviewing location will usually need two or three copies of the materials so that multiple interviewers can work at once. If products are being tested in audio or video formats, cassette players or VCRs will need to be available at each interviewing location and sufficient copies of the questionnaire and any other supporting materials (cards with response categories, etc.) must be available.

Step 3: Set up the interviewing process. There are three main ways of doing this: (1) hiring a commercial firm, (2) contracting with a college or university, or (3) conducting the interview yourself.

Hire Commercial Firms. There are a number of commercial market research firms that conduct mall-intercept interviews; some will also conduct them in other locations. The American Marketing Association's *GreenBook* provides the names, addresses, and phone numbers of commercial firms. Some firms operate only in a local area; others have outlets in a number of malls across the country and can recommend specific locations based on the target audience's demographic characteristics. These firms can conduct fieldwork (interviewing) only, or they can conduct the fieldwork, input the data, and provide cross-tabulations (termed *field and tab*). Some can also prepare reports, although asking for samples before relying on them is wise. The major disadvantages to using a commercial firm are cost and lack of control over quality. The major advantages are ease of interviewing in multiple locales, speed, and management: These firms are set up to do precisely this type of project. They already have the interviewers and the facilities, and they can manage the fieldwork and data processing.

Each component of the project is usually priced separately; a bid from a mall-intercept supplier will include the cost per interview (CPI), the costs for the respondent incentives (also termed *co-ops;* usually a nominal sum, such as $2 or $3 per person, or a lottery ticket or movie pass), the data entry costs, and the tabulation costs. The CPI is calculated based on incidence (the percentage of the overall population that matches the characteristics of the people you want to interview) and length of the interview. Some firms also charge rental fees if VCRs and monitors or audiotape players are required.

Contract with a College or University. Some colleges and universities have survey research centers set up that can conduct and analyze in-person interviews. Good starting points to locate them are the colleges or divisions of political science and journalism or mass communication. Another possibility is professors of marketing or communication research classes; often they will be willing to make such a study a class project. Using a college or university often ensures a more rigorous interviewing and analysis process; for example, the questionnaire will likely be pretested (commercial firms will do this for an extra charge). As with commercial facilities, the college or university will manage the fieldwork and data processing for you. However, using student labor usually significantly increases the time the study takes: It might take an entire semester, versus a few weeks if contracted out to a professional firm. In addition, questionnaires that will be administered by a university often have to be approved by human subjects committees or institutional review boards, and sensitive topics (e.g., sexual behavior) are likely to be rejected.

Conduct the Interviews Yourself. If you are planning to conduct your own central-site interviewing project, as a first step you will need to obtain the necessary approvals from the site management. Many "public" places people gather (e.g., shopping malls, sporting events, grocery stores, schools, etc.) are either privately owned or covered by local ordinances restricting their use. Next, you will need to locate a source of interviewers. Voluntary organizations may be able to rely on their pool of volunteers. Other sources include college students, respondents to an ad in a local newspaper or a community organization's newsletter, or respondents to flyers placed where people congregate. Once a sufficient number of interviewers have been recruited (to calculate how many are needed, consider how quickly the project needs to be done, how long each interview will take, and about how long it will take to find people meeting the study criteria), they will need to be trained to administer the questionnaire.

In general, good interviewers are outgoing enough to be comfortable approaching people they do not know, capable of quickly putting others at ease, and articulate without dominating conversations. They should also be patient and capable of following instructions. The latter traits help ensure that they will let respondents complete their answers and that they will be able to consistently and accurately administer the questionnaire. Exhibit 16–3 provides some suggestions for training interviewers.

Step 4: Conduct interviews. People at the interviewing site who appear to meet the screening criteria (e.g., correct gender, race or ethnicity, or age) are approached and the interviewer asks the screening questions. Those who do not meet the screening criteria are "terminated": The interviewers politely explain either that they have already talked to enough people possessing that criterion or that they want to talk to people who possess the criterion the person does not have (e.g., "I'm sorry, we need to talk to people who do most of the shopping for their household").

Those who meet the criteria are asked if they would be willing to review the materials and answer a few questions. After each interview, the questionnaire should be reviewed by the interviewer for completeness; it should then also be reviewed by a field supervisor.

Exhibit 16–3 Tips for Training Interviewers

---

1. Begin by explaining the project and its purpose.
2. Provide interviewers with a copy of the questionnaire and all supporting materials.
3. Demonstrate an interview.
4. Explain the process, covering details such as
   - the number of times (or length of time) respondents should view materials
   - the need to read each question exactly as written each time (if interviewers start reciting from "memory" the wording will change significantly over time)
   - how to record responses to each question, especially those for which the respondent may have multiple answers
   - the need to review each questionnaire for completeness immediately after the interview
   - What to do with completed questionnaires
5. Have interviewers role play: One administers the questionnaire to the other. The act of administering the questionnaire allows the interviewer to identify questions—and get answers—before they come up during a "live" interview.
6. Discuss any additional questions.

Step 5: Input and analyze data. If you contracted out the interviewing, the organization that did the interviewing probably will handle this process for you. If you are doing the project yourself, you can often find a graduate student to handle this task or you can train someone on your staff.

The most popular analysis of central-site interviewing data involves cross-tabulations, usually referred to as *cross-tabs* or *stub and banner tables*. The answers to each question are presented as a separate table, and the columns of the table are different groups of people. These columns are often termed *banner points*.

The first step of analysis is setting the banner points or determining what groups to examine. The first banner point is usually the total sample; the others are subgroups of interest, such as men and women, different interviewing locations, and so forth. If the same questions were asked for different ads, the ads themselves may be the banner points, so that differences between them can be quickly seen. For example, perhaps 70% of respondents correctly understood the main message of the first ad, but only 40% understood it in the second ad.

Most statistical software can handle a total of 16 to 20 banner points, and commercial suppliers charge the same regardless of how many banner points are included, provided the maximum is not exceeded. If demographic groups are being included in a banner, often it is helpful to examine the frequency distribution (also termed *marginals)* before setting the banner points. Sometimes it is useful to combine two or more groups if few respondents fall into each category. Similarly, looking at the frequency distribution provides an opportunity to combine response categories where it makes sense to do so. Central-site interviews often include questions for which the interviewer can write down any "other" response a participant has. These responses can often be combined into groups to facilitate analysis.

If the interviewing was conducted at multiple locations, most researchers include location in the banner so that they can look at the pattern of responses and determine if there are differences between one interviewing location and another. Sometimes this is the result of true differences in respondent reactions, but other times it indicates a difference in how the questionnaire was administered and warrants further investigation.

Although most central-site interview questionnaires are relatively straightforward, it is a good idea to have someone trained in data analysis review the tables to ensure that they were set up properly.

Step 6: Prepare the report. After the tables have been prepared, it is time to review and interpret the results. Although many managers would like rules of thumb by which to judge pretest scores, the reality is that a number of factors influence how pretest results should be interpreted, including the type of material being tested, the format and situation in which it was tested, and the original communication objectives.

If the material being tested is an ad or something like an ad (i.e., a poster), then its "main message" score should be relatively high because it should have only one main message. Longer materials, such as videos or booklets, may have multiple messages.

As discussed earlier, materials can be tested in a variety of formats. Generally speaking, video products will score higher if they are shown as animatics or live action, rather than as storyboards. All materials will score higher for message recall if they are shown alone rather than embedded in other material. Materials that were developed based on a clear communication strategy and one objective will generally test higher than those with multiple objectives.

If different ads were tested at the same time, it should be possible to compare their scores and assess their relative strengths and weaknesses. To interpret results in absolute terms, for advertisements that are tested alone (i.e., not embedded in other ads or programming), a good rule of thumb is that at least 70% of respondents should recall the main message and understand the call to action (what they are being asked to do). Any source of confusion, dislike, or other concern mentioned by more than 15% to 20% of participants should be addressed during revisions.

Omnibus Surveys

If messages are being tested independent of materials, sometimes it is possible to test them by adding questions about them onto a local or national telephone *omnibus survey.* Such surveys are so named because they are conducted by research vendors who include questions from a number of different organizations. Omnibus surveys have the advantage of being projectable to the population, relatively inexpensive, and (for national studies) fast. For example, questions can be submitted to the vendor on Thursday and go into the field on Friday, with data back as soon as the following Tuesday or Wednesday. Many universities and local commercial firms also offer omnibus studies of a state or metropolitan area; however, these may be conducted relatively infrequently (once a quarter or twice a year is not unusual).

When To Use

Omnibus surveys are appropriate if the target audience is a sufficiently large segment of the general population and if the messages can be understood when expressed as simple statements with minimal (or no) background information. For example, omnibus studies can be an ideal way of assessing how voters will react to alternative ways of framing a message about an issue coming up for vote. If the message requires a substantial amount of education before it will be understood, omnibus surveys are a poor choice of testing methodology.

Process

Step 1: Determine the characteristics of the sample. Most national omnibus surveys interview 1,000 adults, who represent the general public. However, you can develop screening questions to identify those people meeting your target audience criteria (e.g., registered voters, women over 40, or parents with children in grades K–12) and instruct the vendor to administer your questions only to those people. Although omnibus surveys are not an appropriate choice if the target audience is a small proportion of the general public, if the vendor conducts regular surveys (some conduct national studies weekly or more often), your questions can be included on more than one "wave" of the omnibus to increase the number of respondents fitting your target audience criteria.

Step 2: Design questions. The questions should be written by someone trained in survey questionnaire design. There are any number of factors to take into account to properly write survey questions and response scales. Most questions should be closed ended; it is possible to ask precoded or open-ended questions, but they are significantly more expensive. At the current time, omnibus questions cost approximately $750 for closed-ended questions and $1,200 to $1,400 for completely open-ended (no precoded responses) questions. The Pretesting Messages section at the beginning of this chapter provides some suggestions for question design.

Step 3: Identify vendor. There are a number of research vendors that conduct national omnibus surveys, including ICR/International Communications Research (EXCEL), Market Facts (TeleNation), Opinion Research Corporation (CARAVAN), and Roper Starch Worldwide (Limobus). As noted earlier, vendors and universities also conduct local surveys in many major metropolitan areas.

Steps 4 and 5: The research vendor will handle conducting the interviews, inputting the data, and producing cross-tabulations according to your instructions. In addition to the questions you ask, you will be provided with complete demographic information on respondents (age, gender, marital status, education, whether they reside in metropolitan or nonmetropolitan areas, region of the country, household income, presence of children, etc.). More sophisticated analyses can also be performed for additional cost. As with central-site interviews, the answers to each question are presented as a separate table; the columns of the table are different groups of people. These columns are termed *banner points* and must be specified by you. The discussion of banner points in the Central-Site Interviews section of this chapter is also relevant to omnibus survey analysis.

Step 6: Prepare the report. After the tables have been prepared, it is time to review and interpret the results. Research vendors can provide this service at additional cost, but often it is best to have a trained communication researcher who is familiar with the initiative review the data and develop conclusions and recommendations based on the results.

Theater-Style Testing

In this type of pretesting, members of the target audience are brought to a central site to view PSAs or short educational videos embedded in other programming. The audience can either complete a self-administered questionnaire after viewing, or more sophisticated audience response systems can be used. In the latter, respondents press a button when something captures their attention.

The advantages of theater-style testing are that large numbers of people can view the ad or program at the same time and the research team can control administration of the questionnaires more carefully than with central-site interviews. Disadvantages include high production costs (the video must be final or very nearly final) and limitations on the type of people who can participate (those with limited literacy skills may not be able to complete a self-administered questionnaire accurately or at all). Additionally, theater-style testing at a commercial facility is likely to be significantly more expensive than mall-intercept interviews because people will have to be prerecruited and will want more compensation for their time than is necessary with the minimal time commitment involved with a central-site interview. Alternatively, you can set up a theater-style test yourself; an appendix to the National Cancer Institute's *Making Health Communication Programs Work* (National Cancer Institute, 1989) provides detailed instructions for doing so.

When To Use

Theater-style testing is appropriate when video products need to be produced in near-final form to be accurately pretested, or for longer products such as training videos or dramatic programs that are initially produced with the knowledge that they will have to be revised prior to final production.

Process

The process for theater-style testing is similar to that for in-depth interviews; however, some modifications are required due to differences in how participants are recruited and how the questionnaire is administered.

Step 1: Determine the locations(s) where pretests will take place and number and characteristics of participants. The location can be a commercial market research facility that contains a sufficiently large viewing room, a school auditorium, or another room of adequate size.

Participants can be recruited by the commercial facility or through other means, such as an ad in a local newspaper or community groups. As with central-site interviews, ideally 60 to 100 people will participate. A good rule of thumb is to assume about 20% of those recruited will not show up and overrecruit accordingly. To look at differences between subgroups (e.g., based on gender or age), you can either conduct one large theater-style test or convene several sessions.

Step 2: Design the questionnaire and prepare the materials. Because the questionnaire will be self-administered, it will look somewhat different from a central-site interview questionnaire. Many of the questions will be the same, but open-ended questions will not have a list of precoded responses. Also, questionnaires for theater-style testing of advertisements often begin with questions about the programming in which the ad was embedded or with a question asking which ads the respondent can remember. To partly control the order in which participants answer questions, it is sometimes helpful to divide the questionnaire into sections and include a note at the end of each section instructing participants not to proceed until asked to do so.

Step 3: Administer the questionnaire. The questionnaire is generally distributed to participants after they view the video. If a particular ad is being tested, respondents often answer a question abcut which ads they remember, then they are shown the ad being tested again, and then they answer additional questions.

Steps 4 through 6: Data entry, analysis, and reporting. These steps follow the same process outlined under the Central-Site Interviews section.

In-Depth Interviews

When To Use

In-depth interviews can be used if getting audience members to a central site is not feasible or would be cost prohibitive. The process can be very similar to that used for central-site interviews, except the interviewer goes to the interviewee rather than vice versa. This technique is often used with target audiences such as health professionals or policy makers. Sometimes the participants receive an honorarium; at other times the interviewer may compensate the participants in another way, by paying for a standard office visit, for example, or by making a charitable donation on the participant's behalf. In some instances, no compensation is necessary. For example, informal in-depth interviews might consist of meeting with legislative staff to assess their reactions to various regulatory proposals.

When it is desirable to pretest materials with audience members located across the country, in-depth interviews can be conducted over the phone. Participants are sent the materials to be pretested, and then the interviewer calls and schedules an appointment to review the materials and administer the pretest. To control length of exposure, sometimes participants are asked not to open the package of materials until they are on the telephone. Obviously this approach works only for print materials; testing audio or video materials in this fashion would be logistically challenging.

Alternatively, participants may be sent the materials and a review form. They can be instructed to mail back the review form or an interviewer can call to collect their responses. Implementation of this approach is discussed in more detail under the Professional and Field Review section of this chapter.

If highly trained interviewers are used, in-depth interviews provide an opportunity to explore why participants react in a particular way as well as how they react. The disadvantages of in-depth interviews are primarily high cost, timing, and sample size. Labor costs can be much higher because the interviewers are usually more senior than those used for central-site interviews, the length of the interview tends to be longer, and analysis is more labor intensive. Additionally, in-depth interviews can take much longer to field than central-site interviews because they usually involve fewer interviewers (often only one or two) and the process involves locating a list of potential participants, then scheduling the interviews and conducting them. Because of the cost and timing issues, sample sizes for in-depth interviews tend to be smaller.

Process

Step 1: Determine number and characteristics of people to be interviewed and identify source of names. At least 15 to 20 in-depth interviews are needed; each subgroup should include at least 10 respondents, and 15 to 20 would be preferable.

Step 2: Draft the questionnaire. The in-depth interview questionnaire will cover many of the same topics as a central-site interview questionnaire, but probes—questions to elicit insight into the participant's response—are included.

Step 3: Arrange interviewers. Sometimes in-depth interviews are carried out by program staff (if they have appropriate interviewing skills). (The tips on training interviewers provided under the Central-Site Interviews section of this chapter can help bring novices up to speed.) Initiatives with more resources may contract the interviews out to researchers at communications or market research firms. Market research firms often price such projects on a cost-per-completed-interview basis. They may or may not charge separately for the cost of obtaining names, addresses, and phone numbers of potential participants and for report preparation. Communications firms most often quote an estimate for the total project. If they do not provide one, ask to see a breakdown of their anticipated costs, including labor hours, so that you can assess whether they have a good grasp of the scope of the project.

Step 4: Conduct fieldwork. In-depth interviews for pretesting can be coordinated a number of ways. It is usually best to call potential participants and schedule the interview first. If the interviews will be conducted over the phone, you can then send the packet of materials and call back for the interview at the scheduled time. Participants can be asked to review the materials before the interview or to wait until the interview to open the package. For in-person interviews, a packet of materials can be sent ahead if they will take a while to review, or the interviewer can present the materials during the interview. Whenever participants are reviewing materials ahead of time, a self-administered questionnaire can be enclosed; detail on its construction is discussed in the Professional and Field Review section of this chapter. Tips on conducting in-depth interviews were provided in Chapter 11.

Steps 5 and 6: Analysis and reporting should be conducted in accordance with the principles detailed in Chapter 11. For example, unless large numbers of interviews are conducted, results should not be reported in percentages.

Focus Groups

Focus groups tend to be used for pretesting more often than advisable. They are not an appropriate way to test final copy, but they can be a useful way of gathering information on overall reactions to lengthy materials—particularly if there is some reason to expect that people are likely to discuss the material—and ideas on how the materials might be distributed or used. Conducting a focus group in order to pretest materials is similar to conducting a focus group for any other purpose; details of the methodology were presented in Chapter 11.

Focus groups allow information to be gathered from several people at once, but do not provide as many respondents as central-site interviews or theater-style tests. The results are by nature more subjective and open to interpretation than methodologies involving more people or one-on-one questioning. Reporting the percentage of participants who gave a particular response is not possible.

When To Use

For long materials, such as booklets, focus groups are likely to be the most economical way to pretest the information. Often, scheduling in-depth interviews to review the material with each participant would be cost prohibitive: Far more hours of moderator or interviewer time are required, and if participants are recruited by a commercial facility and the interviews are conducted at its location, facility rental charges will also be much higher than for focus groups because the facility will be used for so much longer. Central-site interviews are often not feasible for such materials because of the time required to review the material and then answer questions.

Focus groups are inappropriate when the material to be tested is brief and target audience members would not be likely to discuss it with others if they encountered it during their daily life. For example, most people do not discuss ads that they see with others unless the ads are particularly provocative. By showing ads and then forcing a lengthy discussion, even the best ad is likely to be torn to shreds, and much of the feedback will not be helpful because the group setting is unrealistic.

Process

Step 1: Determine number of focus groups and characteristics of people to be included in them. As with all focus group projects, at least two groups should be conducted with each type of participant. If the groups will be conducted in different cities, usually at least two should be conducted in each city. Different types of participants should be placed in separate groups whenever combining them is likely to hinder discussion. For example, men and women are often separated, as are people of difference races, ages, or socioeconomic status. However, it is important not to get carried away with dividing up participants or you will end up with an unmanageable number of groups. Always assess whether different characteristics will truly hinder discussion. Generally, the more sensitive the topic, the more cause for concern.

Step 2: Prepare instruments and materials. Instruments for focus groups generally include a participant recruitment screener and a moderator's guide. Chapter 11 discussed preparing both. For pretests in which participants are sent materials ahead of time, a self-administered questionnaire that participants complete prior to the group can also be useful; developing it is discussed later in this chapter under the Professional and Field Review section.

Materials for focus group testing are generally produced in formats similar to those that would be used for mall-intercept interviews. If they are to be sent to participants beforehand, they will need to be reproduced in sufficient quantities to send each participant a copy. If they are to be shown in the groups, often only one or two copies are produced, unless the materials are long or participants are supposed to look them over and respond individually.

Step 3: Arrange a meeting place and moderator(s). Most major metropolitan areas have one or more commercial focus group facilities; the previously mentioned *GreenBook* provides listings. Alternatively, you can handle the logistics yourself and conduct the groups in hotel meeting rooms, office conference rooms, or classrooms. Details were provided in Chapter 11.

Step 4: Conduct focus groups. Materials can be sent to participants beforehand so that they have a chance to review them in detail. Alternatively, material can be presented to participants during the course of a group; however, some amount of time must be allotted to let them review it. Having participants complete a self-administered questionnaire at the beginning of the group will provide individual reactions to the material. The group can then be used to discuss overall reactions and topics such as how the material will be used, where participants would expect to obtain it, and who should be providing it.

Steps 5 and 6: Analysis and reporting should be conducted in accordance with the principles detailed in Chapter 11. If a self-administered questionnaire was used in conjunction with the focus groups, the analysis of it generally should be presented in a separate section of the report.

Professional and Field Review

Methods of conducting professional review include sending materials and a review form to each reviewer or convening a meeting at which materials are presented.

When To Use

Asking other professionals to review proposed messages or materials serves a number of purposes. Their review helps to ensure that the information presented is sound, enhances the credibility of the messages or materials with other stakeholders, and can help obtain buy-in from others likely to be overseeing program components that communication activities need to integrate with and support.

Some of the approaches used for professional review can also be used in other pretesting settings where it is desirable to have gatekeepers or target audience members review the materials and complete a self-administered questionnaire assessing the materials and how they could be used.

Process

Step 1: Determine the review process and number and identity of reviewers needed. Will you need to mail out the review forms, or will the review take place in conjunction with a meeting? It is often difficult to get all reviewers to return review forms.

Step 2: Prepare the questionnaire and materials. Exhibit 16–1 includes the types of questions that are often found on professional or field review forms. In addition to the questions, the forms should include a brief description of the materials and what they are for and, most importantly, the address to which they should be returned and the date they are due (unless this information is unnecessary because the review will be conducted as part of a meeting). Reviewers are often instructed to write directly on the materials, in addition to filling out the review forms.

Step 3: Arrange a facility if necessary. If reviewers will be gathered together, arrange a meeting room or time on the agenda of an existing meeting, as needed.

Step 4: Conduct fieldwork. The first step of conducting the fieldwork is to mail the packages containing review forms and materials, or to set up the meeting if that is how the review will take place. If the review forms have been mailed, you may have to follow up with reviewers in order to get the forms returned in a timely manner. The effort you put into follow-up depends in part on how important it is to have the reviews returned. If you asked for reviews simply to avoid later accusations that you did not provide an opportunity for others to comment prior to finalizing materials, then no follow-up may be necessary. If, on the other hand, you sincerely need the comments to finalize the materials, you may need to send a reminder post card or make reminder phone calls. Another technique that is often equally or more effective is to remind before the pretest is sent: Send a post card or call reviewers to let them know the material is coming and remind them that their feedback is very important.

Step 5: Analysis. The approach to analysis depends in part on the number of reviews received. A small number can be tallied by hand on a blank review form, particularly if most questions were closed ended. The aid of a computer will be helpful with a larger number of reviews, particularly if there is any desire to break out different types of respondents (e.g., to compare health professionals with teachers).

Open-ended responses or other comments can be handled two ways. The main themes can be summarized in the report, or the reviewers' comments for each question can be compiled. The latter approach is a useful way of consolidating all comments.

Step 6: Reporting. A report on professional or field review generally includes an introduction (background on the project, descriptions of materials to be tested, and pretesting objectives), methodology (number of reviewers, how they were selected, etc.), findings, and conclusions and recommendations. It is often useful to include a marked-up copy of the materials that were tested, with all of the reviewers' comments written on it. This allows managers to see all of the comments together.

CONCLUSION

Pretests provide an opportunity to refine materials prior to final production by assessing how target audience members and gatekeepers will react to materials. A properly designed pretest can assess whether materials are understandable, attention getting, memorable, and relevant to target audience members. It can also identify any sources of confusion or offense.

Answering the following questions will help you design and conduct a successful pretest.

What is being tested? For example, if an ad is being tested, a focus group setting is unrealistic. People usually do not see an ad and then spend 2 hours discussing it with a group of people. A one-on-one interview provides a more realistic setting: The interviewer can show the material to the participant for a fixed amount of time (e.g., take back a printed piece after 1 minute or play a video or audiotape once) and then ask him or her a series of questions about it. Although this situation is still unrealistic because it forces participants to think more about the material than they otherwise might, it is less unrealistic than forcing them to discuss it with others.

Why is it being tested? Do you want to assess overall communication effectiveness, or are there concerns about particular aspects of the material, such as content, voices, music, and so forth? Is it important to know how participants will obtain, use, or distribute the material as well as how they react to it? The answers to all of these questions help shape what is included in the questionnaire.

With whom does it need to be tested? Are you interested in target audience reactions? Gatekeeper reactions? Both? Is your audience a group that can easily be recruited at a central location, such as a shopping mall? Some low-incidence populations, such as recently diagnosed adults with asthma, may be recruited most easily by working with a clinic. Perhaps an option is to interview people at a clinic while they wait for their appointment.

In what geographic locations does it need to be tested? If the material is for a local program, this question may not arise. For regional or national programs, sometimes it is important to obtain reactions from people in different parts of a state or of the country. This may affect your choice of methodology or your choice of vendors.

When are results needed? Obtaining results by mail usually takes the longest amount of time, particularly if packages are sent and returned via regular mail rather than by express services or fax. Individual in-depth interviews can also take a long time: Once the questionnaire has been developed and potential participants have been identified, interviews usually take at least 2 to 3 weeks to schedule and conduct, and analysis can easily take an additional 2 weeks. Results from mall-intercept interviews can be available as quickly as a week after the questionnaire and materials are ready if the population is relatively large, although mall-intercept firms usually prefer to have at least two weekends to field a questionnaire and may need longer depending on the population. Focus groups normally take about 2 weeks to recruit (once participant characteristics have been determined), although they can be pulled together within a week if the target audience is easy to identify, but it may take 4 to 6 weeks if the target audience is small and difficult to identify. Top-line results can be ready a few days after the groups, but a more thorough report will take 4 to 6 weeks.

What are you going to do with the results? If the material will need to go through a formal clearance process subsequent to the pretesting, is there particular information you can include in the pretest to facilitate clearance? For example, have others raised concerns that you can address through questions in the pretest? Have you included questions that address the types of refinements you could make? If you are going to develop a distribution plan, could the pretest participants provide you with helpful information on where to distribute the final products?

REFERENCES

Doner, L. (1995). USDA's Team Nutrition: The audience and the message. Unpublished manuscript.

National Cancer Institute. (1989). *Making health communication programs work: A planner's guide* (NIH Pub. No. 89-1493). Bethesda, MD: Author.

Sample Central-Site Interview Questionnaire

John Killpack and Associates

Public Service Advertising—Mall Intercept Test

Prepared May 3, 1996

DATE: _____

ID: _____

INTERVIEWER: _____

LOCATION: _____

Hello, I'm (NAME) from (FIELD SERVICE). We're conducting a short study with people in the mall today. Do you have a few minutes to answer some questions?

1. What is your age?

   Under 50 1   [THANK AND TERMINATE.]
   50–64 2   [CONTINUE—50% OF SAMPLE.]
   65 or older 3   [CONTINUE—50% OF SAMPLE.]
   Refused 9   [THANK AND TERMINATE.]

2. RECORD GENDER OF RESPONDENT.

   Female 1   [50% OF SAMPLE]
   Male 2   [50% OF SAMPLE]

I'd like to show you some advertisements that have been produced as a public service and get your reaction to them. I'm not trying to sell you anything. As a way of thanking you for your participation, we'll give you $3. Would you please come with me to our viewing room?

Source: Reprinted with permission. Copyright © 1996, American Association of Retired Persons.

ROTATE ORDER (CIRCLE ORDER USED):

1—"Mr. McBride," "Mrs. Miller," 800 number, print

2—"Mrs. Miller," "Mr. McBride," 800 number, print

3—Print, "Mr. McBride," "Mrs. Miller," 800 number

4—Print, "Mrs. Miller," "Mr. McBride," 800 number

TELEVISION ADS

I'd like to show you the first television ad and then ask you a few questions about it.

[SHOW AD.]

I didn't have anything to do with creating the ad, so please be honest in your answers—you don't have to worry about hurting my feelings.

1. What was the main idea the ad was trying to get across? Anything else?

	First mention (Circle only one)	All other mentions (Circle all that apply)
Fraudulent telemarketers are criminals.	1	1
You can be robbed by a telemarketer.	2	2
Telemarketers who send couriers are fraudulent.	3	3
Prize companies who ask for credit card numbers are fraudulent.	4	4
Other	5	5
Don't know	8	8

2. What is the ad asking you to do?

	First mention (Circle only one)	All other mentions (Circle all that apply)
Don't fall for a telephone line.	1	1
Be wary/suspicious of telemarketers.	2	2
Hang up on telemarketers.	3	3
Don't give money to couriers for telemarketers.	4	4

Don't give credit card number out.	5	5
Avoid telephone contests.	6	6
Avoid investment opportunities over the phone.	7	7
Other	8	8
Don't know	9	9

3. What, if anything, about the ad did you especially like? Anything else?

	First mention (Circle only one)	All other mentions (Circle all that apply)
Everything	1	1
Nothing	2	2
Liked message in general	3	3
New information	4	4
I could relate to ad.	5	5
Ad/content was realistic.	6	6
Words on screen	7	7
Other	8	8
Don't know	9	9

4. What, if anything, about the ad did you especially dislike? Anything else?

	First mention (Circle only one)	All other mentions (Circle all that apply)
Everything	1	1
Nothing	2	2
Message was difficult to follow/understand.	3	3
Voices were hard to understand.	4	4
Type was hard to read.	5	5
Words on screen went too fast.	6	6
Words on screen went too slowly.	7	7
I could not relate to ad.	8	8
Ad/content was not realistic.	9	9
Other (specify: _____)	10	10
Don't know	11	11

5. Was there anything confusing or hard to understand? Anything else?

	First mention (Circle only one)	All other mentions (Circle all that apply)
Nothing	1	1
Don't understand what makes caller/telemarketer a criminal	2	2
Didn't know telemarketers were criminals	3	3
Don't know what's wrong with asking for credit card	4	4
Didn't know sending a courier was wrong	5	5
Didn't understand the "telephone line" pun	6	6
Type was hard to read	7	7
Hard to read and listen at the same time	8	8
Other (specify: _____)	9	9
Don't know	10	10

6. Which of the following statements best describes what the ad was saying: [READ STATEMENTS AND SHOW SCALE.]

   ROTATE:

   All telemarketers are fraudulent. 1
   Some telemarketers are fraudulent. 2
   Don't know [DON'T READ.] 8

7. What does "Don't fall for a telephone line" mean to you?

   Nothing 1
   Don't be taken in by or lose money to fraudulent
      telemarketers/con artists. 2
   Don't trip over the telephone cord. 3
   Other 4
   Don't know 8

8. Who was the sponsor of the ad?

   AARP/American Association of Retired Persons 1
   Other 2
   Don't know 8
   Refused 9

9. I'm going to read you a set of statements describing the ad you just saw. For each statement, please tell me whether you strongly agree, agree, neither agree nor disagree, disagree, or strongly disagree with the statement. [READ STATEMENTS AND SHOW SCALE.]

ROTATE:

	Strongly Agree	Agree	Neither Agree nor Disagree	Disagree	Strongly Disagree
The ad was believable.	1	2	3	4	5
The ad was scary.	1	2	3	4	5
The words were hard to read.	1	2	3	4	5
The ad was interesting.	1	2	3	4	5
I learned something from the ad.	1	2	3	4	5
The message was relevant to me.	1	2	3	4	5

10. Is this ad offensive to anyone?

Yes 1
No 2
Don't know 8

IF "YES" TO Q.10:

10a. Who?

Everyone 1
Legitimate telemarketers 2
Me 3
Other (specify: _____) 4
Don't know 8

PRINT ADS

These are ads that might appear in a newspaper or magazine. They are in the process of being developed, so the illustrations aren't final yet and all of the text hasn't been written.

[PLACE ADS IN FRONT OF RESPONDENT.]

1. Please pick up the ad you would be most likely to look at. [INDICATE WHICH AD RESPONDENT PICKED UP; REMOVE OTHER ADS.]

   A 1
   B 2
   C 3

2. What interests you in this ad? Anything else?

   Picture/drawing 1
   Headline 2
   Particular information 3
   Other (specify: _____) 4
   Don't know 8

3. What is the ad asking you to do?

	First mention (Circle only one)	All other mentions (Circle all that apply)
Don't fall for a telephone line.	1	1
Be wary/suspicious of telemarketers.	2	2
Hang up on telemarketers.	3	3
Get the caller's telephone number.	4	4
Call the National Fraud Information Center/ the 800 number.	5	5
Other (specify:_____)	6	6
Don't know	8	8

4. [PUT OTHER ADS BACK OUT.] Looking at all of the ads, what, if anything, is confusing or hard to understand? Anything else?

	First mention (Circle only one)	All other mentions (Circle all that apply)
Nothing	1	1
Don't understand what makes caller/telemarketer a criminal	2	2
Didn't know telemarketers were criminals	3	3
Didn't understand "telephone line" pun	4	4
Type was hard to read	5	5
Other	6	6
Don't know	8	8

5. What, if anything, is hard to believe? Anything else?

	First mention (Circle only one)	All other mentions (Circle all that apply)
Nothing	1	1
Telemarketers are fraudulent.	2	2
Fraudulent telemarketers are criminals.	3	3
That there are so many fraudulent telemarketers	4	4
Content is not realistic.	5	5
Other	6	6
Don't know	8	8

6. Which of the following statements best describes what the ads are saying: [READ STATEMENTS AND SHOW SCALE.]

ROTATE:

All telemarketers are fraudulent. 1
Some telemarketers are fraudulent. 2
Don't know [DON'T READ.] 8

7. Are these ads offensive to anyone?

Yes 1
No 2
Don't know 8

IF "YES" TO Q.7:

7a. Who?

Everyone 1
Legitimate telemarketers 2
Me 3
Other (specify: _____) 4
Don't know 8

8. How likely would you be to call the 800 number in the ad if you got a suspicious telemarketing call? Would you say . . . [READ SCALE.]

Very likely 1
Somewhat likely 2
Not very likely 3
Not at all likely 4
Don't know [DO NOT READ.] 8

DEMOGRAPHICS

These last few questions are for statistical purposes only.

1. What is your marital status?

   Married 1
   Divorced/separated/widowed 2
   Single (never married) 3
   Refused 8

2. Within the past year, about how many times have you responded to offers from organizations you were previously unfamiliar with by sending money or giving your credit card number to purchase something, enter a contest, make an investment, or donate to a charity?

   Enter number .... _____
   Don't know 8888

3. Please stop me at the range that includes your annual household income: [READ SCALE.]

   Less than $15,000 1
   $15,000–$25,000 2
   $26,000–$35,000 3
   $36,000–$50,000 4
   $51,000–$75,000 5
   More than $75,000 6
   Refused [DO NOT READ.] 8

4. Of the following, which best describes your race/ethnicity? Are you: [READ SCALE.]

   African-American 1
   Caucasian 2
   Hispanic 3
   Asian 4
   Other 5
   Refused [DO NOT READ.] 8

Assessing Progress and Making Refinements

Marketers view evaluation as a tool to improve their programs. Consequently, they place enormous emphasis on formative and process evaluation and are much less concerned about outcome evaluation. However, they have sales data to tell them pretty much anything they want to know about outcomes. In contrast, the standard emphasis in public health is on outcome evaluation. Often there is an expectation that social change interventions will be evaluated using the same techniques and definitions of success that a clinical scientist uses to evaluate a vaccine. Unfortunately, that type of evaluation model can limit the power of the social change initiative and does not adequately address the assumptions underlying how social change occurs.

Process and outcome evaluations can encompass a wide range of activities depending on the complexity of the social change effort. In this section we discuss some of the more common process evaluation activities used in monitoring and refining an initiative. We also highlight the challenges of adequately evaluating social change outcomes and present some approaches that are of use.

CHAPTER 17

Monitoring and Refining Implementation: Process Evaluation Tools

Building process evaluation measures into an initiative's tactics provides an important set of management tools. By using process evaluation data to regularly monitor an initiative's progress, timely refinements can be made to programs, products, materials, and distribution channels. Unfortunately, process evaluation is often overlooked or used solely to document an intervention rather than improve it. This chapter discusses how process evaluation data can be used to monitor and refine implementation, presents a general description of how process evaluation studies fit into program planning and implementation, and gives examples of some common process evaluation techniques and how they are used.

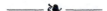

The monitoring information provided by process evaluation can serve as a powerful management device. As Andreasen (1995) noted, "commercial sector marketers crave data. They want to know how they are doing. They want to correct things before it is too late. . . . The major use of monitoring data is for *control*. In its ideal form, control will be a cybernetic self-correcting system that constantly looks at what is happening, diagnoses why it is happening, and takes corrective action as needed" (p. 128). Thorough process evaluation documents actual implementation and compares it to planned implementation, but the primary purpose for doing so is to make improvements in the future.

As activities are implemented, process evaluation is used to document implementation and provide feedback on the activity's progress, allowing the individual components and the overall initiative to be refined on an ongoing basis. Process evaluation typically tracks and documents implementation by quantifying what has been done; when, where, and how it was done; and who was reached. For program components involving mass media, process evaluation provides information on the number of opportunities there were to be exposed to the program messages and the extent to which messages appearing in editorial coverage were consistent with the communication strategy.

For multifaceted interventions, process evaluation is often piecemeal, because data are gathered separately—often using different techniques—for each component and often each tactic. Process evaluation works when it draws together the results of diverse program activities and provides an opportunity to systematically examine overall performance. It should tie together information on the implementation of different program components, providing managers with an overall picture of the effort and actionable recommendations for refinement.

PLANNING AND CONDUCTING PROCESS EVALUATION STUDIES

To be most useful, process evaluation needs to be built into an initiative's activities. It can be much more difficult and expensive to gather data retrospectively, and information collected after the fact is likely to be of little value in managing implementation. The following steps outline the general course of process evaluation activities.

Step 1: Set evaluation objectives and design evaluation plans. Data from process evaluation can be used in many ways. Three of the most common are

1. making decisions about refining the initiative's products, services, or activities.
2. documenting and justifying how resources have been spent.
3. making a compelling case for continued or additional funding.

Some initiatives will need to address all of these issues and others will not. Determining the ways in which process evaluation data will be used prior to designing the system(s) to collect them can save endless headaches later. However, making these determinations requires thinking about future needs, and this can be difficult, especially for new initiatives. The "backward research" approach developed by Andreasen (1985) can be helpful in identifying the questions that process evaluation data will need to answer. The steps involved in the approach are as follows (Andreasen, 1995, p. 101):*

1. Determine what key decisions are to be made using the research results and who will make the decisions.
2. Determine what information will help management make the best decisions.
3. Prepare a prototype report and ask management if this is what will best help them make their decisions.

Source: Copyright © Alan R. Andreasen.

4. Determine the analysis necessary to fill in the report.
5. Determine what questions must be asked to provide the data required by the analysis.
6. Ascertain whether the needed questions have already been asked.
7. Design sample.
8. Implement research design.
9. Write report.
10. Implement the results.

The key is to identify what decisions will need to be made and justifications prepared and what data will be most helpful in making those decisions. Referring to the initiative's goals and objectives is a useful starting point and can help to avoid the common pitfall of collecting information that is easy to collect, rather than information that will help manage the initiative. As Andreasen (1995) noted,

> thus social marketers may be tempted to keep track of how well they are doing by looking at the number of brochures distributed, the number of advertisements run, the number of people attending various events, or the extent of distribution of the products involved in the behavior. The difficulty with this approach is that the data may or may not bear any relationship to the program's objectives and goals. For example, large numbers of distributed but unread brochures accumulated by illiterate audience members should not be taken as a sign that the program is on target. Nor should television advertisements run at late-night hours with little or no audience. (p. 128)

Tracking the number of brochures distributed or the number of advertisements aired will help document the initiative (which is often necessary), but it will not help manage implementation in any meaningful way (beyond ensuring that the brochures do not run out). To make sure process evaluation data also serve as a management tool, a good starting point is to look at the initiative's objectives and think about how progress against them will be measured and what information will be needed to make improvements. For example, if an objective is to frame the public debate through media coverage, to what extent is that happening? Answering this question involves collecting media coverage on the issue and analyzing its content. If an objective is to persuade audience members to get more information through a hotline, how many are calling and where did they hear about the hotline? If a clinic is trying to increase use of a service, how can the service be improved? What important client needs are not fully met?

The nature and duration of the initiative will drive the type of process information needed and the frequency with which it will be needed. For example, if a referendum is on a ballot, a bill is coming up for a vote, or a regulatory agency is about to issue a rule, a campaign to impact the policy change will likely be of relatively short duration (almost certainly less than a year; often 3 to 6 months and sometimes only a few weeks). In contrast, initiatives to change individual behavior may be in place for years, assuming funding sources continue. The policy change initiative would require constant monitoring and refinement (with reports as often as weekly); the behavior change initiative might be managed very well with monthly or quarterly reports, depending on the level of activity.

Once evaluation objectives have been set and an overall approach has been determined, they should be outlined in a plan that contains

- the recommended methodological approach and its associated strengths and limitations
- the proposed study design (e.g., sample sizes, sampling procedures, and respondent specifications, if relevant)
- data collection instruments (and whether they exist or will need to be created)
- an analysis plan
- a timeline (including recommendations for frequency of reports)
- a budget
- staffing needs

The plan ensures that everyone involved with the activity understands and is in agreement as to what information the evaluation will provide. It also facilitates management of the program by providing information on the timing and amount of upcoming resource needs.

Step 2: Design data collection instruments. The instruments used to collect data will vary depending on the methodological approach employed, but may include

- questionnaires, either interviewer- or self-administered. For example, interviewer-administered questionnaires might be used if a telephone survey is used to track public awareness, or by operators answering calls to a toll-free number. Self-administered questionnaires might be used by materials recipients or by visitors to a World Wide Web site.
- recruitment screeners and topic guides for in-depth interviews or focus group discussions.
- tracking forms, used to monitor inventory, track aspects of product or service delivery, record the type of requests received or questions asked, or record details of media placements.

Some types of process evaluation do not require a data collection form but do require other types of preparation. For example, tracking airplay of television products (advertisements, video news releases, satellite media tours, etc.) may require encoding the master tapes prior to dubbing and distribution.

Often the data collection instruments will be distributed with particular program components (e.g., bounceback cards containing short questionnaires might be distributed with public service announcements). Instruments that do not need to be distributed with the component should be ready for use prior to its implementation.

Step 3: Implement and report on evaluation activities. Data collection normally begins in tandem with program implementation. Data should be periodically analyzed using techniques suitable for the data, and the research questions and results should be presented in a report format appropriate to the activity. Often, results are summarized in tabular form on a weekly or monthly basis, with a more detailed analysis prepared quarterly, semiannually, or annually. These more detailed analyses compare planned versus actual implementation, identify strengths and weaknesses in the implementation, and make recommendations for refinement of program components and distribution mechanisms.

COMMON PROCESS EVALUATION ACTIVITIES

Process evaluation can be simple or it can be complex. It encompasses an enormous number of activities and methodological approaches, far too many to adequately address in one chapter. The remainder of this chapter discusses some common process evaluation methodologies and how they apply to various program components, particularly those related to promotional campaigns and tracking reactions to products or services. Many of the approaches discussed here can also be used as needs assessment tools when refinements to a program are being planned. For an excellent discussion and illustration of process evaluation applied to a public health initiative, review the 1994 *Health Education Quarterly* supplement devoted to "Process Evaluation in the Multicenter Child and Adolescent Trial for Cardiovascular Health (CATCH)" (Stone, McGraw, Osganian, & Elder, 1994).

Bounceback Cards

Bounceback cards, also called *business reply cards,* are short questionnaires on the back of a post card. The post card is addressed to the sponsoring organization and includes the sponsor's business reply permit information (hence the name). They can be included with any material distributed to gatekeepers, intermediaries, or target audiences, such as public service advertisements (PSAs), booklets, or videos. They provide an inexpensive way of obtaining feedback on the material and can be a means of obtaining basic information about the recipient.

When distributed with other materials, such as patient, professional, or public education materials, bounceback cards provide an inexpensive mechanism for assessing reactions to the publication and can serve as a mechanism for recipients to order additional copies of the same material or other relevant materials.

Bounceback cards can also be distributed with PSAs as a way of obtaining information from the public service directors who determine whether (and how often) an ad will air. They provide a way to get a sense of how important the topic of the PSA is to the station and to monitor changes in topic and format preferences over time.

Exhibit 17–1 provides examples of the topics that can be included on bounceback cards.

The downside of bounceback cards is their low response rate; for example, when they are distributed with PSAs even many stations who air the PSAs do not return them. Studies to assess nonresponse bias can be prohibitively expensive and may not be permitted (e.g., privacy regulations may preclude follow-up contact of people who have requested materials). However, the methodology does

---

Exhibit 17–1 Topics for Bounceback Cards

Education materials (target audience member responds):
- How much of this booklet/video did you read/watch?
- Did you think it was . . . too long, too short, about right?
- Did you think it was . . . hard to understand, about right, too simple?
- (For printed materials) Was the print . . . too large, about right, too small?
- (For audio/video materials) Was the information presented . . . too quickly, about right, too slowly?
- Were you looking for any information that was not included? If so, what?
- Where did you get this booklet/video?
- How might this booklet/video be improved?
- Ordering information for the same publication or others that are relevant?

Public service advertisements (public service director responds):
- How important is (TOPIC) to your viewers/listeners/readers . . . very, somewhat, not very, not at all? Alternatively, list your topic and other important social topics and instruct the respondent to rank them from most important (1) to least important (5). This approach gives you a sense of the competition.
- Format preferences (e.g., ½" or VHS for TV; compact disc or cassette for radio; camera-ready slicks or computer disk for print)
- Length preferences (e.g., 60-second, 30-second, 15-second for radio and TV; sizes for print)
- Compared with other ads you receive, is the production quality of this ad . . . much higher, somewhat higher, about the same, somewhat lower, or much lower?
- How often do you plan to air this/these ads? (ask for it to be expressed in the unit of time you will analyze—per day, per week, or per month)
- For how long will you use this/these ads? (ask for it to be expressed in the unit of time you will analyze—per day, per week, or per month)

provide insights into how the issue and the materials are perceived. And because of the difficulties encountered with tracking radio, bounceback cards frequently are the only means for programs covering a large geographic area to track radio PSA usage.

Inventory Tracking

In addition to ensuring that adequate quantities of materials are in stock at all times, inventory tracking provides an opportunity to learn where materials are going, which ones are likely to be reaching the most people, and which ones are the most (and least) popular. A simple way to set up an inventory tracking system is to design a database or log where the following information is recorded each time material is distributed:

- date of distribution
- name of material distributed
- quantity
- geographic location distributed to (name of organization or event, if distributed on site; if mailed, ZIP code for a metropolitan area or regional program; city and state for larger programs)

These types of forms can be modified for use in a variety of situations. For some types of materials, it may be helpful to include information on the type of requestors (e.g., is the requestor an intermediary or an individual) and how they heard about the material. The latter information can be obtained in a number of ways. If requestors call to order the materials, they can be asked how they heard about the material when they call. If requestors complete an order form, a few pertinent questions can be included on the form, or order forms that are printed in other publications can be coded so that the publication can be identified. If requestors write in for materials (e.g., in response to an ad or story in the mass media), fictitious department numbers or names can be included in the address they are given to allow identification of the tactic that triggered the response. For instance, the July 1997 media materials might instruct respondents to write to Department 797.

Once the inventory tracking system has been established, it can be analyzed to gain insights into a number of aspects of program implementation. For example,

- the number of requests can be plotted by date and compared with when program activities took place to provide insights into what activities are generating the most requests. Popular activities could be repeated more often or conducted in additional locales. Less popular activities can be examined in more detail: Does it seem likely that these activities are reaching relatively few audience members and therefore should be discontinued? What are the differences between more and less popular activities? Is there a way to alter the latter to increase their utility?

- geographic locations of requestors can be mapped. Regions where requests are light can be targeted for more intensive program activities.
- if some materials are requested far more often than others (or others are rarely requested), a follow-up study can be conducted by contacting people who have requested the materials and asking them what they found appealing (or unappealing) and how they are using the materials.

Service Delivery and Client Satisfaction

For public health programs that include service delivery, monitoring delivery is essential. Such tracking can provide information on how to improve the service and can help determine whether delivery is carried out as designed, whether it is reaching the intended target population, and whether the implementation is helping to achieve program objectives as planned. Delivery data can also be important in evaluating the value of a new product or service and whether it should continue to be offered.

The type of data collected depends on the type of product or service. For example, a public health initiative could easily include training sessions or workshops, a new telephone hotline service for referrals or to order information, health services such as screenings or immunizations at sites other than traditional service delivery sites (i.e., health fairs, sporting events, mobile mammography vans, flu shots at the drug store, etc.), or services within a traditional public health setting (i.e., counseling and testing, prenatal care, etc.).

Monitoring the number and type of people using these services, as well as their satisfaction with them, is an important part of implementation. It facilitates midcourse adjustment, resetting of goals and objectives, administrative planning, and resource utilization. It also "allows program administrators to put into context their own subjective observations and those of others on the success or failure in the implementation of various program components" (Centers for Disease Control and Prevention [CDC], 1993).

The specific service delivery information to be collected needs to be determined based on what is needed to assess whether program objectives are being met and to make necessary refinements. Common information to collect includes

- number of people served (or number of visits or calls)
- characteristics of people served (to assess what percentage are members of the audience the program is trying to reach)
- quantity of services utilized and characteristics of people using each

- peak usage times (to assess staffing and adjust if necessary)
- additional services of interest to clientele (to plan for the future)

In addition to collecting this type of usage information, an invaluable part of assessing service delivery is assessing client satisfaction with the service(s), the facilities, and the personnel. Exhibit 17–2 presents some aspects of each that can be important.

Approaches to measuring client satisfaction can be divided into three basic categories:

1. *Unsolicited client responses,* such as suggestion or comment boxes. This approach is the least rigorous and, as Lamb and Crompton (1992) noted, is limited by its lack of generalizability (the views of those who comment may be very different from the views of those who do not) and inability to assess degree of satisfaction; provided services meet some minimal satisfaction level, people may not make an effort to complain but may not be highly satisfied either.

2. *Observation,* by directly interacting with clients either informally or formally. Informal observation might involve a manager visiting a facility and talking to a few clients about their likes, dislikes, and suggestions for im-

---

Exhibit 17–2　Some Components of Client Satisfaction

Services:
- Cost
- Waiting time after arrival (how long it takes to be seen)
- Waiting time to make an appointment

Facilities:
- Transportation (i.e., adequate parking? Convenient to public transportation?)
- Waiting room—too crowded? Enough chairs? Enough things to entertain children?
- Exam/counseling rooms—Temperature? Privacy?
- Hours—convenient?
- Telephone experiences (i.e., amount of time on hold; number of times transferred)

Personnel:
- Demeanor (i.e., friendly or rude; rushed or patient)
- Knowledge
- Whether questions are answered
- Whether issues are explained clearly

proving products or services. More formal observation can be conducted using qualitative research techniques, such as periodic focus groups or in-depth interviews with current and former clients.

3. *Surveys,* ideally of both current and former clients. This approach has the advantage of being generalizable to the population served if probability sampling techniques are used and the questionnaire is constructed appropriately.

The last two approaches play an important role in developing a complete picture of client satisfaction: Quantitative methods measure the percentage of clients who use particular services and are satisfied or dissatisfied with particular aspects of the services themselves, the facilities in which they are delivered, and the personnel who deliver them. Qualitative studies can shed light on the reasons underlying service usage and satisfaction or dissatisfaction (CDC, 1993). Chapter 11 discussed issues to consider when designing qualitative studies.

Designing, implementing, and analyzing quantitative surveys is a complex endeavor. A good introduction to many of the issues involved with sampling, instrumentation, data collection, data processing, and analysis is provided in *The Survey Research Handbook*, by Alreck and Settle (1985). At a minimum, the following five factors warrant consideration.

Questionnaire Design

Andreasen (1995) and Lamb and Crompton (1992) recommended measuring two dimensions of satisfaction: *how important* each aspect of a program is to the client as well as the typical *how satisfied* the client is with it. First, respondents rate their satisfaction with various aspects of the program on a numeric scale (Andreasen suggested a 10-point scale; Lamb and Crompton used a 7-point scale ranging from *extremely unsatisfactory* to *extremely satisfactory*) and then rate each aspect's importance to them using a similar scale. Andreasen recommended using the resulting information to create a performance–importance matrix by plotting it on a two-dimensional graph.

Knowing how important various aspects of a product or service are to clients can help managers make more informed decisions about changes to make. For example, if clients are relatively unsatisfied with the waiting room but it is not that important to them, changing it may have little or no effect on clinic usage. In contrast, if their satisfaction with clinic hours is moderate, but the hours are most important to them, changing the hours may result in substantial changes in usage.

Sampling

For some services, such as training sessions, it is relatively easy to ask everyone to fill out an evaluation form. For others, such as clinic services or hotline calls, it would be tremendously burdensome to ask each person to fill out an evaluation following each visit or call. The logical option is to sample participants in some way. If a probability sample is used, the results can be assumed to represent the population from which the sample was drawn. A sample is a probability sample if (1) all members of a population have a known (usually equal) chance of being selected and (2) participants are selected randomly. Alternatively, a convenience sample can be used; for example, every person using the service one specific day of the week or week of the month could be sampled. To minimize bias, the day or week should be rotated in case there are differences among people who use the service at different times. Convenience samples are more limited than probability samples but can be considerably easier to construct.

Data Collection Method

Self-administered questionnaires can be confidential and will work even in situations where identifying information, such as names, is not collected. However, they only work for relatively literate audiences. Alternatively, participants could be interviewed in person immediately after using the service, but they may not be willing to cooperate due to concerns about time or confidentiality. Telephone surveys overcome the literacy hurdle but have problems of their own: Many low-income residents do not have a phone, and in order to conduct a phone survey at all clientele phone numbers are needed. In some instances, calling clients may jeopardize their feelings of confidentiality.

Reliability

If clients are asked the same question multiple times, their answers should be substantially the same each time. Reliability depends in part on the nature of the questions asked. The more concrete and easy to answer accurately, the more reliable they are likely to be. Other factors that can affect reliability include differences in the situation in which the questionnaire is administered (e.g., consider what might happen if a client was verbally interviewed about satisfaction in a waiting room full of other clients versus privately), differences in how it is administered, and even differences in the mood of the person completing it (Rossi & Freeman, 1993).

Validity

Does a question measure what it is intended to measure, and are the measures accurate? For example, self-reported information on behavior is often inaccurate because people tend to report what they think they should do rather than what they actually do. There are many potential threats to validity. Rossi and Freeman (1993) outlined four criteria that social scientists used to assess validity: *consistency with past usage* (a new scale or question should not contradict the usual ways the concept has been used previously), *consistency with other measures* of the same concept (the measure should produce substantially the same results as other measures), *internal consistency* (i.e., if several questions measure the same concept, each should produce similar results), and for measures that attempt to predict future attitudes or behavior, *consequential predictability*—in other words, a measure of "propensity to use clinic services" in fact predicts subsequent usage of clinic services. For a measure to be considered valid, it must meet one of these criteria.

Media Coverage Analysis

The term *media coverage* refers to all mentions of a topic that appear in the mass media as something other than an advertisement. Tracking and analyzing both the amount and the content of media coverage of a topic serve a number of purposes. Specifically, they help

- calculate how many opportunities there were for people to be exposed to stories containing information about the topic of the initiative.
- identify which placement tactics are working best.
- identify what messages are appearing in the media and what ones are not, allowing assessment of the extent to which the issue was framed from a policy perspective and providing guidance for tailoring future content of media outreach efforts.
- monitor competing messages, again providing guidance for tailoring future efforts to frame the issue.

Analyzing media coverage can play important roles during other phases of an initiative. For example, it can be used when an initiative is being planned, to assess how the issue is currently being framed, and to calculate baseline measures of media coverage, as discussed in Chapter 10. Its insights into how different reporters and media cover a particular issue can also provide a foundation to use when building relationships with the media, as discussed in Chapter 15.

Terminology

Before attempting to analyze media coverage, it is helpful to understand some of the terms commonly used in conjunction with it.

Circulation and Audience Size. Circulation and audience figures are used to estimate how many people may have seen each story. *Circulation* is the number of copies of a newspaper or magazine that are paid for, either through subscriptions or individual purchases. Because each copy of a newspaper or magazine may have multiple readers (consider the magazines in a physician's office or the many newspapers and magazines that are read by more than one person in a household), circulation does not equate to number of readers. *Audience* is sometimes used to describe the number of readers. *Audience size* is used in conjunction with television and radio. It can refer to the number of viewers or listeners during an average quarter-hour or the cumulative (*cume*) number of viewers or listeners for the program or part of the day. (Obviously, cume figures are larger.) With television, audience size can be expressed in terms of the number of people or the number of households.

Gross Impressions, Reach, and Frequency. Taking all of the stories on a topic and summing their circulation or audience size figures results in a number the industry terms *gross impressions*. Gross impressions are not the same thing as the number of people who were "reached" by the coverage. Why not?

1. Gross impressions do not account for frequency, or the number of times a specific individual was reached. Most people are exposed to multiple magazines, radio stations, and television programs, and some newspapers or magazines may run more than one story on the same topic.
2. Not everyone reads every story in every issue, watches every program, or listens to every news item.

Gross impressions provide an estimate of how many opportunities there were for messages to be seen. To know how many people were "reached" (i.e., actually saw the message) requires a survey of the population, and that approach is fraught with measurement difficulties as well, as discussed later in this chapter. Gross impressions are quite useful; for example, if program objectives include generating a certain amount of media coverage, they allow progress to be measured against those objectives. And, perhaps most importantly, they can be used to estimate how much coverage particular tactics generated and track coverage over time. Both types of information help managers determine when tactics should be changed.

Gross impressions are often misinterpreted and used to make statements that are, at best, hyperbole. For example: "We've reached over 350 million people with our message." Considering that the population of the United States is around 269 million people (199 million adults), apparently the program in question has gone international.

Because newspaper and magazine gross impressions are usually calculated from circulation figures, some practitioners multiply the final number by some amount (2.5 is common). Their rationale for doing so is that circulation figures do not account for pass-along readership (people who read the publication but do not buy it). This is true, but on the other hand not everyone reads every story, and the average number of readers per copy differs greatly from one publication to another. For example, recent estimates of magazines' readers per copy ranged from around 1.4 to over 15 (Mediamark Research, Inc., 1997). Although multiplying circulation by a pass-along readership factor makes the number a lot more impressive, doing so is difficult to defend because it accounts for possible additional impressions without adjusting for people who did not read the stories. Those who want to calculate magazine audience size more exactly can refer to the studies conducted by market research firms such as Mediamark Research, Inc. (MRI). At the time of this writing, MRI's current magazine audience estimates were available free of charge on their Web site (http://www.mediamark.com). For newspapers in the largest 60 metropolitan areas, Scarborough Research Corporation calculates overall readership (average issue and cumulative audience) and readership of specific sections (news, business, sports, food, etc.).

Advertising Equivalencies. Advertising equivalencies are used to estimate the value of media coverage by calculating how much comparable amounts of advertising would have cost. Advertising equivalencies have limitations to keep in mind, particularly if part of a program includes paid advertising.

- The dollar amount that the vendor calculates is based on the total length of the story. Particularly in print media, program messages may have occupied a very small amount of the story. Consequently, a one-paragraph discussion of a topic in a two-page story will wind up being valued at what a two-page ad would cost.
- The price of advertising space is extremely variable and volatile, particularly in television and radio. It is like pricing hotel rooms or airline seats: The more unsold space there is close to the deadline, the more the price drops. In advertising placement, location is everything. Different publications or programs cost different amounts; different locations within them also vary enormously in price. Using the standard advertising unit cost (or average) can grossly under- or overestimate the "worth" of various placements.

The Process of Monitoring Media Coverage

Tracking news coverage of a public health initiative involves contracting with various vendors, sometimes different ones for each medium. Stories that appear in newspapers and magazines can be obtained through a major national clipping service such as Burrelle's or Luce's. Both attempt to subscribe to all U.S. publications targeting the public. However, they do not include trade publications or academic journals; it is best to monitor these publications directly by subscribing to those that are relevant.

Some services also monitor some amount of network, cable, and major local television and radio coverage. Alternatively, such coverage can be obtained by contracting directly with vendors such as Video Monitoring Service. When monitoring television and radio coverage, be aware that the services' coverage of local radio is extremely limited and their television coverage does not include all markets. Television usage of information distributed by your initiative (i.e., video news releases, satellite media tours) can be tracked electronically if the material is encoded before it is distributed to stations.

On-line Resources. Print media coverage can also be obtained using electronic services such as Nexis, Dialog, and ProQuest. (See Appendix 11–D in Chapter 11 for contact information.) They often offer coverage of trade publications and academic journals as well (and some coverage of television and radio news programs). Their disadvantage is that they do not include all publications, do not provide information on circulation (or audience size for broadcast media) or comparable advertising cost and generally do not capture any pictures or graphics that accompanied the story. Increasingly, media coverage can be monitored by looking at the Web sites of the individual media (for campaigns covering a relatively small geographic area) or by using a Web search engine (i.e., Excite, Alta Vista, etc.). However, most media do not put all of the stories that appear in their printed or broadcast editions on their Web sites, and many smaller media may not put any content on the Web.

Clipping Services. Clipping services identify clips by having people read through each publication looking for specific terms and topics. Each reader is responsible for a specific set of publications, but is looking for a large number of issues in those publications. The readers work from reading lists provided by clients. When they encounter a story that meets a client's criteria, they will clip out the page and attach a tag indicating publication, date, and circulation. The clipping service can also provide periodic reports that list this information for each clip and calculate what the equivalent amount of space would have cost if it had been purchased for an advertisement. These reports can include a rudimentary identification of a few messages contained in the story, based on a predefined message list. Although not a substitution for the comprehensive content analysis discussed later, this basic coding can be used to get a general sense of what the stories contain.

Construction of the reading list is a critical part of monitoring media coverage: The list needs to be as specific and concrete as possible. Developing reading lists for social change efforts is often quite difficult because it is not as simple as looking for mentions of a specific product or service. Often the subject is messages about some particular health behavior. The trick is to construct a reading list that is broad enough to capture stories of interest but narrow enough to exclude most of those that are irrelevant. As an example, consider someone managing a cancer prevention and control initiative. Asking for all stories mentioning the word *cancer* would result in many mailboxes full of obituaries as well as stories of interest.

Clipping services usually ship clips to clients every 3 to 4 weeks, although (for a large fee) they can be faxed the day they appear in major publications. These services usually charge a flat monthly fee for monitoring and then charge per clip for each clip sent to the client. Reports summarizing the information are available at an additional cost. Those running local initiatives or those who are interested only in coverage in major media may find acting as their own clipping service to be faster and less expensive.

Alternative Monitoring Methods. As with a print clipping service, vendors tracking radio and television coverage work from a topic list and scan all programming to locate appropriate stories and return transcripts or air checks (copies of the segment on tape), accompanied by information on the station and market in which it aired and an estimate of the audience size reached. Additionally, for television materials such as video news releases (VNRs), satellite media tours, and electronic press kits, tracking reports are often provided by the vendor distributing the material. Many vendors use Nielsen Media Research's SIGMA tracking service, which picks up the electronic code of the material each time it is aired. Reports usually indicate, for each time the VNR is used, the station, market, time, date, story length, and estimated cost if an ad of similar length was placed at that time. For an additional fee, air checks or transcripts can be obtained. Transcripts are inexpensive and useful for content analysis; air checks are expensive but useful for documenting implementation and showing others what the program has accomplished.

As an alternative to contracting with a vendor for monitoring, if program staff know that a relevant story appeared during a particular television program, on a particular radio station, or in a particular newspaper or magazine, the resources used by commercial advertisers can be used to determine how many people are likely to have been reached and an approximation of how much the placement would have cost if it had been paid advertising. Some of these resources are listed in Table 17–1.

Subscriptions to the services shown in Table 17–1 can be quite expensive, particularly if only local information is needed. Many advertising agencies and some public relations firms subscribe to some or all of them; provided requests are reasonable, they may be willing to provide information or access to it on a pro bono basis to support the efforts of community organizations or other small nonprofits. In addition, some university libraries carry some of these resources. Alternatively, the information can be gathered by obtaining rate cards from individual stations and publications.

Analyzing Content

With editorial coverage, it is often desirable to go beyond the information provided by the tracking and clipping services. Because reporters generally use various information sources to prepare their stories, it is necessary to content analyze the coverage to determine the extent to which the coverage is on strategy (i.e., if it includes key messages and frames the issue as intended) and to identify any areas of confusion or negative coverage. The content analysis process involves reading each clip and coding it according to a previously developed message list, then

Table 17–1 Selected Sources of Media Information

Source	Information Available
Arbitron (http://www.arbitron.com)	Radio station audience size estimates and profiles
Mediamark Research, Inc. (http://www.mediamark.com)	Magazine audience estimates and profiles
Nielsen Media Research (http://www.nielsenmedia.com)	Television audience size estimates and profiles; SIGMA tracking data
Standard Rate and Data Service (http://www.srds.com)	Newspaper and magazine profiles and ad pricing; television, radio, and outdoor profiles

examining the number of stories and estimated audience reach for each message. This analysis reveals what messages from program materials are being used, what ones are not, and how often conflicting messages appear, providing guidance for future media relations efforts.

Exhibit 17–3 presents an example of media analysis conducted to support the 5 A Day for Better Health program.

Tracking Advertising Placement

If an initiative relies on public service placement of its ads, tracking that placement is the only means of determining who had an opportunity to be reached by a campaign, and the only means of calculating gross impressions, reach, frequency, and what the placement would have cost had it been paid. For initiatives that pay for placement, tracking placement is far less critical; reach and frequency are normally estimated when developing the media plan that lays out where, when, and how often to run the ads. Even if these calculations were not made, they can easily be made using audience estimates supplied by each station or publication. Many commercial advertisers track placement of their own ads to verify that they actually ran as requested; few social change initiatives have such resources available. Advertising tracking services can also be used to keep an eye on competitors' advertising spending and media schedules.

For initiatives relying on public service placement, tracking data also allow managers to

- compare ads to determine which ones receive the most play.
- thank stations that are "heavy users" of materials, and potentially explore the opportunity for station promotions around the issue.

Exhibit 17–3 Analyzing Media Coverage: The 5 A Day for Better Health Campaign

---

BACKGROUND

The goal of the national 5 A Day for Better Health program, cosponsored by the National Cancer Institute (NCI) and the Produce for Better Health Foundation (PBHF), is to encourage Americans to eat five or more servings of fruits and vegetables daily to decrease their risk of developing cancer. The program today is a complex web of activities conducted at the national, state, and local levels by government agencies, nonprofit organizations, and the private sector.

Both NCI and PBHF conduct media campaigns to disseminate messages encouraging increased consumption of fruits and vegetables. Both organizations monitor the quantity of coverage on an ongoing basis; in addition, NCI periodically analyzes the content of the print media coverage. This case study draws from NCI's initial media analysis report (Eisner, Loughrey, & Davis, 1994) to illustrate how the process works. The report analyzes print media coverage appearing from July 1992 (when NCI's media campaign was launched) through October 1993.

The National Cancer Institute employed a number of tactics to generate media coverage of 5 A Day messages. Regular contact with the media was accomplished through the quarterly distribution of 5 A Day media newsletters to newspaper and magazine food editors. The newsletters contained story ideas, recipes, infographics (Figure 17–1), and camera-ready art; the materials were also available on an accompanying disk or could be downloaded through two computer services.

This regular contact was supplemented by a variety of special events and additional media contacts. The 5 A Day media campaign was launched in July 1992 with a press conference featuring U.S. Department of Health and Human Services Secretary Louis Sullivan, M.D., and National Institutes of Health Director Bernadine Healy, M.D.; the launch was also supported by a video news release featuring press conference footage and Olympic swimmer Matt Biondi. In addition, media activities were conducted in conjunction with the launch of 5 A Day week in September 1993, radio and print public service announcements were produced and distributed periodically, and a magazine media tour was conducted.

Beyond NCI's activities, PBHF, produce manufacturers, and retail stores sponsored many additional media activities.

METHOD OF ANALYSIS

To assess the 5 A Day print media coverage, newspaper and magazine placements published from July 1992 through October 1993 were collected by a national clipping service. The clipping service attempted to clip all daily and weekly newspapers in the United States, as well as nearly 7,000 consumer, trade, and professional magazines and newsletters. However, as would be expected with any clipping service, it is doubtful that all stories resulting from the campaign were obtained because no clipping service covers all publications in the United States, and all services inevitably

continues

Exhibit 17–3 continued

GETTING THE FACTS ON **5 A DAY**
How Americans are doing when it comes to fruits and vegetables

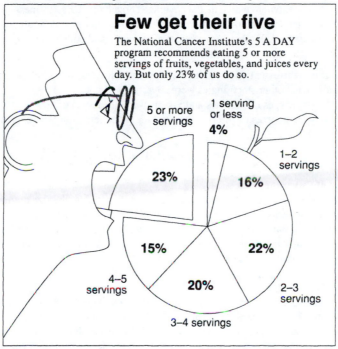

Few get their five

The National Cancer Institute's 5 A DAY program recommends eating 5 or more servings of fruits, vegetables, and juices every day. But only 23% of us do so.

5 or more servings **23%**

1 serving or less **4%**

1–2 servings **16%**

2–3 servings **22%**

3–4 servings **20%**

4–5 servings **15%**

A National Cancer Institute Graphic

Figure 17–1 Infograph from the 5 A Day Campaign. *Source:* Reprinted from National Cancer Institute.

miss some placements. Nonetheless, the clipping service collected 7,625 stories published during the time period.

The first stage of the analysis involved estimating gross impressions by summarizing circulation figures and estimating worth by summarizing advertising dollar equivalencies. To evaluate the content of the coverage in a timely and cost-effective manner, a representative sample was drawn. Sampling was conducted by first grouping the clips by the distribution schedules of their publications—weekly, daily, or monthly. Clips from daily publications were grouped further by the day of the week on which they were published. Proportional samples were drawn based on the per-

continues

Exhibit 17–3 continued

centage of clips in each category (e.g., weekly, monthly, Monday, Tuesday, etc.). The sample included 1,103 clips.

The goal of the content analysis was to improve future media placement efforts by (1) assessing the extent to which media coverage contained NCI's key messages and (2) identifying tactics (in terms of type of information and delivery strategies) that were most successful. To that end, each story was read and coded using a message list that had been constructed with the following objectives:

- Determine the extent to which media coverage reflected NCI's key messages.
- Identify what other story angles were covered.
- Assess what types of statistics and visuals were used most often.
- Assess what sources of information (including spokespeople) were used most often.

Some highlights of the analysis are presented below.

Quantity of Coverage

Circulation of the total 7,625 clips was 396,145,875; based on the size of the clips, the equivalent advertising value was estimated at $5,925,354. Coverage was highest the month the campaign was launched (889 clips with a corresponding circulation of more than 52 million) and the month 5 A Day week was launched (820 clips with a corresponding circulation of more than 40 million).

Content of Coverage

Content analysis of the stories revealed that the vast majority (89% of the 1,103 articles analyzed) contained one or more of NCI's key messages. However, some messages received far more coverage than others. For example, 77% of the articles reported that people should eat a minimum of five servings of fruits and vegetables per day—one of the key messages to increase knowledge. However, only 12% of the stories included another knowledge message—that five servings is a minimum, not a maximum, recommendation.

Messages designed to build skills by focusing on specific actions people could take to increase their consumption of fruits and vegetables received relatively limited coverage, with 28% of the stories including messages such as a suggestion to add two servings each day or more specific actions people could take to add servings (such as having fruit or juice in the morning and having fruit and/or vegetables as a snack).

Messages focusing on the health benefits of eating five or more servings of fruits and vegetables each day received greater coverage: 41% of the placements mentioned a specific health benefit related to this level of consumption, with the association with reduced risk of some forms of cancer being mentioned most often (it appeared in 40% of the stories). Relatively few articles (5%) discussed the barriers to eating 5 A Day, such as seasonality, cost, or preparation time.

continues

Exhibit 17–3 continued

> The analysis also examined the extent to which the coverage included other story angles of interest to NCI. Just over one-fourth (27%) of the articles discussed 5 A Day in conjunction with food (e.g., recipes, food preparation tips, a specific fruit or vegetable, or a Mediterranean diet). Details and background on the 5 A Day program were mentioned in 16% of the clips; about 5% mentioned an organization or group that had joined the 5 A Day program. About 8% of the articles discussed children and 5 A Day, usually in terms of the value of eating produce. Very few (2%) of the sampled articles mentioned a concern about pesticides used on fruits and vegetables.
>
> **Tactics Used**
> Nearly half (47%) of the sampled articles used materials and/or information that could be identified as coming from the National Cancer Institute. About one-fourth (26%) used information from the July 1992 launch materials; 10% used information from the media newsletters; 11% used information from NCI but the precise source could not be identified. About one-fourth of the articles (26%) mentioned an NCI-provided statistic. Current fruit and vegetable consumption was the most frequent focus; 21% of all stories mentioned that Americans currently eat 3.5 servings of fruits and vegetables daily or that only 23% of Americans eat 5 or more daily servings. Thirteen percent of the sampled articles used visuals; 5 A Day infographs were used most often, followed by art from the newsletter and photographs.
>
> *Source:* Data from E. Eisner, K. Loughrey, and K. Davis, 1994, *the National Cancer Institute's 5 A Day for Better Health Program: Analysis of Print Media Placements—July 1992 through October 1993.* Bethesda, MD: National Cancer Institute Office of Cancer Communications.

- refine distribution lists based on who is and is not using program materials.
- discern any need for follow-up studies with nonusers to identify why they are not using the ads and determine if there is anything that can be done to increase their usage.

Sources of PSA Placement Information. PSAs that appear in magazines or newspapers can be obtained through the same clipping services described in the media coverage section of this chapter. The sponsor provides a copy of the ads to the clipping service; when the readers come across the ads in publications, they clip out the page and attach a tag indicating publication, date, and circulation (these pages are sometimes referred to as *tear sheets*). Regional and other specialized editions of magazines make it difficult to obtain all PSA placements (often a PSA will run in one edition that had unsold advertising space but not in all editions). If PSAs are being sent to professional publications, it is often wise to subscribe directly to the publications to ensure PSA placement does not get overlooked.

Television PSAs can be tracked using SIGMA, Nielsen Media Research's electronic tracking service. To use SIGMA, the sponsoring organization contracts with a service provider that encodes the master tapes prior to duplication and release. This encoding uniquely identifies each PSA and is broadcast with the PSA, but it is not visible to the audience. Nielsen's computers identify this code each time a spot is aired. Airplay reports can be customized but typically include, for each airing of the spot, the station and market in which the spot aired (or network if it ran on a network), the date and time it aired, some basic audience composition information (including estimated audience size), and the approximate cost of the time if it had been purchased for commercial advertising. Because the price of television time is subject to extreme fluctuations, this last item is only a rough estimate. Radio PSA play in major markets can also be tracked electronically; however, doing so is extremely expensive, and many areas of the country are still missed.

Additional information on PSA placement can be obtained through a few different mechanisms:

- Commercial verification reports. Broadcast stations and print publications generally send these to commercial advertisers to verify that their ads ran as requested. Some stations and publications automatically send these reports for PSAs; others will do so if asked. The reports typically list the name of the program airing when the PSA ran and the date and time it ran.
- Follow-up phone calls with stations and publications. Phoning public service directors to see if they plan to use a particular spot is labor intensive but can be quite useful, particularly if this technique is limited to priority gatekeepers, or those for whom it will be difficult to collect other information, such as radio stations.
- The resources listed in Table 17–1. Local initiatives that know when and where their ads ran can consult these sources to estimate gross impressions, reach, and frequency.
- Including phone numbers or addresses in PSAs. If a PSA includes a hotline number or an address, information on who was reached and motivated enough to respond by requesting more information can be collected.

Monitoring Policy Changes

The way in which a policy change can be monitored depends on what type of change it is and who has the power to make it. For example, if a change is taking the form of a referendum, bond issue, or proposition that requires citizens to vote, tracking voter opinion can be critical, as is discussed later in this chapter. If private organizations are being asked to make the change, contact with their public affairs personnel or decision makers within the organizations may be the only way to monitor change. Many policy and funding decisions are made by governments at the local, state, or national level. This section provides some suggestions for monitoring these types of policy changes.

At the local level, attending city council meetings and maintaining contact with decision makers can be critical in tracking policy changes. Some activities, such as agendas for upcoming meetings and hearings, can also be monitored through contact with local government agencies or through the Internet. World Wide Web search engines such as Yahoo can help identify the Web sites of local governments, and the Library of Congress THOMAS site (http://www.thomas.loc.gov) provides a number of gateways to local sites.

At the state level, it is increasingly possible to monitor the introduction and progress of bills through legislative Web sites. Most sites can be accessed from the state's main home page, which is generally located at the following URL: http://www.state.xx.us, where the state's two-letter postal abbreviation is substituted for xx. Additionally, staff of the legislator sponsoring a bill (or legislators opposing it, as appropriate) can provide valuable information on the "behind the scenes" progress. States vary in how regulatory agencies operate, but many states have "government in the sunshine" laws that mandate access to some of the proceedings.

At the federal level, legislation can be monitored through the previously mentioned Library of Congress Web site (http://www.thomas.loc.gov). This site provides the complete text of bills as well as information on their status, sponsors, referrals to committees, and so forth. It also provides access to the *Congressional Record* (also available through the Government Printing Office [GPO] in hard copy or on its Web site at http://www.gpo.gov) and to committee reports. Once legislation is passed and signed into law, often an executive branch agency has to issue new regulations to implement the law (e.g., when the Nutrition Labeling and Education Act was signed into law, the Food and Drug Administration then had to issue regulations stipulating the format and content of the label). At this point, the *Federal Register* can be useful. It is also available in hard copy or on its Web site. When an agency is planning to issue a rule (regulation), it first publishes the proposed rule in the *Federal Register* and solicits comments; the notice will stipulate where comments should be sent and the length of the comment period. Sometimes it is useful to go back to the Congressional committee reports and compare the proposed rule with the apparent intent of the legislators; many such reports can be accessed through THOMAS. The *Federal Register* also publishes final agency rules prior to their being added to the *Code of Federal Regulations,* as well as a variety of other notices from federal agencies, such as notices of hearings and investigations, committee meetings, agency decisions and rulings, and issuance or revocation of licenses.

TRACKING TARGET AUDIENCE AWARENESS AND REACTION

The primary focus of this chapter thus far has been on how to measure messages being sent out by a program, but not how to measure the extent to which those messages are received. There are some practical methods of obtaining information about who was reached by building active response mechanisms into the dissemination effort itself, such as a telephone number or address to write to for more information. Quantitative tracking studies provide a means of monitoring reactions among the population as a whole.

Active Response Mechanisms

Active response mechanisms provide information on those people reached who are sufficiently motivated to respond. They can take many forms. Examples include telephone hotlines and coupons or having participants write in for additional information.

Telephone Hotlines

Both automated hotlines (those answered by a recording) and live-operator hotlines can provide a wealth of data. Analysis of call volume by date can be compared with other process data, such as dates of media coverage or community events, to craft a more detailed picture of what tactics are having the greatest impact. If the hotline system is more sophisticated and captures area codes and prefixes, or if callers leave their addresses, this information can be mapped and areas of high and low response can be identified. If live operators are available, a profile of who is asking for more information can be obtained by asking callers a few standard questions. For example, asking where callers heard about hotline numbers provides insights into what tactics are generating the greatest response. Learning basic demographics about callers enables program managers to assess the extent to which the callers' profile matches that of the priority population of interest, and may provide insights into how to adjust communication or delivery strategies to better focus them. If the population has been segmented using a stages of change approach, asking callers a few questions can determine what stage they are in. Materials designed for people in that stage can then be sent, if they are available.

Coupons/"Write for More Information"

Including a coupon with print advertisements or information on where to write for more information on press releases, story ideas, and TV and radio PSAs can provide additional opportunities to learn who is being motivated by the message. Although this approach does not provide information about the participants other than geographic location, it does provide information on the number of people reached. Geographic information also can be useful, as discussed earlier regarding inventory tracking systems.

The coupon idea can also be used creatively by public health initiatives that include partnerships with local businesses. For example, if local movie theater owners agree to include a slide about the program or a PSA or video clip in their premovie entertainment, viewers could be told on the slide (or video) that ticket stubs from the movie theater could be redeemed for some amount off of a screening test or other examination. Or they could be redeemed at another partner; for example, at a local grocery store or restaurant for some amount off of a specific healthier food purchase, at a pharmacy for some amount off of a smoking cessation kit, at a health club for one free visit, at a sporting goods store for some amount off of athletic equipment, or at a department store for running or walking shoes or exercise clothes. Collecting and counting the ticket stubs provides information on how many people were reached and, more important, were motivated enough by the message to take action.

Quantitative Tracking Surveys

Quantitative tracking studies, usually in the form of public opinion polls, can be used to support implementation of social change initiatives seeking to bring about changes in individual behavior or policies, or seeking to promote public health as an institution. They provide a means of monitoring levels of knowledge, awareness, and self-reported behavior among the population.

For policy change initiatives, opinion polls provide an excellent way to determine whether the issue has obtained prominence on the public's agenda (Wallack & Dorfman, 1996), monitor public reactions to various ways of framing the issue, and adjust the framing strategies accordingly. The public opinion data can also be used to help persuade journalists to cover a particular aspect of an issue, and to illustrate public support for (or opposition to) a change to policy makers. Most important, they can identify the need for fast action and can be used to rally additional financial support if needed.

An example of how public opinion tracking data were used quite successfully is the 1994 campaign against California's Proposition 188 (described in more detail in Chapter 11). Proposition 188 was a ballot initiative (sponsored by Philip Morris) that would have repealed all local antismoking ordinances as well as the state's law eliminating smoking in workplaces with weak statewide smoking restrictions (Macdonald, Aguinaga, & Glantz, 1997). The anti-188 campaign coordinated grass-roots advocacy, media advocacy, and paid advertising to deliver a common message. To monitor progress, the health coalition conducted periodic public opinion polls during the 3-month campaign. About 2 months before the vote, poll results showed voters were about equally divided on the proposition. In response, the coalition produced television ads featuring former U.S. Surgeon General C. Everett Koop and paid to air them in major media markets the last week of the campaign, using contributions provided by the American Cancer Society and American Heart Association in response to the poll results (Macdonald et al., 1997).

Initiatives focused on individual behavior change can use tracking data in two ways: to monitor progress and as a news hook to gain additional coverage. In some instances, they may want to "feed back" tracking data illustrating the population's progress in their future media messages, thus providing social reinforcement for the change. In comparison to policy change initiatives, those focusing on individual behavior change are likely to conduct tracking studies less often. Many organizations conduct them once a year, often after their major media push and in time to feed into strategic planning for the coming year. Others have the resources to conduct them more often, perhaps as often as quarterly.

Initiatives that successfully use tracking studies often incorporate one or more of the following approaches into their study designs:

- Collect data periodically, not just at the end when outcomes are assessed. Periodic information is necessary to refine messages and improve delivery.
- Ideally, collect data immediately after major public events; awareness is likely to be highest then and thus easier to detect.
- Include questions that ask where participants learned or heard about the program or its key messages, to help identify what tactics are working best.

Public opinion polls can be too costly for small organizations, but can be extremely cost-effective for larger initiatives. For example, adding questions to a nationally projectable omnibus poll costs about $1,000 per question (less for closed-ended questions, more for those with open-ended answers); tabulation of the question against demographic information collected as part of the study is included in the cost. (See Chapter 16 for more information.)

As Chapter 18 will discuss in more detail, when public opinion polls are used to track the reach of an initiative's messages, it can be difficult to assess change over time because of the magnitude of difference needed to conclude statistical change. If the issue is very much on the public agenda, changes in awareness and opinion may be easy to track, but if coverage has been relatively limited, it can be much more difficult to detect, either because such a small percentage of the population was exposed to the message or because the change was subtle. A change of 1 or 2 percentage points will be washed out in sampling error. The issues discussed in the client satisfaction section of this chapter are relevant to designing and conducting public opinion polls.

CONCLUSION

Adequately tracking and monitoring implementation is a fundamental aspect of the marketing approach. Process evaluation plays a critical role in ensuring that program components are constantly monitored and refined to improve their performance. Unfortunately, it is often overlooked or compromised in favor of outcome evaluation. Appropriate process evaluation mechanisms can be built into every program tactic. With a little creativity, many tactics can be designed so that they not only provide information on how often the message was sent out, but they also provide information on who was motivated enough to do something as a result of exposure.

REFERENCES

Alreck, P.L., & Settle, R.B. (1985). *The survey research handbook.* Homewood, IL: Irwin.

Andreasen, A.R. (1985). "Backward" marketing research. *Harvard Business Review, 63*(3), 176–182.

Andreasen, A.R. (1995). *Marketing social change: Changing behavior to promote health, social development, and the environment.* San Francisco: Jossey-Bass.

Centers for Disease Control and Prevention. (1993). *Planning and evaluating HIV/AIDS prevention programs in state and local health departments: A companion to program announcement #300.* Atlanta, GA: Author.

Eisner, E., Loughrey, K., & Davis, K. (1994). *The National Cancer Institute's 5 A Day for Better Health Program: Analysis of print media placements—July 1992 through October 1993.* Bethesda, MD: National Cancer Institute Office of Cancer Communication.

Lamb, C.W., & Crompton, J.L. (1992). Analyzing marketing performance. In S.H. Fine (Ed.), *Marketing the public sector: Promoting the causes of public and nonprofit agencies* (pp. 173–184). New Brunswick, NJ: Transaction Publishers.

Macdonald H., Aguinaga, S., & Glantz, S.A. (1997). The defeat of Philip Morris' "California Uniform Tobacco Control Act." *American Journal of Public Health, 87,* 1989–1996.

Mediamark Research, Inc. (1997). *Magazine audience estimates, Fall 97.* Available: http://www.mediamark.com.

Rossi, P.H., & Freeman, H.E. (1993). *Evaluation: A systematic approach* (5th ed.). Newbury Park, CA: Sage.

Stone, E.J., McGraw, S.A., Osganian, S.K., & Elder, J.P. (1994). Process evaluation in the multicenter child and adolescent trial for cardiovascular health (CATCH). *Health Education Quarterly,* (Suppl. 2).

Wallack, L., & Dorfman, L. (1996). Media advocacy: A strategy for advancing policy and promoting health. *Health Education Quarterly, 23,* 293–317.

CHAPTER 18

Issues in Outcome Evaluation

Outcome evaluation of social change initiatives can play a number of roles, depending on the nature of the effort being evaluated and the reason for the evaluation. This chapter introduces some of the ways in which outcome data are used to shape policy and to refine individual initiatives. However, because the outcome evaluation models used for public health initiatives have increasingly become the focus of debate in recent years, our emphasis is on presenting some of the key issues involved with evaluating such initiatives. In response to the weak effects seen in some large community-based intervention trials and the inherent problems with evaluating initiatives that do not have a control group, practitioners and evaluators have begun asking whether the outcome evaluation models that are often used are appropriate for social change initiatives.

———— ❧ ————

THE ROLE OF OUTCOME EVALUATION

Outcome data may be collected for any number of reasons. At its most basic, outcome evaluation shows whether a project had the effects it was planned to have. Depending on its scope, it can serve as a management tool by helping to identify how objectives, target audiences, strategies, and implementation might be revised and improved. This type of outcome evaluation is often conducted after a project is finished, but may occur periodically throughout the life of a program. For policy change initiatives, outcome studies may be conducted periodically following implementation of the policy change to monitor its effect and identify any unintended consequences.

In addition to serving a useful monitoring function, sometimes the results of outcome studies can be a powerful tool for future social change initiatives. One of the more striking examples is a study of the sales impact of local ordinances mandating smoke-free bars and restaurants (Glantz & Smith, 1994). The study compared restaurant sales in the 15 cities that first enacted such ordinances with sales in 15 matched cities without ordinances for the period from 1986 to 1993. It found no impact on revenues during the period following enactment of the ordinances. It makes such a convincing argument that the tobacco industry has tried to dismiss the study as "fatally flawed" and has tried to sue Glantz's employer, the University of California, on charges of scientific fraud (Susser, 1997). The study has been peer-reviewed twice, once before its original publication and again in response to an unpublished critique cited by the National Smokers' Alliance; both times, all reviewers agreed that the work was sound (Susser, 1997).

Sometimes policy outcomes are tracked after the fact, when it appears that a new policy may have inadvertently created a new danger to the public's health. Airbag regulations are a current example. As of November 1, 1997, there were 87 confirmed airbag-related deaths; of these, 49 were children (National Highway Traffic Safety Administration [NHSTA], 1997). After the deaths began occurring, the National Highway Traffic Safety Administration (NHTSA) and other organizations responded with widespread efforts to educate the public about steps they could take to lessen the likelihood of airbag injury (e.g., never put a rear-facing child safety seat in the front seat; put children in the back seat when possible; if they or small adults are in the front seat, push the seat back as far as possible). Ultimately NHTSA issued a rule allowing dealers and other car repair businesses to install manual on–off switches for airbags in vehicles owned by or used by people whose requests for switches are approved by NHTSA (NHTSA, 1997).

EVALUATING SOCIAL CHANGE INITIATIVES: THE ROLE OF EXPERIMENTAL DESIGNS

The preceding paragraphs introduce some of the many ways in which outcome data can be used. Because practitioners and evaluators have increasingly begun questioning the appropriateness of the outcome evaluation models that are often used for social change initiatives, the purpose of this chapter is to help program managers think through outcome evaluation issues. It starts with randomized trials and presents some of the limitations inherent in using this to evaluate social change initiatives. It then presents a framework for planning outcome evaluations, highlighting some key issues to consider. Finally, it describes some potentially useful evaluation designs in greater detail.

Most evaluators consider a randomized experiment to be the "gold standard" approach to outcome evaluation. With such an approach, members of the population of interest are randomly assigned to one of two or more groups. One group does not receive the program intervention and is labeled the control group. The other group(s) receives the intervention (or variations of it, if there are multiple groups). Because participants are randomly assigned to the groups, one group should not differ in any significant way from the other group. Therefore, assuming that nothing differentially affected each group during the intervention time period, any observed differences in outcomes can be assumed to be the result of the intervention. Other approaches to evaluation establish less clear-cut cause and effect, but they can assess the degree to which change occurred during the intervention time period. Later sections of this chapter highlight some of the strengths and limitations of various evaluation designs when they are applied to social change initiatives.

Although randomized experiments are the ideal and are useful in a wide array of settings, they can be problematic when used to assess public health initiatives for social change. Program managers, particularly those working in research institutions, often face tremendous pressure to use randomized trials because they are the designs by which other programs in their organizations are judged and with which their managers are most familiar.

Limitations of Randomized Designs When Evaluating Social Change

Randomized trials are based on the premise that the intervention is the only thing that could cause a change in the treatment group because it is the only thing that is different between the treatment and control groups. This premise works very well when testing a vaccine in a laboratory, as Bill Smith (1997) of the Academy for Educational Development observed. However, as he noted, public health interventions are not vaccines, and trying to assess them as though they were creates all kinds of problems. Vaccines and social change initiatives are developed using two fundamentally different models. As Smith (1997) described it, "the vaccine model is linear. It says we hypothesize something. We test it. We evaluate it and then we put it into practice" (p. 13). In comparing this vaccine model with the models used in clinical practice and in marketing, he noted, "the clinical/marketing model is circular. It says research and action are interrelated. We need to assess things first, make some plans based on that assessment, test out that planning in real life, go to scale, and then look at and monitor the thing because we're going to be making mistakes all over the place. Then we'll make some adjustments. And when we make adjustments, we're right back at the beginning" (p. 13).

The problems with thinking of social change initiatives as vaccines and then using randomized case-control trials to evaluate them are threefold:

1. The intervention cannot be adjusted to changing conditions.
2. Randomized trials are appropriate only if there is a true control group, which secular trends often eliminate.
3. The effect sizes required to demonstrate statistical change are often unrealistic.

We discuss each of these issues in more detail in the following pages.

Inability To Adjust the Intervention

Social change efforts need to be dynamic, responding to changes in the environment and the audience. It is not reasonable to set out to develop a program that will be implemented in exactly the same way at different locations at different times. If the program is used somewhere else, some adjustments will have to be made to delivery mechanisms if nothing else. Many traditional outcome evaluation designs force the entire intervention to be implemented exactly as initially planned, and never changed, in order to answer the question, "Did it work when it was implemented the way we planned it?" Because the intervention will never be implemented exactly that way again, one can question the utility of the answer.

Rather than thinking of social change programs as a vaccine, let us think of them as a plan to replace a roof. The plan is implemented: The new roof is put on. It is supposed to last for 20 years. One year later, the roof starts to leak over the living room. Do the owners leave it that way for the next 19 years, because they put the new roof on according to their original plan and they want to see if it will magically correct itself? Of course not. The answer is obvious: It is not holding up, and it needs to be fixed. In the process of fixing it, the owners probably will ask their roofers to examine what went wrong and fix that same problem elsewhere on the roof, so they do not get more leaks. But by fixing it, they increase the complexity of outcome evaluation. If, after 20 years, they ask the question, "How did the roof perform?" there is no simple answer. From one perspective, it failed: It leaked. But from another perspective, it taught them something very valuable. They got the leak fixed, they applied the same fix elsewhere to prevent future leaks, and no leaks happened. Therefore, to fully assess how the roof performed, one must assess the original plan and subsequent adjustments to it.

Similarly, with social change efforts, it is important to assess what changes were made along the way, and to document why those changes were made—what they were designed to fix—so that we begin to get a sense of the conditions under which combinations of services, message appeals, delivery mechanisms, and so forth, work best. The goal of evaluating a social change program should not be to determine if the program worked as initially envisioned or if it is stable enough to use somewhere else. It is not stable, nor is it intended to be. The goals should be to determine how much progress was made toward objectives and to assess how the implemented program differed from that originally planned and why the changes needed to be made. This information will help us determine the value of the intervention and also put together a picture of the circumstances under which various approaches work best.

As Smith (1997) noted, one of the reasons some of the large community intervention trials may appear to fail is because the interventions are not altered to meet changing conditions. Discussing the 22-community, 4-year Community Intervention Trial for Smoking Cessation (COMMIT), he observed that "because it was a case control program, there were a lot of things that occurred during the four years that the interventionists could have changed because they found out they weren't working as well. But they didn't change them because there were testing a 'vaccine' and the vaccine can't be changed in the middle of the test" (p. 12).

Inadequate Control Groups

Using randomized trials to evaluate social change often violates one of the assumptions of a randomized design—that there is a control group. With community-based interventions, there rarely is a true control: The control group may not be receiving the program's intervention, but it probably is receiving some intervention, in the form of secular trends if nothing else. Public health initiatives usually do not come into existence until there is a movement within society to make a particular change. "Science does not operate in a vacuum; the forces that operate to justify large, expensive community intervention studies also are operating among the general public to get them to accept the evidence and act on it even before the scientific establishment does" (Feinlaub, 1996, p. 1697).

These secular trends can have a devastating impact on evaluation. As Rossi and Freeman (1993) noted in their classic evaluation text, "relatively long-term trends in the community, region or country, termed *secular drift*, may produce changes in gross outcomes that enhance or mask the net effects of a program" (p. 224). Secular trends combined with the need to keep an intervention "stable" may create a situation in which the control group has access to more state-of-the-art information and tools than the treatment group over the life of a multiyear program. A number of practitioners and evaluators have argued that secular trends may be why some very large community trials, where interventions take place in one set of communities and other communities are "matched" to these and treated as a control group, fail to show an effect.

Discussing COMMIT, Smith (1997) said "a strong secular trend was affecting both intervention and control communities. Change occurred in both communities; everybody was getting better at decreasing smoking rates. The study showed that the intervention did not produce an effect any stronger than a very strong secular trend. Much of what was going on in the intervention group was going on in the control group as well" (p. 12). Another example comes from the Stanford Five-City Project, a large-scale community-based intervention designed to test whether a comprehensive program of community organization and health education produced favorable changes in cardiovascular disease risk factors, morbidity, and mortality. Authors of one study concluded that "the net intervention effects were modest. This is due, in part, to the strong secular trends in both health promotion and risk factors" (Winkleby, Taylor, Jatulis, & Fortmann, 1996, p. 1778).

Also discussing the effects of secular trends, Hornik (1997a) warned, "local activities build on a spine of national programs that work together. Don't evaluate, don't try to compare treatment and controls that are geographically defined unless there is really going to be a difference in exposure to messages. Don't accept trials as negative evidence until you look hard at the evidence for differences in exposure between the so-called treatment and control areas" (p. 59).

Need for Large Effects

Social change initiatives do not take place in a lab with 50 participants. They take place in communities and states. Sometimes they take place across the whole country. Unlike the lab, we have little control over exactly who receives the intervention and almost no control over exactly how much of it they receive. Yet our field's evaluation standards demand statistically significant change before we can conclude the intervention had an effect. As Fishbein (1996) noted,

> given the nature of our statistical tests and our tendency to use relatively small samples in experimentally controlled studies, this usually means that a public health intervention will be considered a success only if it produces an effect of at least medium size (e.g., a mean difference of at least half of a standard deviation, or about a 20%-to-30% change in a proportion), or, often, an even larger effect size (e.g., a mean difference of a full standard deviation, or a 50%-to-60% change in a proportion). One might ask whether such expectations are either realistic or warranted. That is, can we really expect a usually brief, relatively inexpensive public health intervention to produce medium or large effects? . . . Rightly or wrongly, we appear to be bound by the requirement to demonstrate statistical significance even though we seldom have the resources to evaluate our interventions with sample sizes necessary to detect a small effect. (p. 1075)

To put these effects sizes in context, the Stanford Five-City Project described earlier in this chapter—much more intensive than many population-based public health initiatives—estimated that the adults in the project's treatment communities would have been exposed to around 5 hours of education per year (Farquhar et al., 1990). Is it reasonable to expect even a 20% change—the low end of the range just described—as a result of 5 hours of education over the course of a year? Most public health interventions deliver a much lower dose of education.

If we compare social change initiatives with commercial marketing campaigns, which are another type of initiative seeking to induce widespread population change, we see very different standards for measuring achievement. Commercial marketers conclude that their "interventions" are a great success when market share increases 2% or 3%. Writing about this phenomenon Fishbein (1996) remarked, "Thus, while a condom manufacturer would be more than happy if an advertising campaign increased the company's share of the market by 3% or 4%, a public health intervention that increased condom use by the same 3% or 4% probably would be considered a failure" (p. 1075).

Why are the standards for the two fields so different? Although there may be many reasons, two in particular probably play a part. First, expectations about appropriate effect sizes were carried over from expectations about appropriate effect sizes for clinical studies, with no adjustment made for differences in intervention intensity. As Kristal (1997) noted, "the effect size for clinical interventions is large and hopefully fast. In a public health intervention, it's small, and at best, it's gradual" (p. 39). Second, public health evaluators are forced to rely on samples, which are a considerably less exact measure than market share or, for that matter, many of the measures available in clinical studies. As Kraemer and Winkleby (1997) noted in a response to Fishbein's comments in the preceding paragraph, "if the same condom manufacturers lacked data from the entire population and needed to estimate the market share of the campaign, they might commission a survey research group to sample representative sites within the market area. If the survey research group concluded that the market share was somewhere between 2% and 6%, the condom manufacturers would be uncertain about the effect of the campaign and might be quite dissatisfied with the survey" (p. 1727).

There are two other questions to consider when thinking about effects sizes for social change initiatives:

1. What outcomes are reasonable to expect, given the structure of the intervention?
2. What magnitude of effect is needed to make a difference to public health?

Both questions give rise to all sorts of policy debates, but at the end of the day the answer to either of these questions will be an effect size far smaller than what most outcome evaluations will be able to detect. The answer to the second question, in particular, can make outcome evaluation particularly challenging, because in some instances the magnitude of effect needed to make a difference to public health can be quite small. As Beresford and colleagues (1997) noted in discussing population-wide efforts to change eating habits, "the public health model, or population strategy, consists of shifting the entire distribution of a risk factor, including the mean, down. The diminution in risk for a given individual is typically small and may not even be clinically important. Nevertheless, because the entire distribution is affected, the impact on morbidity and mortality can be substantial" (p. 615).

Citing Prentice and Sheppard (1990), they went on to note that "a 1% reduction in dietary calories from fat made population wide could result in about 10,000 deaths saved in the United States in a year" (Beresford et al., 1997, p. 615). That 1% reduction would not be detectable at the community level using most available evaluation methodologies, and even if it were detected, it could not be said to be statistically significant because of sampling error.

CONSIDERATIONS WHEN PLANNING EVALUATIONS

The issues we have raised in this chapter illustrate some of the many pitfalls of designing useful outcome evaluations for public health interventions. Planning the evaluation in tandem with the initiative eliminates some potential problems and often results in a strong intervention as well as a stronger evaluation. This section outlines some questions to consider when developing outcome evaluation plans.

What Kind of Intervention Is It?

As noted earlier, most population-based public health interventions targeting individual behaviors can expect small, gradual changes. However, there are some exceptions. Hornik (1997b) argued that "straightforward substitution of behaviors, when possible, may allow more rapid change than attempts to introduce new behaviors" (p. 55), citing as examples interventions to prevent Reye's syndrome (by using an aspirin substitute rather than aspirin) and sudden infant death syndrome (by putting babies to sleep on their backs rather than on their stomachs). He noted that both of these behaviors were very easy to change and adopting the new behavior "sharply reduced the risk of a rare but devastating event" (p. 55). We would add that in both situations, adopting the new behavior was linked to a core human value: caring for children.

How Is the Intervention Expected To Work?

Rossi and Freeman (1993) defined an impact model as "an attempt to translate conceptual ideas regarding the regulation, modification, and control of behavior or conditions into hypotheses on which action can be based" (p. 119). They went on to note that "the absence of a well-specified impact model severely limits opportunities to control a program's quality and effectiveness (Freeman & Sherwood, 1970). . . . Even if a social program is successful in delivering services and achieving the objectives set for it, without an explicitly documented impact model there is no basis for understanding how and why it worked or for reproducing its effects on a broader scale, in other sites and with other targets" (p. 120).

Wallack and Dorfman (1996) provided an example of specifying how an intervention is expected to work when they outlined how policy change initiatives using a media advocacy strategy are expected to work. The expectation is that if the issue is appropriately framed in terms of access (to get journalists' attention) and content (telling the story from the policy perspective), it will get on the public agenda through media coverage. Once it is on the public agenda, it will mobilize groups or individuals who influence policy makers, and they, in turn, will put pressure on the decision makers, resulting in the policy being enacted or the change occurring. The airbag example mentioned earlier in this chapter illustrates large parts of this process: The media started covering the airbag-caused deaths of infants and children and NHTSA started getting pressure to allow the airbags to be turned off (car dealers and repair shops normally are not legally allowed to over-ride safety equipment) pending a more permanent solution to the problem.

For public health education interventions targeting individual behavior change, Hornik (1997b) observed the following:

> There are two complementary models of behavior change implicit in many public health education campaigns. One focuses on individuals as they improve their knowledge and attitudes and assumes that individual exposure to messages affects individual behavior. The complementary model focuses on the process of change in public norms, which leads to behavior change among social groups. The models contrast direct effects of seeing mass media materials from indirect effects. The first assumes a viewer sees a public service announcement (PSA) about the role of condoms in safe sex, for instance, and then decides to follow the advice. The second assumes that discussion within a social network is stimulated by PSAs or media coverage of an issue and that discussion may produce changed social norms about appropriate behavior, which affects the likelihood that each member of the social network will adopt the new behavior. If the second model is most correct, if a social process dominates the process of a behavior change, then individuals' detailed knowledge about the benefits of a new health behavior may be less important than their belief that it is an expected behavior. (pp. 54–55)

In Exhibit 18–1, Hornik provides a succinct description of a social change initiative from the viewpoint of a member of the target audience.

As Hornik (1997b) said of this example, "this program is effective not because of a PSA or a specific program in physician education. It is successful because the National High Blood Pressure Education Program has changed the professional and public environment as a whole around the issue of hypertension" (p. 50).

What Outcomes Can Reasonably Be Expected?

Perhaps more than any other question, this question illustrates the need to develop evaluation plans in tandem with the plans for the initiative. The starting point for determining what outcomes are reasonable should be the initiative's objectives. As Rossi and Freeman (1993) and Kotler and Roberto (1989), among others, noted, objectives should operationalize a program's goals, therefore making them measurable. However, they also noted that program objectives often do not do this, rendering evaluation very difficult because the evaluators cannot tell

Exhibit 18–1 Social Change in Action

A person sees some public service announcements and a local TV health reporter's feature telling her about the symptomless disease of hypertension. She checks her blood pressure in a newly-accessible shopping mall machine, and those results suggest a problem. She tells her spouse who has also seen the ads and encourages her to have it checked. She goes to a physician who confirms the presence of hypertension, encourages her to change her diet, and then return for monitoring.

Meanwhile, the physician has become more sensitive to the issue because of a recent article in the *Journal of the American Medical Association,* some recommendations from a specialist society, and a conversation with a drug retailer as well as informal conversations with colleagues and exposure to television discussions of the issue. The patient talks with friends at work about her experience. They also increase their concern and go to have their own pressure checked. She returns for another check-up and her pressure is still elevated although she has reduced her use of cooking salt. The physician decides to treat her with medication. The patient is ready to comply because all the sources around her—personal, professional and mediated—are telling her that she should.

Source: Reprinted with permission from R. Hornik, Public Health Education and Communication as Policy Instruments for Bringing About Changes in Behavior, in *Social Marketing: Theoretical and Practical Perspectives,* © 1997, Lawrence Erlbaum Associates, Inc.

what they ought to be measuring. Even if the goals are operationalized, the resulting objectives may be changes of unrealistically large magnitude.

Another issue to consider when thinking about expected outcomes is how "success" is defined in the initiative's organizational environment. That is, how much of a change will an initiative need to demonstrate in order to be viewed as successful? Can the intervention be structured so that it is of sufficient intensity and duration to achieve this level of success? Can an evaluation be structured to measure it even if it is attained? As discussed elsewhere in this chapter, sometimes a relatively small population-wide change—too small to adequately capture in an evaluation—can have enormous public health consequences. Demonstrating cause and effect can also be problematic. Other factors may influence outcomes, such as activities conducted by complementary or competing organizations. Evaluation may show an association between exposure to program components and increased awareness of or engagement in the appropriate health behavior, for example, but cannot show definitively that the initiative caused the change.

Beyond looking to the initiative's objectives and likely definitions of success for direction, one must consider the preceding two questions as well as issues such as the expected duration and intensity of the intervention. It can take years to see the effects of initiatives targeting individual changes in prevention behaviors. For example, the large decreases in smoking rates and deaths due to cardiovascular disease are seen over a decade or more. Reviewing the results of other initiatives addressing the same or similar topics and using similar implementation strategies may provide some guidance.

The expected outcomes can influence evaluation plans in many ways. For example, if expectations are for small, gradual change, large sample sizes will be required (and still may not attain the needed precision), and it would be wise to wait a sufficient amount of time before attempting to measure outcomes. In contrast, if large, rapid effects are anticipated, sample sizes can be smaller and outcomes measured more quickly.

What Type of Evaluation Design Is Most Appropriate for the Intervention Setting?

Evaluation designs can be divided into three categories:

1. experimental
2. quasi-experimental
3. other

Each category has limitations and underlying assumptions that preclude using it in every setting. In the following sections we present brief descriptions of each type of design and overviews of some of the issues to consider in using them. Those planning an evaluation would do well to consult standard evaluation texts, such as Rossi and Freeman (1993), as well as the classic works on experimental and quasi-experimental design (see, in particular, Campbell & Stanley, 1966; Cook & Campbell, 1979).

Experimental Designs

True experimental designs must have target audience members randomly assigned to treatment and control groups; outcomes are assessed by comparing the treatment group(s) scores with those of the control group. Ideally, both groups are measured before and after the intervention. For public health practitioners, a major limitation of these designs is that they are appropriate only for what Rossi and Freeman (1993) labeled *partial-coverage* programs; that is, programs where the intervention is not delivered to all (or virtually all) members of a target population.

Quasi-Experimental Designs

Experimental designs in this category also compare treatment and control groups; however, assignment to each group is not random (hence the designation quasi-experimental). As with true experiments, outcomes are most commonly assessed by comparing the pre- and postintervention scores of the groups. A major drawback to quasi-experimental designs is what has been termed "the fantasy of untreated control groups" (Durlak, 1995, p. 76). As discussed earlier in this chapter, social change initiatives are usually developed as a result of strong secular trends; it is unlikely that members of the control group are receiving no aspects of the intervention.

A variety of methods can be used to assign target audience members to treatment and control groups. One popular method of assignment with community interventions is selecting communities that match the communities where the intervention is put into place on key variables. This was the approach used in the COMMIT and Stanford Five-City Project community intervention trials mentioned earlier in this chapter.

An alternative approach that works for some types of interventions is to define different groups within a community. For example, schools could be divided into those that receive program materials and those that do not. For mass media components, some commercial advertising methodologies can be used to divide the overall population into two groups. For example, some cable systems can split households, transmitting one ad to half of the households and a different ad to the other half. Some magazines can split press runs in the same way, or they can insert an ad in one edition and not another.

Another technique is to create the control group when outcome data are analyzed, by comparing those who participated in the program (the treatment group) with those who did not (the control group). This approach is rarely an option with community interventions: Because everyone in the community could have been exposed to program messages, even if they do not remember the exposure, there is no way to divide the groups.

Quasi-experimental designs can be used for a number of reasons. They are often used to pilot test an intervention or to evaluate a demonstration project. A true pilot test would normally take place after traditional pretesting but before the planned full-scale implementation. Demonstration projects generally follow the complete program life cycle (e.g., planning, development, implementation, evaluation). The resulting evaluation data can help refine program components and, in some instances, help program planners gauge likely response to or demand for various program elements.

However, expectations of what a pilot test or demonstration project will provide should be carefully considered. Such tests are expensive because materials and products have to be produced in final form and reproduced in small quantities, and the resources required to adequately evaluate the results can far outweigh the costs of development and implementation. Additionally, expectations often are unrealistic because the pilot implementation is qualitatively or quantitatively different from what the future implementation will be. For example, demonstration sites often receive far more training and technical assistance than will be available to other sites when the program is implemented. Test sites may receive materials for free that other sites will have to pay for. The small scale may allow proportionally more resources to be expended, increasing both the total number of people reached by the intervention and the frequency with which they are reached, leading to an overstatement of the likely effects.

Quasi-experimental designs are also used for comparison studies in which two or more implementation strategies are tested against each other. The implementations may differ along such dimensions as types of materials (e.g., different advertisements might be tested against each other) or mix of promotional activities (e.g., one implementation uses only mass media, another uses mass media plus community events, and a third uses only community events).

Other Designs

Rossi and Freeman (1993) called this category *designs for full-coverage programs* because it includes the only types of evaluation designs that are appropriate for programs that are delivered to all members of a target population. Designs in this category include comparisons between cross-sectional studies (independent surveys taken at different points in time, such as were used in the campaign to oppose California's Proposition 188, discussed in Chapters 11 and 17). Some options for cross-sectional studies are provided in the next section.

Many designs in this category make comparisons between the same target audience members before and after the intervention; these target audience members are termed *reflexive controls*. These designs include panel studies (also termed *repeated measures designs* because they involve measuring outcomes multiple times among the same group of people) and time-series analyses, which involve collecting many repeated measures of the same variables prior to an intervention, using them to project what would have happened without the intervention, and then collecting repeated measures postintervention to look at what in fact did happen. Projections are compared with the actual data to estimate the net effects of the program.

Tracking Studies (Periodic Cross-Sectional Surveys). For initiatives tracking outcomes among individuals, conducting a scientifically representative baseline survey prior to implementation and then conducting representative tracking studies periodically thereafter can provide important process and outcome data. Questions typically include self-reported measures of current practice or intent to engage in a behavior (be it increasing physical activity or voting a particular way on an upcoming referendum or bond issue), as well as awareness of the issue and the public health initiative.

Many tracking studies are custom studies; that is, they are designed and conducted specifically to support the initiative. However, some initiatives can minimize the cost of tracking studies by "piggy-backing" onto other data collection activities. For example, federal and state programs can explore options such as the

National Health Interview Survey (for federal programs) and the Behavioral Risk Factor Surveillance System and Youth Risk Behavior Survey (for most states).

Omnibus studies conducted by private research firms and universities provide another cost-effective option for evaluating and refining social change campaigns. A main advantage of omnibus surveys is that they are priced per question, but the price includes access to all the demographic questions asked on the survey. Many national studies are fielded weekly; questions must be provided 1 or 2 days in advance. State and local studies are generally conducted less frequently. Most organizations use multistage probability samples; the standard sample size for national surveys is 1,000 adults, but state or local surveys may use smaller samples. Results are generalizable to all households with telephones in the geographic area in which the study is conducted (95% of U.S. households have telephones). To maximize comparability and avoid bias resulting from other topics on the questionnaire, vendors can be asked to put the public health initiative's questions at the beginning of the questionnaire.

How Will Outcomes Be Measured?

Decisions about measuring outcomes should be made in tandem with selection of evaluation designs. Outcome measures should be driven by the theoretical model used to develop the intervention, and they should be consistent with what the intervention was designed to accomplish. For example, if the intervention was designed to tell people how many servings of fruits and vegetables they should eat, and to convince them to add two servings each day, the outcomes to be measured should be whether the number of people who know how many servings to eat is increasing, and whether people are, in fact, adding two servings per day, not how many servings they are eating.

Beyond problems with measuring outcomes that do not reflect intervention objectives, sometimes outcome measures are not as sensitive to a range of possible changes as they might be. As just one example, consider parts of a commentary by Fishbein (1996) on a community intervention designed to increase the likelihood that young men would engage in safer sex:

> Kegeles [, Hays, and Coates, 1996] evaluated their intervention by looking for a reduction in the proportion of men who engaged in *any* act of unprotected anal sex. The question that must be asked is whether this measure fully captures the effect of their intervention. Not reflected in this outcome measure would be a person who had reduced the number of unprotected acts of anal intercourse from 50 at baseline to 25 at follow-up, or one who went from no condom use to 75% condom use, or who reduced the number of acts of anal sex or the number of partners, or who substituted masturbation or "outercourse" for intercourse. Did the

outcome measures selected by the authors ask too much of their intervention? Was it fair to view a person who reduced unprotected sex acts from 100 to 0 as no more of a success than one who reduced such acts from 1 to none? (p. 1076)

Other challenges arise related to the types of data that can be collected at reasonable cost. For example, for programs focusing on individual behavior changes, self-reported measures are often all that can be obtained at reasonable cost, and these are not always reliable. Sometimes people do not know aspects of their health status (e.g., blood pressure or blood cholesterol levels), and sometimes they do not really know what they do (e.g., how many servings of grains they ate yesterday). At other times, social desirability influences their answer (i.e., they give what they think the answer should be even if it is not what they do). Many researchers attempt to control for this third confounding variable by measuring social desirability traits as part of their studies.

What Was Actually Implemented?

As Orlandi (1986) observed, assessing effectiveness is difficult or impossible without knowing how the program was implemented. Without process evaluation to detail if and how the intervention was implemented, evaluators may make what Scanlon, Horst, Nay, Schmidt, and Waller (1977) termed a Type III error: evaluating a program that has not been adequately implemented or is not measured as implemented (Basch, Sliepcevich, Gold, Duncan, & Kolbe, 1985). Before outcome evaluation is initiated, evaluators should review process evaluation data and determine whether any refinements need to be made to the study design or measures to adjust to a different implementation than was initially envisioned.

How can someone not know if or how a program was implemented? Often outside evaluators are brought in solely to evaluate, and they may not have been involved during implementation. Even if the evaluator is on staff, for many large programs evaluation staff are totally separate from program staff, and they would have no reason to know whether a program had been implemented as planned or not. For multisite programs where collaborating organizations are responsible for much of the implementation, it may be difficult for program managers to truly know the degree to which particular program components have been implemented. Ongoing monitoring and process evaluation activities help ensure this problem does not occur.

CONCLUSION

Evaluators and program managers need to work together to ensure that the evaluation design is appropriate for the intervention model and that the outcomes measured are the outcomes the program sought to affect. Outcome evaluations that emphasize to what degree planned outcomes were achieved and how they were achieved, rather than whether the program as originally planned achieved the outcomes anticipated, will be more useful and will allow the intervention to be adjusted during implementation in response to changing conditions.

There is no question that researchers need to identify the circumstances under which particular types of program components work best and most cost-efficiently. As Walsh, Rudd, Moeykens, and Moloney (1993) observed, "if (as seems reasonable) the question for funders and program designers is whether and under what conditions socially marketed health interventions produce superior results and are more efficient and effective than common alternatives, almost no useful information is available to answer it" (pp. 115–116). However, not every program has to have an evaluation sophisticated enough to address these types of questions. Rossi and Freeman (1993) recommended using the "good enough" rule of thumb when selecting evaluation designs: "The evaluator should choose the best possible design from a methodological standpoint, having taken into account the potential importance of the program, the practicality and feasibility of each design, and the probability that the design chosen will produce useful and credible results" (pp. 220–221).

This chapter has presented a number of factors to keep in mind when determining how the outcome of a social change initiative will be assessed. Foremost among them are the following:

- Choosing an evaluation design appropriate for the intervention in scope, in cost, and, most importantly, in its assumptions about how change will occur. The evaluation should be able to tolerate changes to the program design and implementation.
- Understanding the environment in which the initiative is taking place. Strong secular trends are often present and can mask the effects of an intervention.
- Ensuring that outcome expectations are driven by what is realistic for the intervention and evaluations are designed accordingly.
- Ensuring that the outcomes measured are those the intervention was trying to affect and that the range of possible progress toward those outcomes is adequately captured.

Using traditional randomized designs to assess the outcomes of social change can be problematic in a number of ways. First, the restrictions of the evaluation limit the power of the initiative. As Walsh and colleagues (1993) observed, "the very essence of social marketing is to adapt and change, whereas summative evaluation researchers need a program to stay its course" (p. 115). In other words, traditional outcome evaluation models expect a static, never-changing intervention, but social change initiatives employing marketing principles are designed to be dynamic, constantly adjusting to changing environments and audience needs. Second, large effects may be needed to see statistically significant change, yet sometimes it is not reasonable to expect a large effect and even a small one may have huge public health implications. Third, the outcome data can be difficult to interpret when strong secular trends are also at work.

REFERENCES

Basch, C.E., Sliepcevich, E.M., Gold, R.S., Duncan, D.F., & Kolbe, L.J. (1985). Avoiding type III errors in health education program evaluations: A case study. *Health Education Quarterly, 12,* 315–331.

Beresford, S.A.A., Curry, S.J., Kristal, A.R., Lazovich, D., Feng, Z., & Wagner, E.H. (1997). A dietary intervention in primary care practice: The eating patterns study. *American Journal of Public Health, 87,* 610–616.

Campbell, D.T., & Stanley, J.C. (1966). *Experimental and quasi-experimental designs for research.* Boston: Houghton Mifflin.

Cook, T.D., & Campbell, D.T. (1979). *Quasi-experimentation design and analysis issues for field settings.* Skokie, IL: Rand McNally.

Durlak, J.A. (1995). School-based prevention programs for children and adolescents. Thousand Oaks, CA: Sage.

Farquhar, J.W., Fortmann, S.P., Flora, J.A., Taylor, C.B., Haskell, W.L., Williams, P.T., Maccoby, N., & Wood, P.D. (1990). Effects of community-wide education on cardiovascular disease risk factors. *Journal of the American Medical Association, 264,* 359–365.

Feinlaub, M. (1996). Editorial: New directions for community intervention studies. *American Journal of Public Health, 86,* 1696–1698.

Fishbein, M. (1996). Editorial: Great expectations, or do we ask too much from community-level interventions? *American Journal of Public Health, 86,* 1075–1076.

Freeman, H.E., & Sherwood, C.C. (1970). *Social research and social policy.* Englewood Cliffs, NJ: Prentice-Hall.

Glantz, S., & Smith, L.R.A. (1994). The effect of ordinances requiring smoke-free restaurants on restaurant sales. *American Journal of Public Health, 84,* 1081–1085.

Hornik, R. (1997a). Charting the course from lessons learned. In L. Doner (Ed.), *Charting the course for evaluation: How do we measure the success of nutrition education and promotion in food assistance programs? Summary of proceedings* (pp. 58–61). Alexandria, VA: USDA Food and Consumer Service.

Hornik, R. (1997b). Public health education and communication as policy instruments for bringing about changes in behavior. In M.E. Goldberg, M. Fishbein, & S.E. Middlestadt, *Social marketing: Theoretical and practical perspectives* (pp. 45–58). Mahwah, NJ: Lawrence Erlbaum Associates.

Kegeles, S.M., Hays, R.B., & Coates, T.J. (1996). The Mpowerment Project: A community-level HIV prevention intervention for young gay men. *American Journal of Public Health, 86,* 1129–1135.

Kotler, P., & Roberto, E.L. (1989). *Social marketing: Strategies for changing public behavior.* New York: Free Press.

Kraemer, H.C., & Winkleby, M.A. (1997). Do we ask too much from community-level interventions or from intervention researchers? *American Journal of Public Health, 87,* 1727.

Kristal, A.R. (1997). Choosing appropriate dietary data collection methods to assess behavior changes. In L. Doner (Ed.), *Charting the course for evaluation: How do we measure the success of nutrition education and promotion in food assistance programs? Summary of proceedings* (pp. 39–41). Alexandria, VA: USDA Food and Consumer Service.

National Highway Traffic Safety Administration. (1997). Air Bag On-Off Switches Rule, 62 Fed. Reg. 62406 (to be codified at 49 C.F.R. § 571 and 595).

Orlandi, M.A. (1986). The diffusion and adoption of worksite health promotion innovations: An analysis of barriers. *Preventive Medicine, 15,* 522–536.

Prentice, R.L., & Sheppard, L. (1990). Dietary fat and cancer: consistency of the epidemiologic data, and disease prevention that may follow from a practical reduction in fat consumption. *Cancer Causes Control, 1,* 81–97.

Rossi, P.H., & Freeman, H.E. (1993). *Evaluation: A systematic approach* (5th ed.). Newbury Park, CA: Sage.

Scanlon, J.W., Horst, P., Nay, J.N., Schmidt, R.E., & Waller, A.E. (1977). Evaluability assessment: Avoiding type III and IV errors. In G.R. Gilbert & P.J. Conklin (Eds.), *Evaluation management: A sourcebook of readings.* Charlottesville, VA: U.S. Civil Service Commission.

Smith, W. (1997). Confounding issues in evaluations of nutrition interventions. In L. Doner (Ed.), *Charting the course for evaluation: How do we measure the success of nutrition education and promotion in food assistance programs? Summary of proceedings* (pp. 11–13). Alexandria, VA: USDA Food and Consumer Service.

Susser, M. (1997). Editorial: Goliath and some Davids in the tobacco wars. *American Journal of Public Health, 87,* 1593–1595.

Wallack, L., & Dorfman, L. (1996). Media advocacy: A strategy for advancing policy and promoting health. *Health Education Quarterly, 23,* 293–317.

Walsh, D.C., Rudd, R.E., Moeykens, B.A., & Moloney, T.W. (1993). Social marketing for public health. *Health Affairs,* 105–119.

Winkleby, M.A., Taylor, C.B., Jatulis, D., & Fortmann, S.P. (1996). The long-term effects of a cardiovascular disease prevention trial: The Stanford Five-City Project. *American Journal of Public Health, 86,* 1773–1779.

What Does the Future Hold?

If the public health field is able to adopt a consumer orientation, its future will be bright. This is because there exists "a readily stimulated reservoir of appreciation for the services of public health, within the public in general and among elected officials in particular" (Kroger, McKenna, Shepherd, Howze, & Knight, 1997, p. 274). An overwhelming majority of Americans already attach a great deal of importance to the core functions of public health. The challenge is to define and frame the public health product to tap into this reservoir of support. The existence of strong support for public health services makes marketing public health a great opportunity for the practitioner.

Public health practitioners at all levels of training and public health training institutions must respond positively to this marketing opportunity. Individual practitioners should take advantage of professional education programs to enhance their knowledge and skills in marketing, communication, media advocacy, and public relations. Schools of public health should incorporate these disciplines into their research and training programs, and should provide advanced training in these areas to experienced public health professionals. All public health institutions should seek collaborations with experts in these areas from the private sector, if not incorporate positions in these areas directly into their personnel infrastructure.

The federal government and, in particular, the Centers for Disease Control and Prevention (CDC), should continue to play a lead role in placing an emphasis on marketing public health. The formative research the CDC is conducting will provide the key strategic insights that will allow public health practitioners across the nation to understand target audiences for marketing public health as an institution. But private sector organizations must assist in these research efforts as well, and some level of formative research should be conducted by public health practitioners, even at the local level.

Will public health practitioners abandon the traditional selling orientation and bring a consumer orientation to their work? Will they embrace formative research and learn how to define, package, position, and frame public health behaviors, programs, and policies in a way that satisfies the needs and wants of the consumer and reinforces the core values of their target audiences? Will public health institutions adequately provide for the professional training of new and continuing personnel in the areas of marketing, communication, and media advocacy?

As the public health practitioners of today and tomorrow the future of public health is entirely in our hands. Capitalizing on our opportunity to shape this future will require three accomplishments. First, we must work to restore a unified vision of the mission of public health in society. Second, we must reassert our fundamental role as advocates for the achievement of this mission. Finally, we must turn to the people from whom our charge derives in the first place—the public—and learn how to frame our programs and policies so that their needs and wants are met. Successfully marketing public health requires that we put the public back in public health.

REFERENCE

Kroger, F., McKenna, J.W., Shepherd, M., Howze, E.H., & Knight, D.S. (1997). Marketing public health: The CDC experience. In M.E. Goldberg, M. Fishbein, & S.E. Middlestadt (Eds.), *Social marketing: Theoretical and practical perspectives* (pp. 267–290). Mahwah, NJ: Lawrence Erlbaum Associates.

Hiring Agencies, Contractors, and Consultants

This appendix is designed to provide guidance on (1) determining when to go outside your organization for assistance in developing, implementing, or assessing social change interventions; (2) assessing the options to ensure a good fit between the organization and the agency, consultant, or contractor once the decision has been made; and (3) working with outside firms or consultants. Many of the specific examples are oriented toward selecting firms for marketing communication tasks (usually advertising or public relations agencies) because their services are often used in social change interventions. However, many of the tips would apply when hiring firms for other activities.

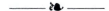

WHEN IS OUTSIDE ASSISTANCE NEEDED?

Social change interventions can include such diverse components as grass-roots advocacy, advertising, special events, media advocacy, continuing medical education modules, train-the-trainer courses, curriculum development, and direct service provision. Organizations rarely have in-house staff trained in all the disciplines that can help develop and implement a social change intervention. Public health organizations turn to outside help for one or more of the following reasons:

- To obtain specialized skills not available internally. For example, few public health organizations employ staff with advertising copywriting and production skills.
- To handle work overflow. Sometimes in-house staff have the necessary skills, but the intervention creates more work than they can handle.

- To obtain an outside viewpoint. Evaluation is most often contracted out for this reason, but outside viewpoints also can be very helpful with strategic planning and message development. And in some situations, the opinions of "outsiders" may have more credibility than the opinions of staff who are trying to get an intervention funded.

TIPS ON SELECTING AGENCIES, CONSULTANTS, AND OTHER CONTRACTORS

Every organization has unique constraints on hiring outside contractors. The process outlined below can be modified to fit your organization's requirements.

1. Determine what in-house staff can do—based on skills and time available—versus what should be contracted out.
2. Group the tasks that must be contracted out based on skills required to perform them—for example, market research, evaluation, advertising, media relations, grass-roots advocacy.
3. Determine how many contractors you will need. Be careful about assuming that one contractor can handle many tasks—or about believing those who say they can. For example, organizing grass-roots advocacy is very different from producing advertising or handling media relations; most firms do not have staff that can handle all of these assignments equally well. If your organization's staff does not have the expertise to assess the types of contractors needed, it may help to convene a search committee that includes in-house staff and outside consultants.
4. Identify potential contractors (firms or independent consultants). Ask colleagues for recommendations, and find out who did work that you think is outstanding. A good next step is to send a short questionnaire to each firm (or consultant) to assess its interest and capabilities. (See Exhibit A–1 for sample questions for advertising and public relations firms. The list of questions in the exhibit is extensive; some questions could be reserved for the written proposals.)
5. Request written proposals or presentations from the firms of interest to you. Make the request in writing, and be clear about what you want done. Convey, at a minimum,
   - basic facts about the program, including goals and objectives.
   - specific services that will be needed.
   - details regarding compensation.
   Giving bidders a ballpark budget helps them tailor their response to your resources.
6. Protect yourself. As part of your initial request or, at the latest, before a contract is signed,

Exhibit A–1 Screening Questions To Identify Potential Communication Firms

GENERAL INFORMATION

1. What were the total annual billings of your firm for each of the last 5 years?
2. List your firm's three largest clients and the percentage of total current agency billings each represents.
3. List three average-sized clients and the percentage of billings each represents.
4. List the accounts your firm has won and lost over the past 2 years and the total billings for each account. Why were the accounts lost or resigned?
5. Describe any experience that your firm and executives have with [SOCIAL CHANGE TOPIC].
6. What experience has your firm had that is pertinent to the marketing, merchandising, and advertising of [SOCIAL CHANGE TOPIC]?
7. (For Advertising Agencies) Approximately what percentage of your last year's billings went into the following media? (List TV, radio, newspaper, magazines, outdoor, other.)
8. Describe your approach to developing communication messages and materials.

ORGANIZATION AND PERSONNEL

1. What is the total number of people employed full time by your agency? Provide a breakdown by department or function.
2. Describe the organization and philosophy of your creative department. What are the agency's capabilities regarding the creation and production of TV, radio, and print advertising?
3. Who is your creative director, and how long has this individual been employed by you? What other agencies has he or she worked for?
4. (For Advertising Agencies) What is the organization of your media planning staff? Describe how they function.

RESEARCH

1. If applicable, describe the organization and capabilities of your research department.
2. How would you describe effective communications?
3. Have you measured the effectiveness of your work for clients?
4. What methods do you use to measure communication effectiveness pre- and post-production?

ADDITIONAL INFORMATION

1. Provide a functional organizational chart of your firm.
2. Furnish biographical information on the people who will work on the account.
3. List your current accounts, approximate billings, and length of time they have been with the firm.

continues

Exhibit A–1 continued

4. Assuming you have no objection, please provide the names, addresses, and tele-phone numbers of several of your clients and principal contacts, preferably at least one large account and one medium-sized account.
5. List any new products or services you have introduced for clients during the past 3 years.
6. In a paragraph or two, describe the attributes of your agency vis-à-vis other agen-cies in [NAME OF CITY/STATE].

Source: Reprinted with permission from D. Zucker, *The Advertising Agency: Your Partner in Communications,* © 1992, The Academy for Educational Development.

- *ask what percentage of time proposed staff are committed to other projects.* Some contractors are notorious for the "bait and switch": They bid staff that have the capabilities you are looking for even though they know they are committed to other projects. Then when they win the con-tract, they substitute other, less experienced staff.
- *include a "key personnel" clause.* This clause states that the contractor cannot remove anyone designated "key personnel" from your project without notifying you first, and that you must approve any "key person-nel" replacements.
- *ask for unit pricing and cost assumptions* (including any additional tasks or materials needed to complete the project that are not in the budget). Both pieces of information help you compare contractor costs. Also, sometimes organizations forget to include particular items in their request (or don't realize they should be included). Scrupulous contractors then find themselves in a quandary: Should they include the necessary steps in their budget, thereby increasing their costs (and possibly causing them to lose the business), or should they assume that the organization will handle the other tasks some other way? (Unscrupulous contractors just ignore the other tasks and materials, wait until the contract is signed, and then bring them up as modifications.) If the contract is for publications or reports that could go through many revisions, ask for the number of anticipated revi-sions to be noted in the assumptions.
- *ask for budgets in terms of labor hours as well as dollars.* This information will help you (1) assess whether the contractor understands the scope of work and (2) compare the level of effort each contractor is proposing (i.e., the total dollar amount might be the same but might buy you vastly differ-ent quantities of professional time).
- *ask for examples of past work done by proposed staff.* Ask that each ex-ample be accompanied by a description of the role each staff member

played in it. When you hire a contractor, particularly for creative products, you are really buying the expertise of the individuals who work on your project. Asking for examples of their work (rather than the firm's) helps ensure that you get what you think was proposed.

- *always get multiple bids or proposals*. Doing so not only helps you compare prices, it helps you assess how clear you were in your instructions—if all bidders have radically different proposals and prices, your scope of work may not have been clear.
- *stipulate that the contractor will incorporate your revisions before finalizing the product*. While most contractors want you to be happy with the final product, it is safest to have all approval points written into the contract.

7. Evaluate the prospects. Exhibit A–2 lists some specific characteristics to assess in communication firms, and Exhibit A–3 lists 10 questions to ask any type of contractor or consultant.

Exhibit A–2 Evaluating Communication Contractors

CORE CAPABILITIES
- *Using research*. It has been clearly demonstrated that the most effective communications programs are based on the ability to understand the true implications of research. Does the firm have a track record of using research to shape effective communication strategies? Does it demonstrate a comfort with research? (Many successful communicators still prefer to go with "gut instincts" or strategies that have worked in the past.)
- *Developing strategy*. Many firms have standardized approaches to developing communication strategies and messages. Does the firm have a specific process it prefers to follow? Is it rigid or flexible? Are the firm's strategies centered on consumer needs or client desires?
- *Innovation*. While traditional approaches to communications and marketing can be comfortably safe and proven, the greatest leaps are often made by those who are willing to take a chance on a new or unproved approach. Can the firm be expected to present fresh approaches? How has it helped other clients become innovators?
- *Execution*. The smartest, most innovative strategy is of course useless if it can't be executed, or isn't executed properly. Does the firm inspire confidence in its ability to get the job done? Can it work "smart" to get the most out of a limited budget?
- *Evaluation*. The success of many communication programs is difficult to measure, particularly when there are no sales figures to examine. How does the firm assess the relative benefit of its work? (Numbers of articles generated or inter-

continues

Exhibit A–2 continued

> views scheduled are not valid measures of success unless those are specific objectives of the program.)
> - *Client service.* Every firm will say that its philosophy is to be a "partner" with its client, but what does that really mean? How does it like to work? Working with a committee can be a challenge: How would the firm suggest approaching the project?
> - *Fiscal responsibility/terms.* What is the firm's preferred method of compensation? Is it familiar with the billing and accounting procedures necessary to work with government agencies?
>
> **CHEMISTRY**
> One of the primary reasons to have individual interviews is to assess the "chemistry" between the committee and representatives from the candidate firms. Provided that all firms are qualified to handle the project, chemistry may be the most valid basis for making a choice. Would it be enjoyable to work with these people?
>
> **INTEREST**
> One of the things that will hopefully become clear in candidates' presentations and/or proposals is their level of interest in the project. If they do not answer the question unprompted, a question to pose is: "Why are you interested in working on the project?"
>
> *Source:* Copyright © John Killpack.

The following are some thoughts to keep in mind as you assess each candidate:
- *Excellent skills are more important than content knowledge in most cases.* Successful contractors get that way by being fast learners. You can teach them what they need to know about your problem, but you can't teach them their discipline. For example, if you have to choose between an advertising agency with great creative abilities but little knowledge of your particular topic and an agency with mediocre creative abilities but lots of content knowledge, go with the former, with one caveat: Agencies that have no experience working with public health organizations often have difficulty working within the scientific constraints imposed by the field and the levels of approval required. Evaluate such agencies carefully to see how willing they are to work within your parameters.
- *Make sure they tell you how they will apply their experience to your problem.* They may have done some great work in the past, but if they can't apply it to your needs, who cares?

Exhibit A–3 Questions for Potential Contractors

---

1. How would you propose working and communicating with us?
2. Why are you interested in this project?
3. How important would this work be to your firm? Why?
4. Tell us about the most personally satisfying project that you've worked on over the past several years.
5. What makes your firm unique?
6. What is your firm's greatest strength?
7. What is the biggest unexpected problem you've encountered on a recent program, and how did you address it?
8. What would you expect from us as a client?
9. Who will be working on our account?
10. What is your preferred/typical method of compensation?

Source: Copyright © John Killpack.

- *Did they follow your instructions?* Contractors are on their best behavior when they are pursuing a business opportunity. If they don't listen to you now, they never will.
- *Don't penalize them if they didn't provide something you didn't ask for.* One contractor may include a great idea that is not part of the services you requested. It is unfair to penalize the others for not proposing the same thing.
- *Make yourself available for questions.* If possible, meet with the candidates before you ask for proposals. You're hiring contractors for their expertise. They may recommend a totally different approach after hearing a little bit about the issue.
- *How's the chemistry?* Do you want to work with them? Contracting relationships are often fraught with tension due to project demands. If you aren't comfortable with the organization, you won't have a good working relationship with that organization, and the project will suffer.

TIPS ON WORKING WITH CONTRACTORS

Once you have selected a contractor,

- make sure you understand how the contractor charges (i.e., hourly, retainer, per project, commission, or some combination) and what the contractor will charge for, including incidentals (such as local travel and phone). Find out how much the contractor charges for services such as photocopying and faxing—these are often moneymakers for the firm and can send your bill much higher than you anticipated. For example, faxing at $2 per page can add up very quickly. Ask if the contractor marks up out-of-pocket costs, and if so, how much (charging 15% or more is not unusual and can add up fast on major expenditures, such as research and production).

- remember that for most contractors time equals money. Don't waste your money by wasting your contractor's time, and don't expect the contractor to give you lots of time for free. Contract staff who bill hourly face enormous pressure to bill as many hours as possible.
- make sure everyone involved understands who is responsible for each aspect of the project. Make sure you understand who your point of contact is for each aspect.
- limit contractor staff at meetings to those who absolutely need to be there (every body is usually costing you money). But make sure that everyone who needs to be there is.
- always give as much direction as possible up front, and be consistent. It usually costs you a lot of money if contractors have to go "back to the drawing board," plus it demoralizes them, so future work may not be as good.
- establish a timeline that includes regular meetings and milestones for you to review the work. Waiting to review a project until it is "finished" is almost always a bad idea because there are too many opportunities for the contractor to go off strategy. But, particularly for creative products, keep the approval process simple and the number of people who must approve small. Good creative almost never emerges from a committee. And, as Roman and Maas (1976) noted, "the best clients are not meddlers. They point out major problems and let the agency find solutions. 'Creative clients' end up with halfway efforts. The agency expects so many changes, it won't try very hard on original submissions" (p. 154).
- ask for estimates of hours for all tasks, and ask for monthly progress reports that account for all hours and expenditures. Monitor them carefully, and discuss any significant discrepancies between estimated and actual costs with the contractor immediately. You don't need to find out halfway through a project that you're out of money.

REFERENCE

Roman, K., & Maas, J. (1976). *How to advertise.* New York: St. Martin's Press.

APPENDIX B

Suggested Readings

Andreasen, A.R. (1995). *Marketing social change: Changing behavior to promote health, social development, and the environment.* San Francisco: Jossey-Bass.

Backer, T.E., Rogers, E.M., & Sopory, P. (1992). *Designing health communication campaigns: What works.* Thousand Oaks, CA: Sage.

Bandura, A. (1986). *Social foundations of thought and action.* Englewood Cliffs, NJ: Prentice-Hall.

Chapman, S., & Lupton, D. (1994). *The fight for public health: Principles and practices of media advocacy.* London: BMJ Publishing Group.

Glanz, K., Lewis, F.M., & Rimer, B.K. (Eds.). (1997). *Health behavior and health education: Theory, research and practice* (2nd ed.). San Francisco: Jossey-Bass.

Goldberg, M.E., Fishbein, M., & Middlestadt, S.E. (1997). *Social marketing: Theoretical and practical perspectives.* Mahwah, NJ: Lawrence Erlbaum Associates.

Green, L.W., & Kreuter, M.W. (1991). *Health promotion planning: An educational and environmental approach* (2nd ed.). Mountain View, CA: Mayfield.

Kotler, P., & Andreasen, A.R. (1996). *Strategic marketing for non-profit organizations* (2nd ed.). Upper Saddle River, NJ: Prentice-Hall.

Kotler, P., & Roberto, E.L. (1989). *Social marketing: Strategies for changing public behavior.* New York: Free Press.

Lefebvre, R.C., & Flora, J.A. (1988). Social marketing and public health intervention. *Health Education Quarterly, 15,* 299–315.

Lewton, K.L. (1991). *Public relations in health care: A guide for professionals.* Chicago: American Hospital Publishing.

Maibach, E., & Parrott, R.L. (Eds.). (1997). *Designing health messages: Approaches from communication theory and public health practice.* Thousand Oaks, CA: Sage.

National Cancer Institute. (1989). *Making health communication programs work: A planner's guide* (NIH Pub. No. 89-1493). Bethesda, MD: Author.

Rogers, E.M. (1983). *Diffusion of innovations* (3rd ed.). New York: Free Press.

Roman, K., & Maas, J. (1992). *How to advertise* (2nd ed.). New York: St. Martin's Press.

Rossi, P.H., & Freeman, H.E. (1993). *Evaluation: A systematic approach* (5th ed.). Newbury Park, CA: Sage.

Rothschild, M.L. (1979). Marketing communications in nonbusiness situations or why it's so hard to sell brotherhood like soap. *Journal of Marketing, 43*, 11–20.

Signorielli, N. (1993). *Mass media images and impact on health: A sourcebook.* Westport, CT: Greenwood Press.

Stone, E.J., McGraw, S.A., Osganian, S.K., & Elder, J.P. (1994). Process evaluation in the multicenter child and adolescent trial for cardiovascular health (CATCH). *Health Education Quarterly* (Suppl. 2).

Sutton, S.M., Balch, G.I., & Lefebvre, R.C. (1995). Strategic questions for consumer-based health communications. *Public Health Reports, 110*, 725–733.

Wallack, L., & Dorfman, L. (1996). Media advocacy: A strategy for advancing policy and promoting health. *Health Education Quarterly, 23*, 293–317.

Wallack, L., Dorfman, L., Jernigan, D., & Themba, M. (1993). *Media advocacy and public health.* Newbury Park, CA: Sage.

Walsh, D.C., Rudd, R.E., Moeykens, B.A., & Moloney, T.W. (1993). Social marketing for public health. *Health Affairs*, 105–119.

Glossary of Terms

Audience segmentation: Dividing the population into groups with the goal of identifying groups whose members are similar to each other and distinct from other groups along dimensions that are meaningful in the context of the program.

Bounceback cards: Short questionnaires on the back of a post card addressed to the sponsoring organization and including the sponsor's business reply permit information. Used as a process evaluation instrument. Also called *business reply cards.*

Business reply cards: See *bounceback cards.*

Coalition: A group of organizations that come together to address a common goal. Most often run by a committee composed of representatives from each (or many) coalition members.

Communication strategy: How the social change will be positioned in the audience's mind. It describes the target audience, the action they should take as a result of exposure to the communication, the key benefit they will receive in exchange, support for that benefit, the image of the action that the communication should convey, and how target audience members can be reached.

Creative brief: A one- to two-page summary of the communication strategy that is given to the creative team to use for guidance when developing materials.

Entertainment–education: Embedding social change messages in entertainment media (i.e., movies, television programs other than news, some radio programs, comic books).

Focus groups: A qualitative research technique that involves 1- to 2-hour structured discussions among 6 to 10 participants, led by a trained moderator working from a list of topic areas or questions. Results are not projectable to the population from which participants were drawn.

Formative evaluation: Studies conducted to assess reactions to proposed messages, materials, or program components so that they can be refined before they are finalized and implemented.

Framing memo: A document that analyzes the ways an issue is framed by proponents and opponents. Its core is a matrix that summarizes, for each framing strategy, (1) the core position, or main argument; (2) the metaphor used (typically a familiar analogy); (3) catch phrases used to describe the argument; (4) symbols; (5) visual images evoked by the argument; (6) the implied source of the problem; and (7) the principle or core values appealed to.

Frequency: The number of times each target audience member is exposed to a particular message or material.

Gatekeeper: An individual or organization through whom a program's components or materials must pass to reach the target audience.

Goals: Translation(s) of a program's mission into specific behavioral outcomes. Distinct from *objectives*.

Gross impressions: An estimate of how many opportunities there were for messages delivered through the mass media to be seen or heard; calculated by summing the circulation and/or audience size associated with each publication of a story or advertisement. Not a measure of number of people reached.

Intermediary: An organization or individual that can or must be used to reach a constituency for you.

Marketing mix: Product, price, place, and promotion; the variables that a marketer can change.

Media advocacy: Bringing about policy changes by using the media to put pressure on policy makers. This is accomplished by placing issues on the media agenda through media relations efforts and/or paid advertising, or seeing that issues already on the media agenda are framed from a policy perspective. The belief is that once issues are on the media agenda, they become part of the public agenda and force policy makers to act.

Message concepts: Statements that present key aspects of the communication strategy to members of the target audience.

Objectives: Quantification of goals; objectives describe the specific intermediate steps to be taken to make progress toward goals. For public health efforts, objectives are often changes in audience behavior over time; levels of participation in specific program activities; or measured changes in attitudes, beliefs, or skills associated with prevention practices, with the expectation that change in these factors will facilitate or reflect change in outcome behavior and ultimately morbidity and mortality. Distinct from *goals*.

Outcome evaluation: Research conducted to determine whether an intervention had the intended effects on behavior. Usually conducted after the intervention is finished, but can be conducted periodically during and after the intervention.

Place: Outlet(s) through which products are available—or situations in which behavior changes can be made.

Price: Cost to a target audience member, in money, time, effort, lifestyle, or psyche, of engaging in a behavior (or purchasing a product or using a service).

Primary research: Studies that are designed and conducted specifically to answer a current research question (as compared with *secondary research*).

Process evaluation: Studies conducted during and immediately after implementation to document what program components, materials, and messages were delivered and to whom, how, when, and where they were delivered; this information can then be used to assess and refine components and delivery strategies.

Product: Behavior, good, service, or program that is provided to a person in exchange for a price.

Promotion: Some combination of advertising, media relations, promotional events, personal selling, and/or entertainment to communicate with target audience members about a product, service, program, or behavior change.

Qualitative research: Provides insights into a target audience; addresses questions of *why* rather than *how many*. Results are not quantifiable and not projectable to the population from which participants were drawn.

Quantitative research: Provides measures of *how many* members of a population have particular knowledge or attitudes, or engage in a particular behavior. If conducted with a probability sample and appropriately constructed questions, can be representative of and projectable to the population from which the sample was drawn.

Reach: The total number of people exposed to a message or material.

Secondary research: Studies that were originally conducted for some purpose other than the current research question(s) (as compared with *primary research*).

Social marketing: Application of commercial marketing technologies to the analysis, planning, execution, and evaluation of programs designed to influence the voluntary behavior of target audiences in order to improve their personal welfare and that of their society.

Storyboard: Used to express ideas for television ads or other video products in cartoon-strip format; separate frames depict the main action above a written description of what the viewer will see and hear.

Strategy: Long-term (usually 3 to 5 years), broad approach(es) that an organization takes to achieving its objectives. Distinct from *tactics.*

Tactics: Short-term detailed steps used to implement a strategy. For example, a community event, a specific training module, or a specific public service advertising campaign are all tactics.

Index

A

Addictive behavior, 34
  unwholesome demand, 34
Adolescent
  autonomy, 46
  control, 46
  freedom, 46
  independence, 46
  individualism, 46
  needs and desires, 46, 47
  self-reliance, 46
  smoking, marketing, 46–47
  values, 46
Advertisement, 158, 159, 162, 213
Advertising, 404–411. *See also*
  Specific type
  principles, 404–405
  promotional activity, 352–354
  public service placement, 408–411
Advertising equivalencies, defined, 462
Advocacy, 37–38
  defined, 93
  inadequate emphasis, 37–38
  lack of expertise, 38
  lack of training, 38–39
  lobbying, compared, 93

  public health, 91
  as role and responsibility, 38
Affirmative action debate, framing,
  325–337, 328–329, 330–331
Agenda-setting research, 350
AIDS, 20, 21
  funding, 143–144
Alcohol abuse, drunk driving,
  program success compared, 59–60
American Cancer Society, 157–158
Antiregulatory sentiment, 88–90
  autonomy, reframing, 134–136
  freedom, reframing, 134–136
Antismoking ordinance, reframing
  example, 146–147
Argument testing, 157
Arizona, tobacco tax, 163–165
  disparity in financial resources, 163
  failed efforts, 163–165
  public opinion poll, 163–165
  tobacco industry, 164–165
Armchair media tour, 398
Asthma, 13
Audience profiling, Five a Day for
  Better Health program, 267–268
Audience segmentation, 265–270
  defined, 506

differential responsiveness, 270
exhaustiveness, 270
general public, 276–277
mass media, 277–278
measurability, 270
mutual exclusivity, 270
policy maker, 275–276
process, 269–270
reachability, 270
segmentation data sources, 266–269
strategy selection, 270
substantiality, 270
types, 265–266
Audience size, defined, 460–461
Autonomy
adolescent, 46
antiregulatory sentiment, reframing, 134–136
drunk driving, 61
framing, rationale for government programs to address poverty, 135–136
value of, 45, 48

B

Behavior change, commercial marketing, 203–204
Behavior segmentation, Five a Day for Better Health program, 266, 267–268
Behavioral Risk Factor Surveillance System, 266
Behavioral risk factors, chronic disease, 9, 10
Block grant, 84–86
legislation to convert entitlement programs, 84–86
Bounceback card
defined, 506
process evaluation, 453–455

Brochure, 384
Budget, program component, 358–360
Bureaucracy, 156
Business reply card. *See* Bounceback card

C

California, tobacco tax, 152–155
arguments in support of tax increase, 153
Californians Against Unfair Tax Increases, 153
Coalition for a Healthy California, 153
crime theme, 154
David/Goliath argument, 154
destination for tax revenue, 153
tobacco industry, 153–154
tobacco industry advertising, 153–154
Californians Against Unfair Tax Increases, 153
Campaign financing reform, 87–88
Cancer, death rates, 7
Cause of death, chronic disease, 6
Centers for Disease Control and Prevention
framing
core American values, 172
strategies, 177–179
funding, 170–182
budget increase, 174–176
floor debate in Congress, 184–192
marketing
case study, 170–182
focus group, 180
public opinion poll, 180–181
threat of uncontrolled disease, 179

new disease, 172–174, 176–178,
180
Centers for Disease Control and
Prevention framing, 177–179
Office of Health Communication,
179
Central-site interview
college or university vendor,
424–425
commercial firm, 424
data analysis, 426–427
interviewer training, 425, 426
materials, 423–424
pretesting, 419–427
process, 420–427
questionnaire design, 423–424
report, 427
sample questionnaire, 438–445
self-conducted, 425
when to use, 420
Change
transtheoretical model of stages of,
201–202, 232–233
constructs, 233
transtheoretical model stages of,
314–315
action, 315
contemplation, 314
precontemplation, 314
preparation, 314–315
Child, poverty, 10
Child safety seat, 209–210
technological approach, 210
Cholera, 141–142
Chronic disease
behavioral risk factors, 9, 10
cause of death, 6
cost, 5
deteriorating social and economic
conditions, 9–17
direct medical costs, 7

disability, 7
effects, 8
epidemic, 5–8
public health practice
implications, 18–21
epidemiology, 5–6
impact, 5
indirect costs, 7
socioeconomic status, 7–8
Cigarette tax, framing, 128–131
Circulation, defined, 460–461
Civil rights, framing, 134
Client satisfaction
components, 457
process evaluation, 456–460
data collection, 459
questionnaire, 458
reliability, 459
sampling, 458–459
validity, 459–460
Clipping service, media coverage
analysis, 463–464
Coalition, 374–378
characterized, 374–375
defined, 506
leadership, 377
operating procedures, 377–378
participation agreement, 376
recruiting coalition members, 375
selecting coalition members, 375
Coalition for a Healthy California, 153
Colorado, tobacco tax, 163–165
disparity in financial resources, 163
failed efforts, 163–165
public opinion poll, 163–165
tobacco industry, 164–165
Commercial marketing
behavior change, 203–204
concepts, 200–217
consumer importance, 204–206
cost benefit exchange, 200–203

marketing mix, four Ps, 206–217
 place, 211–213
 price, 210–211
 product, 207–210
 promotion, 213–215
 social change, marketing
  differences, 198
Communication. *See also* Mass
 communication
 uses, 312–313
Communication contractor,
 evaluating, 500–501
Communication strategy, 213–214,
 313–338
 breaking through inattention, 337
 defined, 506
 development process, 324–332
 development worksheet, 341–342
 emotional appeal, 334
 emotional benefit appeal, 334–335
 framing, 312–338
 heuristic appeal, 334–335
 humorous appeal, 336
 message construction, 332–337
 message content, 332–337
 pitfalls to avoid, 332
 positive emotional appeal, 334–335
 pretesting, 416
 rational appeal, 334
 role of theory, 314–315
 strategic questions for, 315–324
 target audience, 315–316
  benefits, 319–320
  benefits credibility, 320
  channels for reaching audience,
   320–321
  characteristics, 315–316
  current behavior, 316–319
  desired behavior, 316–319
  image, 322–324
  obstacles, 319

threat appeal, 335–336
 types of appeals, 334–336
 uses, 313
Competition, product, 208
Conference, 411–412
Congressional Record, 104th
 Congress, Centers for Disease
 Control and Prevention funding,
 184–192
Consultant, 496–503
 evaluation, 500–501
 need for, 496–497
 screening questions, 498–499
 selection, 497–502
 working with, 502–503
Consumer, determining what
 consumer wants, 49–51
Consumer education, telemarketing
 fraud, 221–224
 community-based activities,
  223–224
 evaluation, 224
 goal, 221
 legislative advocacy, 224
 mass communication, 223
 objectives, 222
 opportunities, 221
 partnerships, 222–223
 promotion, 223–224
 strategy, 222
 target audiences, 222
Contractor, 496–503
 evaluation, 500–501
 need for, 496–497
 screening questions, 498–499
 selection, 497–502
 working with, 502–503
Control
 adolescent, 46
 illness, 43–45
 value of, 45, 48

Coping, 44
Core values, 140–145
    drunk driving, 61
    framing, 123–124, 125, 126
        reframing, 133–134
Cost, print materials, 386–387
Cost benefit exchange, commercial
    marketing, 200–203
Cost-benefit analysis, social change,
    248–251
Countermarketing, 36–37
Creative brief, defined, 506
Crime, health status, 14–15

D

Data collection instrument
    focus group, 285
    in-depth interview, 292
    process evaluation, 452–453
David/Goliath argument, 154
Demand
    demand level states, 32
    for social change, 31–36
Demarketing, 32
Demographic segmentation, 265–266
Developmental marketing, 32
Diabetes, incidence, 7
Diffusion, defined, 230
Disability, chronic disease, 7
Disease
    defined, 43
    illness, distinguished, 43
    societal meanings, 143, 144–145
Distribution, 348
    training, 348
Drunk driving
    alcohol abuse, program success
        compared, 59–60
    autonomy, 61

    core values, 61
    freedom, 61
    public health marketing, 58–61

E

Ebola virus, 21, 172, 173, 174, 176–
    178, 180
Economic change, demand state, 35
Editorial coverage. *See* News
    coverage
Education, health status, 11–12
Elderly patient
    health care access, 18
    quality of care, 18
Electronic media, 387–388
Emerging infections, 21, 172–173,
    174, 176–178, 180
Emotional appeal, 334
Emotional benefit appeal, 334–335
Employer newsletter, promotional
    activity, 354
Endemic infectious disease, 103–108
Entertainment-education, 401–403
    characterized, 401
    defined, 506
    examples, 401–402
    uses, 403
Environmental issues
    framing, 130
    health status, 14
    marketing principles, blame shift
        from corporations to individual,
        121
    special-interest lobbying, 87–88
Ethical issues, partner, 370–373
Evaluation, program component, 360
Exchange process
    defined, 29
    necessity for, 30

Experimental design, 486
  outcome evaluation, 477–482
    inability to adjust intervention,
      479–480
    inadequate control group, 480–
      481
    limitations, 478–482
    need for large effects, 481–482

F

Federal Register, 471
Field review, 434–435
  process, 434–435
  when to use, 434
Five a Day for Better Health program
  audience profiling, 267–268
  behavior segmentation, 266,
    267–268
  media coverage analysis, 466–469
  partner, 216
  place, 212–213
Focus group, 280–290
  analyzing data, 289–290
  characterized, 280
  conducting, 285–289
  data collection instrument, 285
  defined, 506
  in-depth interview, selection
    criteria, 291–292
  logistical details, 285–288
  moderator's guide, 306–309
  participants, 280–284
  preparing report, 289–290
  pretesting, 432–434
    process, 433–434
    when to use, 432–433
  professional moderator, 285, 286–
    287
  recruitment screener, 303–305

research objectives, 284
study design, 284–285
topic guide, 285, 286–287
vendor, 288
volunteer moderator, 285
Food and Drug Administration, 35–36
Formative evaluation, defined, 507
Formative research, 62, 63, 261–294
  concept, 49
  cultural differences, 50
  defined, 49
  determining what consumer wants,
    49–51
  developing strategies and tactics,
    278
  diversity of attitudes, beliefs, and
    values, 50
  framing, 273, 279–280, 281–282
  general public, 276–277
  goal, 49
  health behavior change, 264–273
    audience segmentation, 265–270
    audience selection, 270–273
    shaping intervention, 272–273
  health care reform, 119–120
  HIV prevention, 66–69
  immunization, 262
  importance, 66–69
  information resources, 310–311
  market segmentation, 50–51
  mass media, 277–278
  policy maker, 207, 275–276
  product definition, importance,
    118–122
  public health policy initiatives,
    273–280
    audience segmentation, 273–278
    shaping policy initiative, 278–280
    target audience selection,
      273–278

purpose, 49
role, 261–264
school health, case study, 296–302
shaping intervention components,
    272–273
telemarketing fraud, 220
Framing
affirmative action debate, 325–337,
    328–329, 330–331
antismoking ordinance, reframing
    example, 146–147
autonomy, rationale for government
    programs to address poverty,
    135–136
Centers for Disease Control and
    Prevention
    core American values, 172
    strategies, 177–179
cigarette tax, 128–131
civil rights, 134
communication strategies, 312–338
concept, 123
core values, 123–124, 125, 126
    reframing, 133–134
defined, 122–124
developing public health frames,
    128–131
    objectives, 128
dominant tobacco control frames,
    243
eliminating smoking in restaurants,
    128, 129
environmental issues, 130
examples, 123–124
formative research, 273, 279–280,
    281–282
freedom, rationale for government
    programs to address poverty,
    135–136
importance, 124–128
mandatory seat belt law, 130

needle exchange program, 130
news coverage, 394–396
Norplant, 132–133
reframing public health issues,
    131–136
research, 136
tobacco industry, 124–127
    dominant frames, 243
    level playing field frame, 124,
        131–132
    tuberculosis, 130
Framing memo, 324
    defined, 507
    tobacco policy debate, 240, 241–242
Freedom, 55–56
    adolescent, 46
    antiregulatory sentiment, reframing,
        134–136
    drunk driving, 61
    framing, 135–136
    value of, 45, 48
Frequency, defined, 461, 507
Funding
    AIDS, 143–144
    Centers for Disease Control and
        Prevention, 170–182
        budget increase, 174–176
        floor debate in Congress, 184–
            192
    local health department, 84
    National Institutes of Health, budget
        increase, 174–176
    prevention, 77
    public health
        antiregulatory sentiment, 88–90
        block grant, 84–86
        budget cuts, 83–84
        campaign financing reform,
            87–88
        economic factors threatening,
            83–90

legislation restricting, 85
political factors threatening,
 83–90
special-interest lobbying, 87–88
state public health agency, 84
Funding organization, partner, 371

G

Gatekeeper, defined, 507
General public
 audience segmentation, 276–277
 formative research, 276–277
Geoclustering, 266
Geodemographic segmentation, 266
Goals, defined, 507
Gross impressions, defined, 461, 507
Group A ("flesh-eating")
 streptococcus, 21

H

Hantavirus pulmonary syndrome, 21
Health
 price of, 30–31
 value, 43–45
Health advocacy group, 92–93
Health behavior change, formative
 research, 264–273
 audience segmentation, 265–270
 audience selection, 270–273
 shaping intervention, 272–273
Health belief model, 201
Health care access
 crisis, 17–18
 elderly patient, 18
 Medicare, 18
 quality of care, 17–18
Health care delivery, changes, viii
Health care reform
 formative research, 119–120

public health
 differences, 78
 illusion of reform as solution, 78
 relationship, 78
Health insurance
 lack of coverage, 17
 poverty, 17
Health status
 crime, 14–15
 education, 11–12
 environmental hazards, 14
 factors, 9–17, 19–20
 housing, 12–13
 hunger, 11
 poverty, 9–11
 social support, 15–17
 socioeconomic status, 9–11, 77
 unemployment, 13
 violence, 14–15
Health threat, characterized, 173
Heart disease, mortality rates, 7
Heuristic appeal, 334–335
HIV, 21
 formative research, 66–69
Homicide, 7
Housing
 asthma, 13
 health status, 12–13
 lead poisoning, 13
Humorous appeal, 336
Hunger, health status, 11
Hypermedia, 388

I

Identity, mass communication,
 383–384
Illness
 control, 43–45
 defined, 43
 disease, distinguished, 43

independence, 44
  subjective meaning, 48
  uncertainty, 43–44
Image
  print materials, 386–387
  strategic marketing, 53–54
Immunization, formative research, 262
Impact model, 483
Implementation, monitoring and
  refining, 449–475
Independence
  adolescent, 46
  illness, 44
  value of, 45, 48
In-depth interview, 290–293
  analyzing data, 293
  data collection instrument, 292
  focus group, selection criteria, 291–
    292
  logistics, 292–293
  preparing report, 293
  pretesting, 430–432
    process, 431–432
    when to use, 430–431
  research objectives, 290
  study design, 290–292
  vendors, 292–293
Individual autonomy, 134
Individualism, adolescent, 46
Infectious disease
  mortality rate, 20
  reemergence, 20–21
Innovation, defined, 230
Innovation diffusion, 230–232
  characteristics affecting, 231
Intermediary, 378, 379
  characterized, 378
  defined, 507
Internet, 388–392
  characteristics, 355–356
Interview. See In-depth interview

Interviewer training, central-site
  interview, 425, 426
Inventory tracking, process evaluation,
  455–456

K

Knowledge-attitudes-behavior
  paradigm, 203

L

Lead poisoning, housing, 13
Leadership, coalition, 377
Legal issues, partner, 370–373
Legislation, vii
  monitoring, 470–471
Level playing field frame, reframing,
  131–132
Lifestyle change, unfavorable state of
  demand for, 34–35
Lobbying
  advocacy, compared, 93
  defined, 93
Lobbying regulations, public health
  organization, 100–101
Local health department, funding, 84
Lyme disease, 21

M

Magazine
  characteristics, 355–356
  coverage opportunities, 397
Maintenance marketing, 32
Malaria, 178–179
Malaria Control in War Areas, 178
Mall-intercept interview. See
  Central-site interview
Mammography program, objectives,
  253

Managed care
 goals, 81–82
 incentives, 81–82
 public health
  differences, 79–83
  illusion of managed care as
   opportunity for public health,
   79–83
  managed care as danger to public
   health, 82–83
  mission, 79–80
  relationship, 78
 underlying values of, 80–81
Mandatory seat belt law, framing, 130
Market segmentation, formative
 research, 50–51
Marketing. *See also* Commercial
 marketing
 applying marketing principles,
  197–218
 Centers for Disease Control and
  Prevention
  case study, 170–182
  focus group, 180
  public opinion poll, 180–181
  threat of uncontrolled disease,
   179
 defined, 29, 43
 extensive research in, 199
 new marketing strategy for public
  health, 137
 as process, 199
 public health practitioner
  opportunity, 117–145
 social change, 197–199
  principles, 198
 tobacco tax
  campaign spending, 152
  case study, 151–168
  failed campaign characteristics,
   166

 successful campaign
  characteristics, 166
 using theory, 229
Marketing mix
 commercial marketing, four Ps,
  206–217
 defined, 507
Marketing research, state cigarette
 excise tax, 120
Mass communication, 223, 381–413.
 See also Specific type
 assessing proposed materials and
  activities, 383
 identity, 383–384
 planning development time, 382–383
 use of, 381–382
Mass media, 392–413. *See also*
 Specific type
 audience segmentation, 277–278
 formative research, 277–278
 health behaviors framing, 350–351
 nontraditional, 354
 promotional activity, 350–354
  options, 352–354
Massachusetts, tobacco tax, 157–163
 advertisement, 158, 159, 162
 American Cancer Society, 157–158
 argument testing, 157
 maximum tax, 157
 political consulting firm, 157
 public opinion poll, 157–158
 reframing, 160
 tobacco industry, 158–163
 tracking poll, 160
Media advocacy, 215
 defined, 507
Media coverage analysis, 460–470
 clipping service, 463–464
 content analysis, 464–465
 Five a Day for Better Health
  program, 466–469

monitoring process, 462–464
on-line resources, 463
sources of media information, 463–
    464, 465
terminology, 460–462
tracking advertising placement,
    465–470
Media training, 361
Mediamark Research, Inc., 268–269
Medicaid, restructuring, 84–86
Medical sociology, 43
Medical treatment
    immediate benefits, 109
    misunderstanding importance of,
        74–78
Medicare
    health care access, 18
    quality of care, 18
Meeting, 411–412
Message concepts, defined, 507
Montana, tobacco tax, 155–157
    bureaucracy, 156
    public opinion survey, 155, 156–157
    revenue use, 155–156
    tax *vs.* health issue, 156
    telephone tracking survey, 156
    tobacco industry, 156
Mortality
    causes, 75
        shift in, 75, 76
    decline due to public health, 74–75
Mothers Against Drunk Driving,
    58–61

N

National Health and Nutrition
    Examination Survey, 266
National Health Interview Survey, 266

National health observance, by month,
    365–366
National Institutes of Health, funding,
    budget increase, 174–176
National Rifle Association, special-
    interest lobbying, 87
Needle exchange program, framing,
    130
New disease, Centers for Disease
    Control and Prevention, 172–174,
    176–178, 180
    Centers for Disease Control and
        Prevention, framing, 177–179
News coverage, 392–401
    building relationships with media,
        393–394
    elements of newsworthy stories, 395
    framing, 394–396
    news-generating tactics, 398–401
    promotional activity, 352–354
    tactics to increase coverage,
        396–397
Newsletter, 385
    promotional activity, 354
Newspaper
    characteristics, 355–356
    coverage opportunities, 397
Norplant, framing, 132–133

O

Objectives
    defined, 253, 507
    mammography program, 253
Observational learning, 234
Omnibus survey, 489
    process, 428–429
    when to use, 428
104th Congress
    characterized, 171

floor debate on Centers for Disease Control and Prevention funding, 184–192
Opposition framing, reframing public health issues, 131–136
Outcome evaluation, 476–492
  defined, 508
  evaluating social change initiative, 477–482
  experimental design, 477–482
    inability to adjust intervention, 479–480
    inadequate control group, 480–481
    limitations, 478–482
    need for large effects, 481–482
  planning, 483–490
    designs for full-coverage programs, 488–489
    evaluation design, 486–489
    experimental design, 486
    impact model, 483
    intervention action mechanism, 483–484
    intervention setting, 486–489
    intervention type, 483
    omnibus study, 489
    outcome measurement, 489–490
    periodic cross-sectional survey, 488
    program implementation variables, 490
    quasi-experimental design, 486–488
    reasonable outcome expectations, 484–486
    reflexive control, 488
    repeated measure design, 488
    tracking study, 488
  role, 476–477
Outdoor ad, 406

Out-of-home media, 406
  characteristics, 355–356

P

Participation agreement, coalition, 376
Partner, 367–380
  aid from, 371–372
  aid to, 372
  appropriate, 370–371
  challenges, 374
  developing appropriate roles, 373
  developing successful partnerships, 369–374
  for establishing credibility, 370
  ethical issues, 370–373
  Five a Day for Better Health program, 216
  flexibility, 373–374
  funding organization, 371
  identifying benefits to, 369–370
  legal issues, 370–373
  partner's activities, 372–373
  program component, 361–362
  regulatory agency, 370–371
  role, 367
  social change, 215–217, 222–223
  types, 368–369
  written agreement, 374
Periodic cross-sectional survey, 488
Personal Responsibility and Work Opportunity Act, 16–17, 86
Place
  commercial marketing, 211–213
  defined, 211, 508
  Five a Day for Better Health program, 212–213
  social change, 211–213

Planning
  outcome evaluation, 483–490
    designs for full-coverage
      programs, 488–489
    evaluation design, 486–489
    experimental design, 486
    impact model, 483
    intervention action mechanism,
      483–484
    intervention setting, 486–489
    intervention type, 483
    omnibus study, 489
    outcome measurement, 489–490
    periodic cross-sectional survey,
      488
    program implementation
      variables, 490
    quasi-experimental design,
      486–488
    reasonable outcome expectations,
      484–486
    reflexive control, 488
    repeated measure design, 488
    tracking study, 488
  process evaluation, 450–453
  promotional activity, 350–354
  social change, 225–259, 227
    analyzing information, 235–252
    analyzing public policy issues
      framing, 239–240
    current science review, 236–237
    evaluation, 230
    goals, 253–255
    identifying complementary and
      competing activities, 237–239
    identifying problems based on
      public health burden, 246–252
    identifying sources of
      information about potential
      target audiences, 240–246
    information collecting, 236–246

    innovation diffusion, 230–232
    leveraging resources and
      relationships, 229
    models of behavior, 230–234
    objectives, 253–255
    principles, 229–230
    prioritizing problems based on
      public health burden, 246–252
    role of theory, 230–234
    situation analysis, 235–252
    situation assessment, 246–252
    social cognitive theory, 234
    strategic plan, 234–235
    strategy importance, 227–228
    transtheoretical model, 232–233
    unified strategic program, 229
  strategic plan, 257–258
Policy change, monitoring, 470–471
Policy maker
  audience segmentation, 275–276
  beliefs about reasons for disease,
    141–142
  formative research, 207, 275–276
  perception of broad societal
    susceptibility, 140–142
  perception of hazards as threat to
    economic stability, 143
  perception that disease is out of
    control of societal effort, 142
  as target audience, 140
  what public health means to, 140
Political action committee, 88
Political consulting firm, 157
Positioning, 122
Positive emotional appeal, 334–335
Poverty
  child, 10
  health insurance, 17
  health status, 9–11
Press conference, 398–399
Press kit, 399–400

Pretesting, 415–437
central-site interview, 419–427
communication strategy, 416
focus group, 432–434
process, 433–434
when to use, 432–433
in-depth interview, 430–432
process, 431–432
when to use, 430–431
materials, 416–418
messages, 416
methodologies, 418–435
role, 415
television advertising, 421–423
Prevention
funding, 77
government's spending priorities, 77
policy implications, 76, 77
socioeconomic status, 77
vs. treatment, 74–78
Price
commercial marketing, 210–211
defined, 210, 508
social marketing, 211
Pricing, 349
Primary research, defined, 508
Primary target audience
defined, 255
selecting, 255–256
Print advertising, 405–406
Print materials, 384–387
assessment, 386–387
cost, 386–387
distribution, 385–386
image, 386–387
purpose, 385
reproduction, 385–386
use, 385
Process evaluation, 449–475
bounceback card, 453–455

client satisfaction, 456–460
data collection, 459
questionnaire, 458
reliability, 459
sampling, 458–459
validity, 459–460
conducting, 450–453
data collection instrument, 452–453
defined, 508
designing evaluation plans, 450–452
implementation, 453
inventory tracking, 455–456
objectives, 450–452
planning, 450–453
reporting, 453
service delivery, 456–460
data collection, 459
questionnaire, 458
reliability, 459
sampling, 458–459
validity, 459–460
types, 453–471
uses, 449–450
Product
commercial marketing, 207–210
competition, 208
defined, 31, 207, 508
ease of adoption, 209
feasibility, 209
perceived psychological price, 211
tangible or intangible, 207
use frequency, 208–209
Product definition, formative research, importance, 118–122
Product development, 348
Professional review, 434–435
process, 434–435
when to use, 434
Program component
briefing partners, intermediaries, and stakeholders, 361–362

budget, 358–360
component fit, 357
component reinforcement, 357
developing concepts, 354–357
development, 360
evaluation, 360
implement, 363
monitor, 363
partner, 361–362
preparing spokespeople and other
    staff, 360–361
refining, 363
stakeholder buy-in, 358
timeline, 358–360
timing, 357–358
tracking mechanisms, 360
Promotion, 227
commercial marketing, 213–215
defined, 213, 508
lack of funds to purchase time and
    space, 214
limited ability to assess impact, 215
limited control over message
    delivery, 214–215
negative demand, 214
social change, 213–215
    communication strategy,
        213–214
types, 213
Promotional activity
advertising, 352–354
employer newsletter, 354
mass media, 350–354
    options, 352–354
news coverage, 352–354
newsletter, 354
planning, 350–354
school system newsletter, 354
Public health
advocacy, 91
challenges, 76–77

common vision of mission and role,
    92
countermarketing, 36–37
decline in mortality, 74–75
delay in implementing reforms, 103
economic boundaries, 105–106
eighteenth century, 103
focus, 18–19
funding
    antiregulatory sentiment, 88–90
    block grant, 84–86
    budget cuts, 83–84
    campaign financing reform,
        87–88
    economic factors threatening,
        83–90
    legislation restricting, 85
    political factors threatening,
        83–90
    special-interest lobbying, 87–88
future directions, 494–495
goals, 81–82, 209
health care reform
    differences, 78
    illusion of reform as solution, 78
    relationship, 78
history, 103–108
hostile marketing environment,
    36–37
inadequate emphasis on advocacy,
    37–38
incentives, 81–82
lost vision of, 90–94
major functions, 20, 21
managed care
    differences, 79–83
    illusion of managed care as
        opportunity for public health,
        79–83
    managed care as danger to public
        health, 82–83

mission, 79–80
  relationship, 78
medical opposition to, 103
most urgent challenge, 6
objectives, 29
personal behavior, 19
principles, 90–92
public responsibility for social
  health and welfare, 90–91
social justice, 90
social policy, 20
threats to authority, vii
threats to survival, 73–94
underlying values of, 80–81
as unique marketing challenges,
  31–39
Public health department, role, viii
Public health marketing
  limited capacity of public health
    practitioners to compete for
    public attention and resources,
    113–114
  public health practitioner challenge,
    102–115
Public health organization
  customer driven, 205–206
  lobbying regulations, 100–101
Public health policy
  formative research, 273–280
    audience segmentation, 273–278
    shaping policy initiative, 278–280
    target audience, selection,
      273–278
  marketing, 57–61
    steps, 57
  target audience
    general public, 274, 276–277
    mass media, 274, 277–278
    policy makers, 274, 275–276
Public health practitioner
  future directions, 494–495

inadequate training in advocacy,
  38–39
limited expertise in advocacy, 38
primary challenge, 42
Public health product
  defining, 59–60
  documentation or support, 57
  framing, 60–61
  packaging, 60–61
  positioning, 60–61
  redefining, 51–52
    central task, 51–52
    importance, 51
    toward core values, 52
  reframing, 53–57
    significance, 53–54
    youth antismoking campaign,
      54–55
  repackaging, youth antismoking
    campaign, 54–55
  repositioning, youth antismoking
    campaign, 54–55
  strategic marketing, 62, 63
    components, 57, 58
Public health program
  benefits
    obscurity, 110–111
    remote connection, 109–110
  hostile environment for marketing,
    111–113
  marketing, 57–61
    steps, 57
  perceived psychological price, 211
  unfavorable state of demand,
    109–111
Public health surveillance, 62, 63
Public opinion poll, 155, 156–157,
  157–158, 163–165, 180–181
Public opinion tracking data, 473–474
Public service announcement,
  placement, 408–411, 465–470

Q

Qualitative research, 50, 263–264
    defined, 508
    gaining insights, 280–293
    methodologies, 280–293
    quantitative research, distinctions
        between, 264
    use, 280
Quality of care
    elderly patient, 18
    health care access, 17–18
    Medicare, 18
Quantitative research, 263
    defined, 508
    qualitative research, distinctions
        between, 264
Quantitative tracking survey, target
    audience, 473–474
Quasi-experimental design, 486–488
Questionnaire, design, 458

R

Radio
    characteristics, 355–356
    coverage opportunities, 397–398
Radio advertising, 406–407
Rational appeal, 334
Reach, defined, 461, 508
Reciprocal determinism, 234
Recruitment screener, focus group,
    303–305
Reflexive control, 488
Reframing, 160
Regulatory agency, partner, 370–371
Reliability, 459
Remarketing, 32
Repeated measure design, 488

S

Sampling, 458–459
Sanitary reform, 103–107
School health, formative research,
    case study, 296–302
School system newsletter, promotional
    activity, 354
Secondary research, defined, 508
Secondary target audience
    defined, 255
    selecting, 255–256
Self-efficacy, 234
Self-reliance, adolescent, 46
Service delivery, process evaluation,
    456–460
    data collection, 459
    questionnaire, 458
    reliability, 459
    sampling, 458–459
    validity, 459–460
Signification, defined, 172
Simmons Market Research Bureau,
    268–269
Smoking, adolescent, marketing,
    46–47
Social advertising, 198
Social change, 31
    challenges to, 257
    commercial marketing, marketing
        differences, 198
    cost-benefit analysis, 248–251
    demand state, 33, 35
    expectations, 229
    initiatives stages, 200
    iterative process, 225
    marketing, 3, 29–39, 42–69,
        197–199
    principles, viii, 198

negative demand, 33
no demand, 33
partner, 215–217, 222–223
place, 211–213
planning, 225–259, 227
  analyzing information, 235–252
  analyzing public policy issues
    framing, 239–240
  current science review, 236–237
  goals, 253–255
  identifying complementary and
    competing activities, 237–239
  identifying problems based on
    public health burden, 246–252
  identifying sources of
    information about potential
    target audiences, 240–246
  information collecting, 236–246
  innovation diffusion, 230–232
  leveraging resources and
    relationships, 229
  models of behavior, 230–234
  objectives, 253–255
  principles, 229–230
  prioritizing problems based on
    public health burden, 246–252
  role of theory, 230–234
  situation analysis, 235–252
  situation assessment, 246–252
  social cognitive theory, 234
  strategic plan, 234–235
  strategy importance, 227–228
  transtheoretical model, 232–233
  unified strategic program, 229
as product, 207–208
promotion, 213–215
  communication strategy,
    213–214
resources, 206

unfavorable state of demand for,
  31–36
unwholesome demand, 33
Social cognitive theory, 234
  environmental changes, 234
  observational learning, 234
  reciprocal determinism, 234
  self-efficacy, 234
Social communication, 198
Social justice, 90
Social marketing
  defined, 198, 509
  price, 211
Social marketing mix, 217
  five Ps, 217
Social norms, government effort to
  change, 134
Social policy
  demand state, 35–36
  public health, 20
Social price, 210–211
Social support
  health status, 15–17
  "welfare reform," 15–17
Socioeconomic status, 141
  chronic disease, 7–8
  health status, 9–11, 77
  prevention, 77
Special event, 412–413
Special-interest lobbying, 87–88
  environmental protection, 87–88
  National Rifle Association, 87
Spokesperson, 360–361
Stakeholder buy-in, program
  component, 358
State cigarette excise tax, marketing
  research, 120
State public health agency, funding,
  84

Storyboard, defined, 509
Strategic marketing
  core values, 53
  desired action, 53
  image-building, 53–54
  product/benefits, 53
  public health product, 62, 63
    components, 57, 58
Strategic plan, 234–235
  outline, 235
  planning, 257–258
Strategy
  construction, 228
  defined, 227, 509
  development, 272–273
Stroke, mortality rates, 7
Suicide, 7
Synchromarketing, 32

T

Tactics
  defined, 227, 509
  development, 272–273
Target audience, 229
  active response mechanisms, 472–473
  communication strategy, 315–316
    benefits, 319–320
    benefits credibility, 320
    channels for reaching audience, 320–321
    characteristics, 315–316
    current behavior, 316–319
    desired behavior, 316–319
    image, 322–324
    obstacles, 319
  coupon, 472–473
  needs and desires, 46, 118
  public health policy
    general public, 274, 276–277

    mass media, 274, 277–278
    policy makers, 274, 275–276
    quantitative tracking survey, 473–474
  selection, 255–256
    factors, 270–272
  telephone hotline, 472
  tracking awareness and reaction, 472–474
  understanding, 256–257
  write for more information line, 472–473
Telemarketing and Consumer Fraud and Abuse Act, 220
Telemarketing fraud, 220–224
  consumer education, 221–224
    community-based activities, 223–224
    evaluation, 224
    goal, 221
    legislative advocacy, 224
    mass communication, 223
    objectives, 222
    opportunities, 221
    partnerships, 222–223
    promotion, 223–224
    strategy, 222
    target audiences, 222
  cost, 220
  formative research, 220
Telephone hotline, target audience, 472
Telephone tracking survey, 156
Television
  characteristics, 355–356
  coverage opportunities, 398
Television advertising, 407–408
  animation, 407
  demonstrations, 407
  pretesting, 421–423
  production, 408, 409–410

slice-of-life, 407
testimonials, 407
Temporary Assistance for Needy
Families block grant, 86
Theater-style testing, 429–430
process, 430
when to use, 429–430
Threat appeal, 335–336
Timeline, program component, 358–360
Tobacco industry, 153–154, 156, 158–
163, 164–165
framing, 124–127
level playing field frame, 124,
131–132
Tobacco industry lobbyist, 92–93
Tobacco policy debate, 241–242
framing memo, 240, 241–242
Tobacco settlement, 92
Tobacco tax
Arizona, 163–165
disparity in financial resources,
163
failed efforts, 163–165
public opinion poll, 163–165
tobacco industry, 164–165
California, 152–155
arguments in support of tax
increase, 153
Californians Against Unfair Tax
Increases, 153
Coalition for a Healthy
California, 153
crime theme, 154
David/Goliath argument, 154
destination for tax revenue, 153
tobacco industry, 153–154
tobacco industry advertising,
153–154
Colorado, 163–165
disparity in financial resources,
163

failed efforts, 163–165
public opinion poll, 163–165
tobacco industry, 164–165
marketing
campaign spending, 152
case study, 151–168
failed campaign characteristics,
166
successful campaign
characteristics, 166
Massachusetts, 157–163
advertisement, 158, 159, 162
American Cancer Society,
157–158
argument testing, 157
maximum tax, 157
political consulting firm, 157
public opinion poll, 157–158
reframing, 160
tobacco industry, 158–163
tracking poll, 160
Montana, 155–157
bureaucracy, 156
public opinion survey, 155,
156–157
revenue use, 155–156
tax *vs.* health issue, 156
telephone tracking survey, 156
tobacco industry, 156
Topic guide, focus group, 285, 286–287
Tracking study, 488
Training, distribution, 348
Transit ad, 406
Transtheoretical model, 232–233
Tuberculosis, 21
framing, 130

U

Uncertainty, illness, 43–44
Unemployment, health status, 13

V

Validity, 459–460
Video news release, 400–401
Violence, health status, 14–15

W

"Welfare reform"
    impact, 16–17

social support, 15–17
World Wide Web, 388–392
    testing, 391–392
    web site design, 389–391
Written agreement, partner, 374

Y

Youth Risk Behavior Survey, 266